Nursing Home Organization and Operation

Nursing Home Organization and Operation

DULCY B. MILLER, M.S.A.M.

Administrative Director
The Nathan Miller Center for Nursing Care, Inc.
White Plains Center for Nursing Care

Instructor, Health Administration
School of Public Health, Columbia University

JANE T. BARRY

Assistant Administrator
The Nathan Miller Center for Nursing Care, Inc.
White Plains Center for Nursing Care

VNR **VAN NOSTRAND REINHOLD COMPANY**
New York

Copyright © 1979 by Van Nostrand Reinhold Company Inc.

Library of Congress Catalog Card Number: 84-3608
ISBN: 0-442-26406-2

Manufactured in the United States of America.

Published by Van Nostrand Reinhold Company Inc.
135 West 50th Street
New York, New York 10020

Van Nostrand Reinhold Company Limited
Molly Millars Lane
Wokingham, Berkshire RG11 2PY, England

Van Nostrand Reinhold
480 Latrobe Street
Melbourne, Victoria 3000, Australia

Macmillan of Canada
Division of Gage Publishing Limited
164 Commander Boulevard
Agincourt, Ontario M1S 3C7, Canada

15   14   13   12   11   10   9   8   7   6   5   4   3

Library of Congress Cataloging in Publication Data
Miller, Dulcy B.
  Nursing home organization and operation.

  Reprint. Originally published: Boston: CBI Pub. Co.,
c1979.
  Includes bibliographical references and index.
  1. Nursing homes—Administration.   I. Barry, Jane T.,
1951—   . II. Title.
RA997.M52 1984   362.1′6′068   84-3608
ISBN 0-442-26406-2

Dedicated to

M. B. M.

Table of Contents

List of Figures   xv
List of Exhibits   xvii
Foreword   xix
Preface   xxi
Introduction   xxiv

1. Administration   1

Introduction   1
Sponsorship and Organization   2
Bylaws   4
Operating Information   5
Management   6
Staffing Pattern   8
Consultants   10
Administrative Policies   12
Administrative Records   16
Communications   17
Government Influence   21
Intra- and Interfacility Relationships   25
Summary   27
Notes   28

2. Personnel   29

Introduction   29
Staffing Pattern   30
Recruitment   31
Part-time Versus Full-time Employment   33
Private Duty Personnel   33
Personnel Policies   34
Personnel Relationships Within and Outside the Facility   38
Records   39

Table of Contents (continued)

Unions   43
Summary   52
Notes   52

3. Medicine and Allied Health Professionals 53

Introduction   53
Medical Direction Alternatives   54
Attending Medical Staff   57
Scope of Responsibility   61
Duties and Procedures   62
Allied Health Professionals   68
Diagnostic Services   74
Pharmacy   74
Pharmacy Policies   80
Financial Arrangements   84
Records   84
Facilities and Equipment   86
Summary   92
Notes   92

4. Nursing 93

Introduction   93
Geriatric Nursing in a Long-term-care Facility   93
Staffing Pattern   95
Patient Care Procedures   104
Records   120
Nursing Department Communications   138
Facilities, Equipment, and Supplies   139
Summary   145
Notes   145

Table of Contents (continued)

5. Infection Control   146

Introduction   146
Infection Prevention   147
Nursing Home Policies   148
Residents   152
Housekeeping   153
Building Structure and Maintenance   155
Dietary   155
Surveillance   156
Summary   160
General References   161

6. Social Service   162

Introduction   162
Staffing Pattern   162
Social Work Programs with Patients and Families   164
Relationship with Community and Government Agencies   180
Records   180
Facilities and Equipment   182
Summary   183

7. Rehabilitation Services   184

Introduction   184
Physical Therapy   185
Occupational Therapy   196
Speech Pathology and Audiology   204
Summary   208
Notes   209

Table of Contents (continued)

8. Activities and Volunteers 210

Introduction 210
Staffing Pattern 210
Program 212
Activities Plan 221
Library 222
Evaluation 222
Religious Activities 223
Volunteers 227
Records 232
Facilities, Equipment, and Supplies 238
Summary 240
Notes 241

9. Consumerism 242

Introduction 242
The Resident as Consumer 242
Residents' Council 247
Resident Advocates 250
Families as Consumers 251
Community Intervention 254
Summary 258

10. Dietary 259

Introduction 259
Unique Aspects of Nursing Home Dietary Service 260
Patient Disabilities 260
Staffing Pattern 262
Diets 266
Menu Planning 269
Resident Meal Service 270

Table of Contents (continued)

Employee Meal Service   272
Records   273
Facilities and Equipment   275
Relations with Families and Visitors   280
Summary   280
Notes   281
General References   281

11. Housekeeping, Furnishings, and Laundry   **282**

Introduction   282
Outside Management Contracts   282
Staffing Pattern   283
Furnishings   287
Housekeeping Procedures   293
Odors   298
Laundry   298
Records   302
Facilities, Equipment, and Supplies   302
Relations with Patients and Families   304
Summary   305
Notes   305
General References   305

12. Building Design and Maintenance   **306**

Introduction   306
Scope of Maintenance   306
Staffing Pattern   307
External Environment   310
Internal Environment   311
Program   315
Energy Conservation   321

Table of Contents (continued)

Surface Transportation   322
Inspection by Government and Insurance Agencies   323
Purchasing   324
Records   326
Facilities and Major Equipment   329
Summary   330
Notes   330
General References   330

13. Safety   331

Introduction   331
Building Criteria   332
Safety Inspections   333
Accident and Incident Prevention   333
Grounds and Building Security   339
Fire Safety Program   342
Evacuation Plan   345
Utility Interruption   346
External Disasters   348
Bomb Threats   349
Civil Disturbance   349
Summary   350
Notes   351
General References   351

14. Business   352

Introduction   352
Definitions and Principles   353
Staffing Pattern   363
Rates   368
Procedures   370
Payroll   372

Table of Contents (continued)

Purchasing   373
Stores Control   375
Insurance   375
Bank Accounts   378
Protection of Valuables   379
Technology   379
Records   381
Facilities, Equipment, and Supplies   384
Summary   384
Notes   385
General References   385

15. Records   **386**

Introduction   386
Staffing Pattern   386
General Records and Forms   388
Health Records   390
Indexes   396
Procedures   397
Facilities and Equipment   398
Summary   400
Notes   400

16. The Therapeutic Organization   **401**

Introduction   401
Team Organization   401
Interdepartmental Cooperation   402
Committees and Meetings   410
Summary   418
Notes   418
General References   418

Table of Contents (continued)

17. Education and Research   419

Introduction   419
Education for Professionals   420
Administrative Support   420
Staffing Pattern   420
Programs for Staff Within the Facility   421
Programs for Staff Outside the Facility   429
Evaluation   430
Records   431
Programs for Families   434
Programs for Volunteers   435
Programs for Students   436
Programs for the Community   438
Budgeting for Educational Programs   439
Reference Material   440
Research   441
Summary   443
Notes   443

Epilogue   444

Notes   445

Index   447

List of Figures

Figure 1–1   Suggested Organizational Pattern of a Skilled Nursing Facility   15

Figure 1–2   Wheelchair-height Telephone   18

Figure 2–1   Staff Party   40

Figure 3–1   Suggested Organizational Structure of the Medical Staff in a Skilled Nursing Facility   58

Figure 3–2   Physician Writing Monthly Orders   66

Figure 3–3   Dental Survey   72

Figure 3–4   Podiatry Treatment   73

Figure 4–1   Family Member Feeding Patient   97

Figure 4–2   Mobile Shower Chair   106

Figure 4–3   Electronic Thermometer   108

Figure 4–4   Monitoring Patient on Intravenous Therapy and Nasogastric Tube Feeding   110

Figure 4–5   Nurse Checking Patient with Restraints   112

Figure 4–6   Medication Cart   119

Figure 4–7   Use of Dual Kardex System   128

Figure 4–8   Patient Using Call Buzzer   140

Figure 4–9   Chair Scale   144

Figure 5–1   Administering a Tuberculin Tine Test   150

Figure 5–2   Handwashing   151

Figure 5–3   Covered Receptacle for Soiled Laundry   154

Figure 6–1   Interview with Family   167

Figure 6–2   Therapeutic Group   178

Figure 7–1   Joint Exercises   186

Figure 7–2   Parallel Bars Assist Ambulation   193

Figure 7–3   Therapeutically Oriented Activity   198

Figure 7–4   Adaptive Card Holder   203

Figure 8–1   Participation in Physical Exercise   214

Figure 8–2   Indoor Gardening   217

Figure 8–3   Bandage-rolling Project   220

Figure 8–4   Religious Services   224

List of Figures (continued)

Figure 8–5   Junior Volunteer   230
Figure 8–6   Volunteer Recognition   233
Figure 8–7   Activity Brought to Patient's Room   239
Figure 9–1   Resident Signing for Receipt of Cash   245
Figure 9–2   Residents' Council Meeting   248
Figure 9–3   Family Advisory Committee   253
Figure 10–1   Off-floor Food Storage   277
Figure 11–1   Worker and Patient Communicating   286
Figure 11–2   Pedestal Tables Accommodating Wheelchairs   289
Figure 11–3   Resident Art as Interior Decoration   290
Figure 11–4   Room without Personal Belongings   291
Figure 11–5   Room with Personal Belongings   292
Figure 11–6   Separate Baskets for Residents' Laundry   301
Figure 12–1   Three Levels of Care   312
Figure 12–2   Repairing Autoclave   317
Figure 12–3   Fire Department Verifying Maintenance of
               Extinguisher   325
Figure 13–1   Caution Sign Marking Hazardous Area   336
Figure 13–2   Maintenance Worker Wearing Protective Gear   338
Figure 14–1   Reviewing Bill with Sponsor   367
Figure 15–1   Ample Space Needed for Records Coordinator   399
Figure 16–1   Nursing and Social Service Planning Patient
               Admission   406
Figure 16–2   Interdisciplinary Clinical Conference   413
Figure 16–3   Personnel Committee Meeting   414
Figure 17–1   Sensitizing Staff to Patient Disability   424
Figure 17–2   Walking Rounds   427
Figure 17–3   Grand Rounds   428

List of Exhibits

Exhibit 2–1   Application for Employment   41
Exhibit 2–2   Employee Reference Inquiry   44
Exhibit 2–3   Employee Performance Appraisal   45
Exhibit 2–4   Personnel Checklist   47
Exhibit 3–1   Pharmaceutical Service Contract   77
Exhibit 3–2   Monthly Physicians' Orders and Progress Notes   85
Exhibit 3–3   Podiatrist Evaluation and Prescription Form   87
Exhibit 3–4   Outpatient Consultation Record   88
Exhibit 3–5   History and Physical   89
Exhibit 3–6   Restraint Prescription   91
Exhibit 4–1   Comprehensive Nursing Assessment   122
Exhibit 4–2   Diagnostic History   126
Exhibit 4–3   Dual Kardex   129
Exhibit 4–4   Attending Physician Reminder   136
Exhibit 5–1   Individual Infection Report   159
Exhibit 6–1   Social Service Summary   172
Exhibit 7–1   Physical Therapy Prescription   194
Exhibit 7–2   Occupational Therapy Prescription   202
Exhibit 8–1   Patient Activity Plan   235
Exhibit 8–2   Patient Report   236
Exhibit 10–1   Nutritional History   274
Exhibit 12–1   Maintenance Work Order   328
Exhibit 14–1   Details of Costs and Expenses   357
Exhibit 14–2   Statement of Income and Expenses   364
Exhibit 14–3   Balance Sheet   365
Exhibit 14–4   Statistical Operational Data   382
Exhibit 15–1   Suggested Periods of Record Retention   389
Exhibit 17–1   Nurses' Orientation Checklist   432
Exhibit 17–2   Lesson Plan Number Two: Temperature-Pulse-Respiration   433

Foreword

Long-term-care administration is an important, emerging profession. Dulcy Miller and Jane Barry help us better understand the nature of this profession's increasingly important contribution to the provision of quality long-term care.

Forty years ago, the United States Bureau of Census reported only around 1200 long-term-care facilities with a capacity of about 25,000 beds. Today there are 22,000 facilities accounting for 1.3 million beds. The dramatic increase in these statistics reflects a number of important trends in American society. For one thing, we are an aging population because we now prefer smaller families and because modern medicine enables us to live longer than ever before. Further, we have become increasingly independent of our family "roots" as our nation's prosperity provides the young with education and employment equaling the highest standards available throughout the world. We decided in the 1930s that our government should insure us against the economic risks of old age, death, and disability, and in recent years we have extended this commitment to include the risks of illness.

These trends will, most certainly, continue. In fact, their effects on the demand for long-term care promise to be even more dramatic in future years. Recent studies on the future of long-term care completed by the Congressional Budget Office, for example, estimate that the demand for long-term-care beds will increase by around 87.5 percent between 1975 and 1985—from 1.6 million residents to 3.0 million residents. Equally dramatic will be the increase in demand for competent people pursuing careers in long-term care—doctors, nurses, therapists, social workers, nursing assistants—people who are familiar with the problems of the elderly and disabled; people who are trained to assist residents in achieving and maintaining their optimal functional levels; people who are closely coordinating their efforts with others in providing a "total living environment" for long-term-care residents.

There will also, of course, be a need for long-term-care administrators. A few years ago, one of the special congressional committees study-

Foreword (continued)

ing problems in nursing homes concluded that the administrator ". . . was the single most important influence on the quality of long term care. . . ." Accordingly, *Nursing Home Organization and Operation* provides students of this profession with a comprehensive foundation of principles in organizing and managing a modern long-term-care facility. Certain appropriate themes are emphasized in this book, including the human side of the long-term-care enterprise, the rehabilitative nature of all care and services, and the important distinctions between long-term-care and acute-care facilities. Most of the field's major problems—shortage of people qualified for employment, social values regarding the elderly, the absence of physicians, negative public attitudes—are directly and candidly confronted. New and important emphasis is given to the benefits long-term care can derive from "consumerism" and from educational and research programs essential ". . . for any organization to remain viable, growing, and productive. . . ."

Indeed, Miller and Barry contribute towards the development of long-term-care administration as a profession. Students of the field and others who seek to better understand the operations of a long-term-care facility will surely profit from studying these pages. Certainly their better understanding will assure that administrators will continue to have a positive influence on the quality of care available to residents in long-term-care facilities.

Robert Burmeister, Ph.D.
Director of Education and Research
American College of Nursing Home Administrators

Preface

Nursing Home Organization and Operation documents the organization and operation of the skilled nursing facility. The title of the first book, *The Extended Care Facility: A Guide to Organization and Operation,* reflected terminology used in the original Medicare legislation, which made "extended care" benefits available to Americans over age 65 in January 1967. Great professional and community interest ensued, and general hospitals, homes for the aged, and public and private agencies participated in the construction of long-term-care units to complement their existing facilities and in the development of new freestanding extended care institutions. In the next decade, facilities increased both in size and in the breadth of professional services offered.

More recently, the term "skilled nursing facility" replaced the original "extended care facility," and the intermediate-care facility came into being for people requiring a supposedly lesser level of care. Although this volume is directed to a 100-bed skilled nursing facility, the concepts, philosophy, and principles are equally applicable to the intermediate-care facility (health-related facility). We are not impressed with these artificial levels of care, as the conditions of sick old people do not remain static and such artifacts serve only to defeat continuity of care. Moving the ill elderly from one setting to another is costly, both in human and financial terms. It is costly in human terms when aged ill people who have sustained losses of spouse, role, health, and home must adapt to new people and new places. And financial expenses mount with ambulance charges and with myriad federal and state regulations associated with each patient's admission and discharge.

There are three units in the model 100-bed skilled nursing facility discussed in the text: a 30-bed concentrated care unit for the severely physically handicapped, a 36-bed unit for the behaviorally and physically disabled, and a 34-bed unit for the more moderately disabled. Although the 34-bed unit presumably could be larger, the number of available patient candidates precludes adding more beds.

Medical care alone is insufficient for institutionalized elderly be-

Preface (continued)

cause of their level of disability and behavioral pathology. Even so, the social components of care without medical care do not address a holistic program for the frail elderly.

While the text is basically objective and informative, we have attempted to make the book realistic and readable by using examples drawn from our experience in administering nursing homes. We have included special forms and photographs to illustrate specific activities peculiar to nursing home management. The factual material is essential for students in health care administration, and the discussion, suggestions, and recommendations should be uniquely helpful to practicing administrators.

We hope that this volume will serve as a guide to those who are responsible for the planning, financing, development, supervision, and management of health care institutions—including governing boards, planning agencies, developers, medical and dental staff, administrators, department heads, unions, and representatives of government agencies, ranging from the Social Security Administration to the various health and welfare departments responsible for certifying skilled nursing facilities to receive Title XVIII and Title XIX patients. Section 1908 of Public Law 90-248, providing for compulsory licensing of nursing home administrators, serves to accentuate the need for text material for educational programs in the field.

We further hope that this book will prove useful to professionals in related disciplines—to the clergy in their work with the institutionalized aged, to hospital administrators contemplating transfer agreements with skilled nursing facilities, and to social workers in family agencies working with the elderly. Third-party payers and fiscal intermediaries can plan appropriate reimbursement formulas only if they are familiar with the daily activities of the skilled nursing facility.

With the projected increase of the over-seventy-five population in the next decades, the availability of long-term services for the aged must grow. We sincerely hope that this book will prove useful as a reference, a

Preface (continued)

---

role definer, and a communications tool to professionals working with the ill aged in long-term-care settings, and to health care administration students in undergraduate, graduate, and continuing education programs.

We are grateful for the cooperative efforts of Jeanne Brimigion, R.N.; Josephine Strachan, R.N.; Robert Quinlan, activities coordinator; Irene Martin, R.D.; Marilyn Frey, physical therapist; Suellen Clifton, O.T.R.; and Harris Rakov, counsel to the board of directors of The Nathan Miller Center for Nursing Care. We would also like to thank Alice Feldman, R.N.; Natividad Gulle, social worker; Janet Saunders, activities coordinator; Patricia Hammer, R.P.T.; William Woodruff, director of maintenance; Franklin Hoffman, R.Ph.; and Nicki Pagidas, R.R.A., of the White Plains Center for Nursing Care; Maurice Singer, C.P.A., of White Plains; and William Breger, A.I.A., of New York. Special acknowledgment is due Susan Beer for her supervision of the sensitive photography of Rae Russell and for her editorial guidance. Lastly and most importantly, we deeply appreciate the stimulation and deep involvement of Michael Miller, medical director, in the development and implementation of the therapeutic organization.

Introduction

During the past few years, for a variety of complex and interrelated reasons, the profession of health services administration has assumed an increasing importance within the health services delivery system. As technology advances, personnel specialize, service modalities change, and costs escalate, the professional health services administrator becomes increasingly visible as the manager of this dynamic process.

Given the dimensions of the changes that are occurring within the delivery system, it is certainly not surprising that academic programs that prepare individuals for the career of health services administration have both expanded and added depth to their curricula. The nature of the problems encountered in the field of practice has caused the addition and/or expansion of program coursework in quantitative methods, planning, financial management, and systems analysis. This adjustment within the majority of curricula has added breadth to the student's perception of the health services system and provided the theoretical basis for many of the management functions that the student will perform in a future administrative career.

However, because curricula now include more content of a conceptual or theoretical nature, and since the time frame for completion of an academic program has essentially remained the same, there has been a concomitant decrease in courses that focus on the more specific requirements of facility administration. Currently the most common method of providing this information is the administrative internship or residency in a health services facility. As one would expect, there is a diversity of opinion on these changes in the curricula of academic programs in health services administration. It is not my intention to elaborate on those opinions. Rather, I wish simply to identify the fact that many students of health services administration today do not receive much exposure to the specifics of facility administration. Those who do are by and large schooled in the realities of a hospital operation. They have little experience with other service components of the health care system.

Introduction (continued)

This lack of experience seems to be the case not only because of the increasing coursework and limited time but also because of a presumption that tends to prevail among faculty that administration is generic, that is, substantially the same wherever performed and that the transfer of skills from one setting to another is somewhat automatic. To a large extent, this is undoubtedly true. Basic administrative skills in planning, organizing, staffing, and financial management are required of an administrator of any health services facility. However, it is equally true that the problems that present themselves reflect the nature of the facility in which they occur and thus determine to a large extent the type of activity in which the administrator will become involved. For example, in the hospital, the primary purpose of which is acute medical care, the administrator is likely to spend a substantial percentage of time negotiating with a large, well-organized medical staff. In the long-term-care facility, where the health problems encountered are chronic and where the physician ordinarily spends very little time, the administrator may be primarily involved in coordinating all professional staff into an interdisciplinary unit that delivers care to the patient. While the administrative skills brought to bear will be substantially the same, the nature of the problem to which they will be applied will differ. It is my opinion that students of health services administration need some exposure to these differences that are prevalent among health care facilities. *Nursing Home Organization and Operation* is one step toward achieving that objective. Dulcy Miller and Jane Barry have prepared a book that reflects their years of experience in the organization and operation of a long-term facility and that will do much to clarify for students of health services administration the nature of the long-term-care facility and the problems to which their administrative knowledge and skill is to be applied.

Much has been said and written during the past few years about the need to emphasize not only the nursing aspect of the nursing home but also the characteristics that contribute to making it a home for the patient/resident. While the levels and modalities of the medical and nurs-

Introduction (continued)

ing services provided in this facility differ to some extent from the same services provided elsewhere in the health services delivery system, it is the emphasis on the social components of care in the nursing home setting that establishes the more significant difference between facilities and that is likely to present to the administrator the more unusual or atypical problems for administrative solution.

Some sections of *Nursing Home Organization and Operation* specifically focus on the creation of a personalized ambience in the long-term-care facility. They address family relationships, group process, activities programming, menu planning, and other dimensions of this aspect of care. More importantly, however, throughout the book the authors have conveyed the message that the patient/resident in the nursing home is of primary importance and that each and every service, whether related to health or social activities, is directed to the benefit of that person and to the creation of an appropriate environment for him. In this context, they describe health and social services in the long-term-care setting and identify problems related to the delivery of those services that differ from the problems that would be present in another health care facility. For this reason, this book will be of great benefit to students of health services administration who are infrequently exposed to the difficulties encountered in the management of an organization that serves a chronically ill population suffering from multiple physical, psychological, and social disabilities.

Two chapters deserve specific mention because they address subjects not frequently covered in texts that describe long-term-care administration. They are Chapter 9, "Consumerism," and Chapter 17, "Education and Research." Chapter 9 provides an overview of the various ways in which a patient's rights may be considered: personally, environmentally, legally, and from a health point of view. It introduces some of the more complex issues to be faced by the administrator as multiple rights interface and offers alternative suggestions for introducing advocates into the nursing home facility.

Introduction (continued)

Chapter 17 (the final chapter in the book) presents the nursing home as an educational facility. This dimension of the nursing home has traditionally not received much attention. The authors, however, in a reflection of their own thoughtful and enlightened views, emphasize the importance of education, both inside and outside the facility: in-service education and the availability of time and financing for staff to participate in educational programs outside the nursing home; the use of the facility for the clinical education of professionals; educational programming for patients/residents and family members and a program of research related to the function of the facility. The communication of this attitude toward growth and improvement will help establish in the minds of health services administration students that the nursing home is a full participant in the community health services delivery system.

Nursing Home Organization and Operation is a book about the specifics of administration in the long-term-care facility. It will be helpful in providing an opportunity for students of health services administration to cast the theory they have learned against the practical reality of day-to-day administration in a long-term-care facility. In addition, and more importantly, it is a text that sees the administrator as the facilitator, the change agent who structures all services and activities to the benefit of the patient/resident . . . a happy and humane change for the image of management.

Patrica A. Cahill
Vice-President and Director
Office of Long-Term Care
Association of University Programs in Health Administration

Administration

INTRODUCTION

A skilled nursing facility should be concerned with providing medical care, nursing care, and rehabilitative services for inpatients who are no longer in an acute phase of illness. Its chief interest should be to help patients recover as fully as possible by assisting them to function physically, socially, and emotionally to the best of their ability. The nursing home must also be concerned with the development of a close working relationship with families of patients, a vital element of a successful rehabilitation program as well as an important aid to families of patients in identifying and resolving problems accentuated by the placement of a family member in an institutional setting.

To achieve this purpose, it is necessary to understand the nature of the patient population. Nursing home residents are generally about eighty years old, white, with eight or fewer years of schooling and an income often below the poverty line. In addition, females outnumber males by three or four to one. The population is characterized by a preponderance of people severely handicapped by multiple advanced physical diseases, behavioral pathology, or a combination of the two. Although only about 4 to 5 percent of the ill aged over sixty-five are nursing home residents, one out of five older persons will spend some time in a long-term-care facility during his lifetime.

The future long-term-care population will be older and probably sicker. They will probably be more affluent, reflecting greater educational opportunities. The number of foreign-born will be smaller, but the number of minority patients will be greater. A large proportion will be high school and college graduates. More probably will have experienced multiple marriages, divorce, and separation. Fewer will be traditionally religious, and more will come from higher occupational levels. It is likely that they will have different values regarding sexuality, the use of relaxation and leisure time, self-determination, and social relationships. They will probably demand more privacy, dignity, and respect. They will have experienced greater mobility and greater leisure than have current nursing home residents. They will probably have less stable and less rewarding family relationships and fewer children. Future long-term-care patients also will have been more accustomed to seeking professional services such as psychiatry and dentistry.

In all probability, the family of future long-term-care clients will be smaller, more geographically mobile, and less apt to have elderly relatives live with them. It is conceivable that the women's rights movement, the increase in the number of working wives, and the weakening of traditional ties will tend to lessen the importance of families in the direct care of their ill, aged relatives.

SPONSORSHIP AND ORGANIZATION

The skilled nursing facility may be organized as a separate and freestanding entity; a branch of a religious, charitable, or fraternal agency; an extension or addition to an existing organization; a satellite of an existing agency; or a link in a chain of organizations. A skilled nursing facility may be a nonprofit organization, a public agency, or a proprietary agency, but it always has a governing body that is responsible for the quality of care provided.

Nonprofit Corporation

A nonprofit corporation is organized according to a written constitution and abides by written bylaws that preclude officers and directors both from receiving pecuniary or material benefit from the institutional corporation and from liability for any debts of the corporation. The governing body is a board of directors. Voluntary agencies are exempt from federal, and usually from state and local, taxation.

Public Agency

A public agency abides by written bylaws that are developed according to the statutes, rules, regulations, and policies that govern the parent government organization, which also may direct the operation. The governing body may be an appointed representative of the parent agency or a specially appointed or elected board of directors. The governing body may not receive any pecuniary or material benefit from the nursing home, and it is not liable for the facility's debts. Public agencies are exempt from federal, state, and local taxation.

Proprietary Agency

A proprietary agency should operate under established rules. A proprietary skilled nursing facility may be run by individuals, by a partnership arrangement, or by a corporation with stockholders. The governing body is the owner(s), who may derive material and pecuniary benefits from the organization and, in the case of an individual or partnership, is liable for the agency's debts. Individuals generally are not liable for debts in a proprietary corporate structure. As a commercial enterprise, a proprietary facility is subject to all forms of taxation.

The Board of Directors

For the most part, voluntary, investor-owned, and public nursing homes are governed by a board of directors or trustees. Government institutions and some facilities owned by religious orders may present a slightly different structure; irrespective of the exact organization, however, there is a decision-making body.

In voluntary facilities, and sometimes in government facilities, boards are generally composed of business and professional leaders in the particular community of the facility. Although these people often are extremely busy, it is thought that they are probably in positions to open doors to top-level government officials, to make helpful contacts for fund raising, and so on. A mix of high-level and non-high-level board members is suggested, for the non-high-level members will have more time to devote to nursing home affairs. Indeed, large corporations often donate company time so that their midlevel executives can participate in community activities that reflect well on the company image. With the growing emphasis on retirement planning, boards should consider recruiting potential or early retirees.

Other suggestions for board members are generalists, including homemakers and consumers who have the time and interest and individuals with particular technical skills such as builders and computer specialists. The appointment of minority members and other representatives of the community is of increasing concern. And families of former and present residents of the facility are a particularly valuable resource for board membership.

Members of public nursing home boards are usually appointed. If the appointments are political, it is desirable that the members have expertise to offer the facility. Often board members are elected to office by the corporation; in this instance, it is also hoped that the successful candidates will be elected for their expertise in managing the nursing home.

In the main, boards tend to be self-perpetuating and tend to serve for extended periods, filling vacancies as they occur. The advantage of self-perpetuating board membership is continuity and a wealth of experience. Some boards have a system of rotation whereby a member serves one term on and then has one term off the board. New board members have the advantages of bringing new ideas and talents, but they need considerable education to the needs of long-term patients and their families as well as the operation of the facility.

Accountability to the community is an important responsibility of the board. Perhaps one board member or a committee should be designated to serve as a liaison with the community.

The governing body will determine its mode of operation, whether it will act as a committee of the whole, or whether it will function with a strong executive committee or via standing committees, ad hoc committees, or task forces.

BYLAWS

The content of the bylaws, or rules and regulations, of the skilled nursing facility may vary, depending on the sponsorship of the agency. Bylaws for any agency address the manner in which the agency is to be governed.

The bylaws must identify the governing body's title and size, the method of its election or appointment, its terms of service, and related issues, such as whether the terms will be staggered to afford continuity and whether a board member may serve consecutive terms.

It is generally thought that an effective governing body should have eight to fifteen members. The governing body would elect or appoint officers in accordance with the bylaws, which would specify the composition of the officers, their terms of office and related issues, and the appointment of members to fill unexpired officer terms. The officers should include a chairperson or president, who presides at all meetings and may serve as an ex-officio member of all governing body committees; the vice-chairperson or vice-president, who assumes the position of chairperson or president with the appropriate authority in the absence of the latter; the secretary, who is responsible for all governing body records and meeting minutes and who notifies members of meetings; the treasurer, who is custodian of all agency funds and ensures proper methods of accounting and reporting of all financial affairs; and other officers sanctioned by the bylaws.

The duties of the governing body, described in the bylaws, include the supervision of the property, affairs, and finances of the facility. The governing body should engage two administrative officers, a medical director and an administrative director, who act on the behalf of the governing body in the daily management of the nursing home.

In the instance of an organized medical staff, the bylaws would describe the process by which the governing body should select and appoint a medical staff, including their qualifications, privileges, length of appointment, and the provision for a hearing if a staff member is not reappointed. The governing body should give the organized medical staff the responsibility for the routine functions of recommending appointments, reappointments, changes of status, and disciplinary action, but it should reserve for itself final approval as well as the right to handle special situations. Finally, the medical director and/or medical staff should be delegated the responsibility for ensuring professional comprehensive patient care and continuously appraising the quality of care.

The bylaws should provide for the specifics of regular and special meetings of the governing body. It is useful to have these meetings at the facility so that members of the governing body have continuing exposure to the nature of the patient population and programs of the facility. The regular meeting should be scheduled toward the middle of the month or later in order to permit the preparation of current reports for presentation. Special meetings may be called by the president of the governing body or at the request of one-third or one-fourth of the entire governing body. A written notice stating the purpose(s) of the meeting should be sent in advance of the meeting. A quorum for meetings should be identified.

The bylaws should specify the number, purpose, members, and quorum of standing committees of the governing body, and the president should appoint special committees to function as long as they are needed. Standing committees should include the executive committee—composed of, at a minimum, the president, secretary, and treasurer of the governing body—which has the power to transact business between meetings, examine monthly finances, and present an annual operating budget. The finance committee, composed of the treasurer and two other members, supervises the proper investment of trust and endowment funds and the proper handling of these moneys in accordance with trust arrangements. If the facility has an organized medical staff, there should be a medical staff committee, composed of three members of the governing body, who make the final determination of medical staff appointments, approve the specific professional area of concern of each medical staff member, serve as the governing body representatives to the joint conference committee, and act as the governing body's representatives in all matters pertaining to the medical staff. The nominating committee has the duty of presenting nominations for vacancies on the governing body. Other standing committees—such as personnel, building, or master plan committees—may also be authorized by the bylaws.

Provisions for amending the bylaws would vary in accordance with the facility's sponsorship.

OPERATING INFORMATION

Permission to operate a skilled nursing facility is received from the appropriate state licensing agency. Approval depends on the submission of certain information. A full disclosure of ownership must be made, identifying all those who have a direct or indirect ownership of 5 percent or more, or who own, in whole or in part, a 5 percent interest in any mortgage secured by the agency. Directors or officers in a corporate structure or partners in a partnership arrangement must be identified. Other required documentation includes a proposed program and staffing plan, policies and procedures to ensure an orderly operation, a duly established constitution or a copy of the constitution of the parent body, bylaws, a copy of the certificate of occupancy, a copy of the certificate of doing business (for a noncorporate organization) or a copy of the certificate of incorporation (for a corporation), and a copy of the lease (if the property is rented). Other material may be requested.

Corporations need a certificate of incorporation from the appropriate state authority to operate. Once granted, this charter can be amended only with the acquiescence of the granting authority. Information requested on the application for the charter would include the corporation's title and location, its objectives and purposes, its status (e.g., nonprofit or proprietary), the size of its governing body, and the method of election and terms of office of its governing body, and its officers. If the corporation is a membership corporation, the qualifications for membership and the plan for membership dues must also be described in the application. When a proprietary agency does not have a corporate structure, a certificate of doing business is required in order to begin operations, to open checking accounts, and so on.

In addition, the skilled nursing facility, depending on its location, may be licensed by other agencies, such as the county or city department of health and the municipal department of public safety. Individual elements in the building—such as the cafeteria, elevators, incinerators, and boilers—require special permits for operation from any of the aforementioned agencies.

MANAGEMENT

One of the newer trends in the management of health care facilities is to contract with a proprietary firm for the overall or departmental management of the facility. This may occur in proprietary, voluntary, and even in public facilities. The goal is more effective and more economical management by more experienced managers. This concept is frequently reflected in the operation of a single department within the nursing home, such as housekeeping or dietary, where an outside company is employed to perform only that department's duties. The rationale is that the specialist in, say, foodservice can run the dietary service more effectively than the health care facility can.

In a long-term-care facility, the organization should be an open system with easy communication to foster the concept of the therapeutic milieu where all persons—staff, patients, families, and volunteers—and even the physical environment interact to provide a remedial atmosphere. Techniques such as management by objectives and organizational development can be helpful in obtaining effective patient care.

Executive Management

The executive management of the skilled nursing facility should be jointly shared by the medical director and the administrative director, and their professional responsibilities should be clearly defined. The functions of the medical director will be discussed in Chapter 3.

The administrative director is charged by the governing body to implement its policy directives and to act as its liaison to the health care community. The administrative director's obligations to the governing body are to be present at all meetings of the governing body, to serve as an ex-officio member on the joint conference committee and the medical board (if applicable), and to keep the governing body informed by presenting periodic and special progress reports concerning the nursing home's activities and finances. If the facility has an organized medical staff, the administrative director prepares letters of appointment as directed by the governing body.

The proper maintenance of the building, grounds, and equipment ultimately rests with the administrative director. Decisions about the purchase of major new equipment must, of course, be the final responsibility of the administrator. Important and costly pieces of equipment will be included in the capital expenditures budget and must have prior approval by the governing body.

One of the more important tasks of the administrative director is to program a staffing plan commensurate with the skilled nursing facility's needs. Specifically, staff members employed in the areas of dietary, housekeeping and laundry, business and administration, maintenance, and activities and volunteers are the administrator's overall responsibility. However, the administrator has the duty of ensuring the development of personnel policies affecting all employees and of interpreting patients' rights to all staff.

The administrative director's share of executive management includes responsibility for the general financial affairs, especially ensuring compliance with the operating budget and the development of a comprehensive insurance program. He prepares the annual budget in conjunction with the department heads, thus assuring their understanding of overall facility needs and the financial expectations and limits of their respective services.

The most encompassing charge to the administrative director is to be knowledgeable regarding the problems encountered in long-term care and to be available to the various staff members to help resolve such problems. Further, he should be alert to changes within the patient population and social and professional trends in order to effect improvements in patient care or nursing home services.

To be current on important issues, the administrative director should serve on several staff committees, including safety, personnel, pharmacy, infection control, patient care policy, interdisciplinary, budget, utilization review, and education.

Finally, the administrative director should be sensitive to the importance of community relations and the interpretation of the skilled nursing facility and its work to the professional and lay community. Involvement in related professional and community organizations is an effective mode of conveying the nursing home's presence in and importance to the community.

The governing body should define and state in writing the order of responsibility in the absence of the administrative and medical directors. When the two executive officers of the nursing home are absent, the affairs of the institution should be the responsibility of the assistant administrator, followed by the director of nursing, the supervisor, and finally the senior charge nurse (with registered nurses taking precedence over practical nurses).

Departmental Management

Each department should be directed by a competent person with leadership ability. Departments may be divided into professional and nonprofessional categories, with the professional services responsible to the medical director. Professional services would include nursing, the matrix of all patient services in the skilled nursing facility; social service, primarily involved in patient admission, adaptation, and discharge planning; the rehabilitative services; diagnostic services; and medicine. Other departments—including dietary, housekeeping and laundry, maintenance, business, and activities and volunteers—are generally considered support services. They are directly responsible to the administrative director.

STAFFING PATTERN

In addition to the administrative director, several staff members come under the administration's purview. The exact number of administrative personnel would depend on facility size; however, for the 100-bed facility, a discussion of the positions of assistant administrator, administrative assistant, secretary, and receptionist will suffice. In some instances, duties could be combined if the work load is not sufficient to warrant hiring a full-time employee.

Assistant Administrator

The assistant administrator is responsible to the administrative director and, in the latter's absence, functions as acting administrator. A variety of duties may be assigned to the assistant administrator, such as serving as director of personnel, preparing regular and special reports for the governing body or government agencies, gathering data for research studies, serving as the administrative director's representative at committee meetings, planning meetings and maintaining minutes, reviewing and amending nursing home policies and procedures, and generally assisting the administrative director in the daily operation of the nursing home. A candidate for this position should be a licensed nursing home administrator with, preferably, a college degree, knowledge of personnel and business management, and familiarity with government codes and regulations and with current trends in long-term care.

Administrative Assistant

An administrative assistant who reports to the administrative director may be employed for the primary purpose of communicating information concerning nursing home activities, policies, personnel, and the like within the nursing home and to the outside community. Specifically, this task would entail planning, writing, producing, and distributing all literature pertaining to the nursing home, including monthly newsletters, an annual report, a periodic professional bulletin, personnel and emergency handbooks, policy and procedure manuals, and press releases. In addition to handling written material, the administrative assistant designs and maintains general and staff bulletin boards involving the posting of current information and visually stimulating displays; prepares artwork and layouts for posters, flyers, invitations, and the like; arranges for a photographer when needed and for the storage and use of nursing home photographs; assists in planning and arranging special nursing home programs involving patients, families, staff, and the professional and lay communities; and represents the nursing home in the community. To perform such a multiplicity of duties, the administrative assistant must develop one-to-one relationships with patients and staff and participate in the residents' council meetings, family group meetings, interdisciplinary meetings, medical rounds, and personnel committee meetings. A college degree or some college background should be required for this position, but any candidate must have experience in writing, some artistic ability, and a knowledge of journalism techniques, printing, and art layout. Above all, a genuine interest in people is required.

Secretary

The services of a secretary are certainly needed, although whether the position is part-time or full-time depends on the volume of work. A secretary is responsible to the administrative director and works closely with all administrative staff to assist them in typing letters, articles, and manuals; preparing stencils; typing meeting minutes and reports; duplicating material reproduced on the premises; relieving the receptionist for lunch and breaks; and generally assisting with other clerical duties. Skill in operating a typewriter, dictating equipment, and other office equipment, and general clerical knowledge should be requirements for this job.

Receptionist

The receptionist holds a key position in the facility, as the first person with whom community visitors, families, physicians, and guests come into contact. This person's competence and friendliness—or lack thereof—can give an overall impression of the nursing home to all who enter. A receptionist must be on duty seven days a week. Arrangements could, therefore, be made either for two part-time receptionists or for one full-time receptionist to work during the week and a part-time receptionist for weekend work. The receptionist, who reports directly to the administrative director, greets and directs incoming visitors to their destinations; maintains a daily revised file of appropriate information on current residents and a list of all staff on duty and where they can be reached; distributes incoming mail and stamps and deposits outgoing mail; helps prepare large mailings, for example, by collating materials and addressing and stuffing envelopes; and makes announcements over the public address system. Unless a switchboard operator is employed, the receptionist may answer telephones and connect calls to the desired party or take messages. Also, positioned near the main door, the receptionist must remain alert to confused residents who may wander outside. A receptionist should be friendly, courteous, and cooperative and have a pleasing voice and telephone manner. Typing skills would be beneficial.

CONSULTANTS

It is always preferable to employ a full-time person in a responsible professional position. However, due to the size of the nursing home or an individual department, consultants are often retained for specialized professional direction or guidance to the organization, to provide direct services to patients and families, to determine unmet needs with respect to the purchase of costly equipment, to assess the functioning of a department or personnel, or to advise the governing body in the development of future plans.

Upon employment, consultants should be required to work at the nursing home on a full-time basis for an appropriate length of time, thus giving them the opportunity to learn the nature of the patient population, the gestalt of the staff, the character of family members, and the expectations and limitations of volunteers. Only after understanding the interrelationships among all these components can a consultant have the basic knowledge to function effectively in the skilled nursing facility. For consultants involved in direct patient care, a half-day per week is the minimum amount of time that should be scheduled.

The nursing home should always execute a written contract signed by the administrator and the individual consultant or consulting firm—in fact, most purveyors providing services to the nursing facility—to clearly define each party's responsibility. The contract should describe the objectives of the service, the nature and quantity of service to be rendered, and the terms of the agreement, including the financial arrangements and conditions under which the contract may be terminated. Sufficient notice—at least thirty days—should be specified in the termination clause to allow the nursing home adequate time to find a replacement. In contracts with consultants providing direct professional services to patients, federal regulations require that the facility assume administrative and professional responsibility for the treatment rendered. With the proliferation of malpractice suits, however, consultants would be wise to carry their own professional liability insurance.

When appropriate, the terms of the agreement should state the consultant's responsibility for submitting periodic written activity reports, including changes in services, recommendations for improvements, and plans for implementation. Because a consultant is traditionally not responsible for implementing these recommendations, the abilities and limitations of the nursing home in terms of financing, staffing, and program planning should be taken into consideration. If the consultant is aware of these factors, suggestions can be directed to areas that may be realistically considered.

External professional consultants may be retained for either long or short periods, depending on the purpose and nature of their activities. Internal consultants appointed on a continuing basis may include a certified public accountant, an attorney, an interior designer, a pharmacist, a dietitian, a social worker, a physical therapist, an occupational therapist, a speech pathologist/audiologist, a dentist, a podiatrist, a clergyman, and a safety expert.

For special situations where an objective point of view would prove useful, external consultants may be retained for a limited period. Professionals such as a systems expert, an administrative nurse, a physician, an architect, or a computer specialist may be considered for such purposes.

Depending on facility size, outside purveyors may be hired to provide services that are not within the scope of the nursing home program. Contracts for such services would be of a continuing nature; however, it is important that the activities or products of outside purveyors be supervised and that their charges be regularly compared with those of other vendors. Some of these outside resources might be exterminators, sanitation companies, linen rental services, elevator maintenance services, window cleaners, gardeners, and possibly pharmacies.

ADMINISTRATIVE POLICIES

For organizational clarity, it is necessary for the facility to have a written statement of philosophy regarding the nursing home goals and patient care. This philosophy should be reflected in the facility's policies. A philosophy for a skilled nursing facility should emphasize the importance of all staff members' awareness of patient care problems.

The purpose of policies is to define a course of action that will guide and determine present and future actions. Written policies are necessary to formalize a prescribed method of action, while procedures expand on this standardization by delineating how to carry out policy statements by following a series of steps.

All facility operations must comply with rules and regulations set forth by various government agencies concerned with overseeing health care facilities. Cooperation is important in maximizing the benefits of the survey process. When government representatives arrive on the nursing home premises, they should be asked for their credentials and referred to the administrative director unless they have made prior arrangements to visit specific departments. After they complete their survey, they should be asked to sign their name, title, and date of visit in a notebook labeled "Records of Inspections."

Where facility sponsorship (e.g., religious or fraternal) does not predetermine admission policies, it is recommended that patients be accepted, staff engaged, and volunteers recruited without regard to race, color, creed, sex, national origin, sponsor, or handicap. Generally, admission of patients should be limited to persons who are over a specified age, who do not suffer from tuberculosis or other communicable or contagious disease, and who do not have a behavioral disorder that would endanger the patient himself or other residents. Patients must be admitted to the facility by physician recommendation.

At the time of admission, it is highly desirable for the patient and/or his family to designate a responsible party, hereafter referred to as the patient's sponsor, with whom all financial transactions should be conducted. In the case of a Medicaid patient, the sponsor with financial responsibility for the patient's stay in the nursing home would be the designated state Medicaid agency. However, this does not preclude every resident, regardless of financial sponsorship, from having a designated responsible representative to whom the nursing home staff may relate on other than financial matters. In the case of a patient with private financial resources, the patient's representative and the sponsor may be one and the same person.

To foster the continuity of care, transfer agreements or affiliations should be developed between freestanding skilled nursing facilities and community general hospitals and home health care agencies. Ideally, such arrangements will redound to the benefit of the patients as cooperative education programs for nurses and rotating internships for medical students expose professionals in all settings to the needs of the chronic ill aged wherever they may be. Upon the admission and discharge of residents, completed transfer information from the referring agency must accompany the patient.

The skilled nursing facility is an integral part of community health services, and as such it has responsibilities to the community as well as responsibilities to residents to help them remain members of the community. This may be enhanced by encouraging local groups to participate in the activities program or to use the nursing home for their own activities and/or meetings. Various communications media should be used to relate to the community and to residents, their families, staff, and volunteers.

When setting visitation policies and hours, the nursing home should consider that visitors may benefit or hinder a patient by their presence. For instance, visitors at mealtime may help make meals a more pleasant and social experience for some residents, while visitors may interfere with this important part of the rehabilitation program of others. Facilities must decide, then, whether they want totally open visitation, limited visitation with prescribed hours, or a combination of both, which will vary according to individual residents or resident units. All residents are entitled to sufficient time each day for their personal care. Under any policy, a more flexible visitation schedule might be allowed for critically ill residents.

Although it is important to encourage continued family and community ties for the individual's well-being, the skilled nursing facility must establish certain guidelines relating to the patient's safety and to the liability of the institution. Written permission from the attending physician should be obtained before a patient is allowed to leave the premises alone or with responsible companions. In addition, the patient's physical capabilities and any limitations regarding off-premises activities should be noted and relayed to the escort.

An off-premises book should be maintained at each nursing station to record the time of a patient's departure and expected time of return, along with the name and relationship of the accompanying person. For an outing sponsored by the nursing home, the patient's representative should be asked to sign a permission and release-of-responsibility form.

The nursing home should maintain accurate and complete medical, financial, and personal records on all patients, staff members, and volunteers in the strictest confidence. The nursing home must determine its policy regarding patient funds, that is, whether the institution, family, or sponsor will have the responsibility for receiving, guarding, and disbursing residents' personal money. If the institution accepts this responsibility, specific procedures must be outlined concerning limits on the amount of money to be kept, accounting methods, placing funds in interest-bearing bank accounts, and regularly reporting balances to residents or sponsors.

Finally, policies and procedures should be developed by various committees of the facility to outline the functions of the facility's departments and services.

Certain operational decisions come under the purview of the administrative director in consultation with the governing body, the medical director, and other executive staff. All staff members must understand the organizational plan, which describes the entire structure of the nursing home services and delineates lines of authority. (See Figure 1-1.)

Complete rate information should always be accessible and available for persons making inquiries. The daily rate may be an inclusive rate providing for total comprehensive patient care, or it may be limited to room and board, routine nursing, activities, religious and social services, with medical care, rehabilitative services, laboratory services, x rays, prescribed drugs, and so on charged separately. Posting rates and giving due notice to patients and/or sponsors before rate changes are effected are good institutional practices.

In addition to certification for Medicare purposes, medical care facilities, including hospitals and nursing homes, may pursue accreditation by the Joint Commission on Accreditation of Hospitals—a national member organization comprising the American College of Physicians, the American College of Surgeons, the American Hospital Association, and the American Medical Association and composed of commissioner representatives of those four organizations plus the American Health Care Association. This body is devoted to the standardization and eleva-

FIGURE 1-1
Suggested Organizational Pattern of a Skilled Nursing Facility

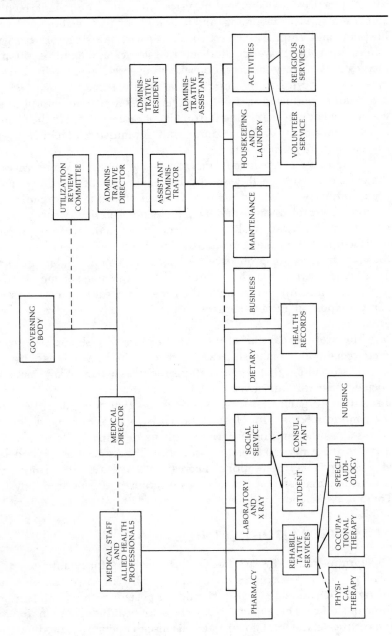

tion of patient care in hospitals and related facilities through defining requisites in the following areas: governing body, administration, personnel practices, management, physical plant and equipment, medical and dental services, laboratory and radiology services, relationships with hospitals and emphasis on continuity of care, nursing services with criteria for patient care, medical records, storage and administration of medications, dietary services, housekeeping services, rehabilitative services, social services, activities, and quality assurance.

Audits conducted by the Joint Commission may be helpful to the governing body in evaluating the quality of care provided in the facility. Indeed, some organizations require Joint Commission accreditation as a prerequisite for membership.

In addition, to remain current with developments in long-term care, the skilled nursing facility should become a member of professional organizations, such as the National Council on Aging, an organization composed of professionals and lay people; the American Hospital Association; the American Health Care Association (predominantly proprietary facilities); the American Association of Homes for the Aging (only for voluntary not-for-profit facilities); and the National Safety Council. These organizations may have certain criteria that must be met in order to gain membership; for example, the American Health Care Association is proposing that all member facilities participate in a peer review program.

The professional staff of the nursing home also should be encouraged to maintain memberships and participate in the activities of professional associations. Such organizations include the American Geriatrics Society (primarily for physicians), the Gerontological Society (an interdisciplinary organization), the National Association of Social Workers, the American Society for Hospital Social Work Directors, the American Nurses' Association, the American College of Nursing Home Administrators, the American Dietetic Association, the Association of Food Service Supervisors, the National Recreation and Parks Association, the American Occupational Therapy Association, the American Physical Therapy Association, and the Association of Directors of Volunteers.

ADMINISTRATIVE RECORDS

The administrative director has the responsibility for retaining certain facility records, particularly those mandated by law. Any license issued to the skilled nursing facility should be posted in the administrative director's office. These may include the state health department operating certificate, the local government license to operate a skilled nursing facility, the state health department controlled substances license, the state health department narcotics license (if there is a dispensing pharmacy on the premises), the Department of Labor permit to pay wages by check, and the Medicare provider number. Reports of surveys conducted by the state agency or the Joint Commission on Accreditation of Hospitals and the certificate of doing business or certificate of incorporation should be housed in administrative files.

Record books that should be located in the administration office are copies of all policy and procedure manuals, bylaws of the nursing home, governing body records and minutes, patient daily census record book (which should also include a breakdown of the daily Medicare, Medicaid, and private patient census), job descriptions book, state health code, Medicare Conditions of Participation ("Skilled Nursing Facilities: Standards for Certification and Participation in Medicare and Medicaid Programs"),[1] interdepartmental committee meeting minutes, visitors' registers, inspection record, departmental reports, and annual report of general and statistical information. In addition, the administrative director may elect to retain financial statements—balance sheets, operating budget, and operating reports.

COMMUNICATIONS

Various types of communications are advisable for the skilled nursing facility to reach staff members, families, and the professional and lay public. Several considerations should be taken when installing telephones, particularly investigating the cost of purchasing equipment in lieu of rental. In the absence of a switchboard, separate telephone lines should be installed for nursing units and other departments so that physicians can speak directly to nurses and calls can go directly to the intended party. Incoming calls for residents may be taken on portable phones so that the residents can receive calls in the privacy of their own rooms. Public telephones should be installed with two purposes in mind—so the staff can use them for making outgoing personal calls and so residents can use them. The telephones should have an appropriate height and dimensions to accommodate wheelchair patients.

Emergency telephone numbers should be available to all department heads and supervising nurses. In addition to the fire department, police, hospital, and ambulance service, these numbers would include the home phone numbers of the medical director and his alternate, administrative director, assistant administrator, director of nursing, staff or community pharmacist, social service director, dietitian, foodservice supervisor, activities director, volunteer services director, physical therapist, occupational therapist, speech pathologist/audiologist, executive housekeeper, and maintenance director. In the absence of the maintenance director and the alternate, telephone numbers for the repair of certain major equipment should be available to key staff on every shift.

FIGURE 1-2
Wheelchair-Height Telephone

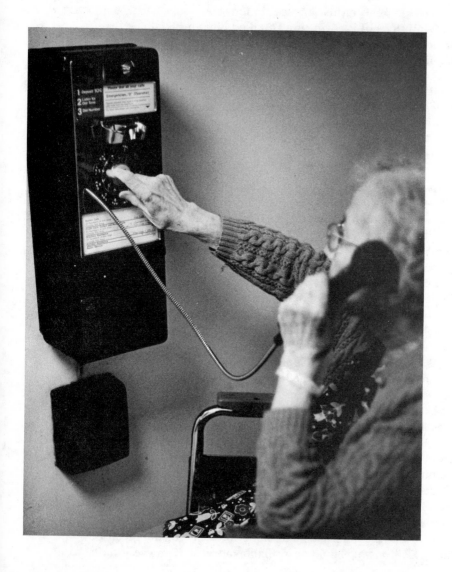

Such numbers would include those of the plumber, electrician, exterminator, and service representatives for the boiler, oil, gas, electric, elevator, air conditioning, freezer, fire alarm, fire extinguishers, incinerator, office equipment, laundry machines, telephones, and automobiles.

It is useful to have an intercom system installed in the telephone system to notify staff of incoming calls or visitors, to hold in-house conference calls, and to allow visitors who arrive after the receptionist has left to announce themselves to the main nursing station. A public address system with microphones located at key offices is an additional system that can be used when staff members cannot be reached via the intercom. A public address system is also helpful in contacting visitors or attending physicians, in giving directions during fire drills or emergency situations, in making announcements for all staff and/or residents, and in playing recorded music.

Several types of communication between patients' bedrooms, lavatories, and bathing areas and the nursing station may be considered for use in a skilled nursing facility. A closed-circuit television system would provide nurses the ability to monitor patients constantly. Different combinations of audiovisual call systems may be installed, dependent on whether the conversational component is appropriate to the specific patient population, for example, the intellectually impaired. Another mechanism is the call buzzer system, with signal codes for distinguishing calls from bedrooms or bathrooms, to summon an attendant to that room.

Written communication may be handled in several ways. Department heads and key administrative personnel may have individual clipboards or centrally located message boxes for the transmission of information. In addition, bulletin boards should be located throughout the facility for different purposes. Each nursing station and department office should have one. A bulletin board in the staff dining room or lounge area should be used for the dissemination of information and posting of notices applicable to all staff. The main entrance area of the facility also should have a bulletin board to display selected news items and the schedule of upcoming activities for the notification of patients, families, visitors, and staff.

Four publications issued by the skilled nursing facility—newsletter, professional bulletin, medical memo, and annual report—can serve as valuable forms of communication with residents, staff, families, and the community. It is advisable for the administrative director to review and approve any written material that will be distributed outside the facility to ensure appropriateness, accuracy, and uniformity of content. A mimeograph machine can most often be used for duplicating, although professional printing may be considered for special projects. Photocopying should be an alternative only for small quantities of duplication. When preparing material to be distributed to residents as the primary audience, the typeface and spacing should facilitate its being read by those with visual disabilities. The administrative assistant should maintain a chronological file of issues of all publications.

A periodic newsletter should keep patients, families, staff, and volunteers abreast of current and prospective programs; exchange personal news items of patients, families, staff, and volunteers; cement relationships with volunteer groups by an enthusiastic description of their activities; invite letters to the editor discussing pertinent topics; and promote the staff's and families' understanding of the nursing center's goals and problems. The administrative assistant should solicit help in compiling material for the newsletter by having staff representatives from each department and/or nursing shift and patient representatives from each unit serve as contributing editors. The newsletter can be distributed to all current patients and selected discharged patients, their families, staff members, persons and organizations mentioned in the bulletin, volunteers, members of the governing body, interested friends in the professional community, and members of the communications media (especially the local newspapers).

A periodic professional bulletin may be compiled, with the administrative assistant serving as editor and members of the professional staff of the nursing home serving as contributing editors. The bulletin should be designed to acquaint the professional community with newer trends in long-term care, results of studies conducted in the facility, and articles written by staff members and published in professional journals. The distribution of such a bulletin ought to include professionals in the local community, professionals involved in health care problems on a national organizational level, representatives of concerned government agencies, and legislators in all levels of government.

A medical memo designed specifically to inform attending physicians, dentists, and allied health professionals of new health code regulations, nursing home policy and procedure amendments, and other items of interest may be published as the need arises. Information to be included should be solicited from the professional services of the nursing home and compiled in a style that discusses the item clearly, concisely, and as briefly as possible. The professional consultants of the nursing home and all attending physicians and dentists should receive copies of the medical memo.

The annual report of the facility should highlight the past year's activities as well as include appropriate statistical and financial information. Material for the annual report may be gleaned from monthly and annual written departmental reports, appropriate material concerning the governing body, newsletters, interviews with selected staff, and various records and reports that include statistical and financial data. The annual report of nonprofit organizations may also include a request for contributions. All interested persons—patients, families, staff, volunteers, members of the governing body, and members of the corporation or shareholders—should receive the report.

Newsworthy information should be sent to the news media. Appropriate material would detail human interest stories such as unusual backgrounds of residents, special events such as the wedding of elderly patients, or the newly found talents of nursing home residents. Descriptions of the facility's programs, especially special entertainment or visitors, new services to be provided, the purchase of major new equipment, future building plans, fund-raising events, and volunteer awards warrant informing the media, as does professional and personnel information such as appointments and awards and material concerning the facility's educational activities and research studies. The administrative assistant should maintain a file containing all newspaper and magazine clippings mentioning the nursing center.

Depending on the facility's size, the administrative director should request that monthly or periodic reports as well as annual reports from each department head become a permanent part of the facility records. Such written reports should include a compilation of statistical data; reports of activities; and material relating to staff, plant and equipment, or expenditures, with specific emphasis on exceptions to normal operating procedures and suggestions for improvements with plans for implementation.

GOVERNMENT INFLUENCE

No discussion of the operation and management of a skilled nursing facility in today's society would be complete without a mention of the influence that government activities have on the nursing home. Prompted by a commitment on the part of legislators to stem the rising cost of health care combined with the notion that every American deserves quality health care, the federal government has steadily increased its participation in the health care sector, particularly in long-term care, during the past decade.

Plans for new nursing care facilities or for service changes, equipment, and/or building improvements costing $100,000 or more in skilled nursing facilities must be approved by the federally mandated Health Systems Agency (HSA) for the region. Created by the National Health Planning and Resources Development Act of 1974, the agencies are responsible for determining how and where health dollars are to be spent, with consumer and provider participation as the cornerstone of the new system. One HSA for each of the more than 200 health service areas throughout the country has been designated by state governors on the basis of such factors as population and the availability of resources to provide necessary health services for residents in the area. Each HSA gathers and analyzes health data and prepares a Health System Plan (HSP).

Health facility structures, and any changes thereto, must always conform with the standards outlined by the Department of Health, Education and Welfare (HEW),[2] should comply with American National Standards Institute specifications,[3] and any further state and local construction standards. In addition, facilities certified for participation in the Medicare and Medicaid programs must meet the criteria of the *Life Safety Code*, a fire safety code regarding physical standards prepared by the National Fire Protection Association.[4]

Medicare and Medicaid

Government influence in the skilled nursing facility is documented by two programs, Medicare and Medicaid, that pay for the cost of care. Medicare (Title XVIII), managed by the Social Security Administration, is a federal insurance program for persons over age 65 or those who have received Social Security disability benefits for at least two years. Medicare is composed of two forms of insurance coverage. The first, Part A, is available to all those who qualify for Social Security and provides hospital insurance and coverage for a stay in a skilled nursing facility for up to 100 days, or up to 100 home health agency visits. To qualify for Part A coverage in a skilled nursing facility, the patient must meet certain criteria: he must require daily skilled nursing care or rehabilitation services as certified by a physician, must be hospitalized for at least three days prior to placement in the nursing home, must be admitted to the nursing home within fourteen days of hospital discharge, and must require treatment in the nursing home for the same condition necessitating hospitalization. Medicare Part A covers the entire cost of the first twenty days of authorized coverage and all except the coinsurance factor for the remaining covered days in a skilled nursing facility. For Medicare Part A beneficiaries, information is constantly gleaned from medical records to determine continuing coverage; Medicare coverage is denied if it is found that the patient no longer requires skilled nursing care or rehabilitative services.

Medicare Part B, medical insurance, is an elective insurance program that requires premium payments and has an annual deductible. Part B pays 80 percent of the allowable cost of covered services, which include but are not limited to doctors' visits, medical supplies, physical therapy, ambulance charges, outpatient services, laboratory studies, x rays, and the services of certain types of practitioners.

Medicaid (Title XIX), the most comprehensive of the health care financing programs, is designed to provide coverage for persons who demonstrate a medical and financial need for assistance. Medicaid will not pay expenses covered by Medicare, but it will reinstate coverage when Medicare benefits are denied or exhausted.

Although funded by federal, state, and local governments, setting the standards for eligibility for Medicaid as well as the payment structure is the responsibility of the individual states, with some federal guidelines. Hence covered services and the payment authorized for each differs from state to state. Additionally, the program is administered under local jurisdiction, which allows for further variations of procedures and implementation of the law.

Participation in the Medicaid and/or Medicare programs has a tremendous impact on the operation of the skilled nursing facility. For a facility to receive payment for the care of Medicaid/Medicare patients, it must be certified as complying with the federal Conditions of Participation, promulgated by the Health Care Financing Administration of the Department of Health, Education and Welfare, which delineate standards pertaining to the building structure, staffing patterns, and patient services. Facilities must be recertified annually by HEW for participation in the Medicare program and by the designated state agency for inclusion in the Medicaid program. The recertification process involves a survey of the facility to ensure continued compliance with the Conditions of Participation.

Facilities accepting Medicaid patients must also undergo the periodic medical review, which entails that a team composed of physicians and other appropriate health and social service personnel review the condition and need for care of each inpatient. The team must review the care being provided, the adequacy of the services available to meet the current health needs and to promote each patient's maximum physical well-being, the necessity and desirability of continued placement of such patients in the facility, and the feasibility of meeting their health care needs through alternate institutional and noninstitutional services. The periodic medical review differs from utilization review in that it requires the evaluation of each individual patient and an analysis of the appropriateness of the specific treatment in a given institution. Utilization review, discussed further in Chapter 16, is often done on a sample basis with special attention given to certain procedures, conditions, or length of stay.

The payment mechanisms for the two programs differ dramatically. The Medicare insurance program functions like any insurance plan and involves the use of a fiscal intermediary to process and pay claims. The skilled nursing facility selects its fiscal intermediary from private insurance companies approved to perform this service, or the fiscal intermediary could be the Social Security Administration itself.

In the Medicaid program, however, the individual states determine the procedure for payment, with this responsibility delegated to a state agency. The nursing home then works directly with the appropriate agency in processing claims. As may be expected when the government is involved in funding a program, extensive auditing of the facility's financial records is yet another example of the government's impact on the nursing home.

The receipt of public moneys is often a dictating factor in the enforcement of federal legislation. In other words, facilities caring for Medicare and/or Medicaid patients must abide by certain federal laws outside the purview of specific health regulations. For example, programs receiving federal financial assistance must comply with Title VI of the Civil Rights Act of 1964, which forbids discrimination in admission, placement, and provision of care for residents and in the selection and termination of employees. Prohibition of discrimination was recently extended by the Rehabilitation Act of 1973, which provides for equal opportunity for handicapped persons who are defined as ". . . any person who (i) has a physical or mental impairment which substantially limits one or more major life activities, (ii) has a record of such an impairment, or (iii) is regarded as having such an impairment."[5] As a provider of service, the skilled nursing facility must ensure that its facilities and programs are accessible to the handicapped and that new facilities to be constructed can accommodate handicapped persons.

Due to the nature of the patient population served, relatively newer long-term-care facilities have been designed with such features in mind. Therefore the major concern for nursing homes is making older facilities conform to new regulations and conducting ongoing reviews of employment and personnel practices. Pre-employment health inquiries are allowed only as they relate to the applicant's ability to perform job-related duties. Employers must make "reasonable accommodations"[6] for the employment of handicapped persons; what is reasonable may vary from facility to facility.

The law requires certain administrative functions. For employers of fifteen or more persons, a grievance procedure must be adopted and a staff member must be designated to coordinate the efforts to comply with the legislation. Another stipulation of the regulation is that facilities must evaluate their entire operation within one year of the law's effective date, which includes consultation with interested organizations representing handicapped persons to ensure that the facilities' programs, policies, and procedures are in accordance with the regulation and, if not, to take remedial action and note same in writing.

To receive federal Medicare and Medicaid funds, a facility must have a licensed administrator. Federal legislation was responsible for the requirement of licensure of nursing home administrators, which effectively created a profession overnight. Once again, however, the implementation of the legislation was assigned to the separate states, hence the state variations in nursing home administrator licensure and relicensure criteria. Most licenses are renewable biannually; the vast majority of states require a prescribed number of hours of continuing education for eligibility for relicensure.

If the candidate has not studied health care administration or its equivalent on a baccalaureate or graduate level, the State Boards of Examiners of Nursing Home Administrators require the successful completion of a 100-hour course in nursing home administration, covering such areas as general and departmental administration, patient care, medical terminology, and the physical environment. In most states, before the candidate can sit for the required examination, he must participate in an administrator-in-training program for a period of up to a year. In some states, only college graduates are eligible for licensure and, with the passage of time, nursing home administrator licensure will require a graduate degree.

In response to the growing professional call for peer review in the determination of quality care, the creation of Professional Standards Review Organizations (PSROs) was mandated in federal legislation and charged with the responsibility for the comprehensive and ongoing review of services provided under Medicare and Medicaid auspices. The program is conducted under physician sponsorship, with an individual PSRO assigned to carry out the review for a specific area. The intent of this review is to determine for purposes of reimbursement whether services in hospitals and skilled nursing facilities are medically necessary; are provided in accordance with professional criteria, norms, and standards; and are rendered in an appropriate setting.

INTRA- AND INTERFACILITY RELATIONSHIPS

Perhaps the most significant role for a facility's administration is the ongoing contact with its various constituencies. Often, an organization's success is measured by those who participate in it by their access to and influence on the chief decision makers. Specifically, these groups are the residents, the families of residents, the staff members, and various segments of the community—lay, civic, and professional. The administration's relationship with any of or all these groups may keenly affect its success and, more important, the success of the nursing home itself.

The administrative staff contact with the different constituencies may be planned or unplanned. In most instances, unplanned contacts entail such chance encounters as meeting patients, staff, or family members throughout the building while following a daily routine; making telephone calls; conversing with staff members during lunch or coffee breaks; and accidentally meeting people outside the nursing home at social engagements. Even though the contact may be informal, the administrative director and the administrative staff must be aware, as must all people in leadership roles, of opportunities to foster relationships both on a personal basis and as a representative of the skilled nursing facility. Attentiveness offered by the administrative staff during such meetings can do much to reaffirm the individual's or group's importance to the effectiveness of the operation.

Formal contacts with these groups will vary, depending on the purpose of the contact and the group that is addressed. Residents are met during the course of medical rounds and at meetings of the residents' council, which is designed specifically to develop a dialogue between the resident population and the administration. In addition to confirming the administration's responsiveness during a council meeting, the administrative director, assistant administrator, and administrative assistant should also use this opportunity to relay requests, discuss problems, solicit suggestions, and describe improvements or changes in services to the entire resident population, thus utilizing the council as an important tool in the therapeutic community.

Relationships with families are greatly influenced by planned affairs such as family group meetings, which may be called to discuss not only problem areas or the necessity of increasing charges, but also to seek counsel from family members whose different viewpoints and individual expertise should be a resource for the administration. Formal communication with families and sponsors may also be achieved via personal letters, group mailings, and the newsletter.

The administration's customary methods of communicating directly with staff members include announcements over the public address system, notices on the bulletin boards and in paycheck envelopes, and discussion during an organized function such as a committee meeting, especially personnel committee meetings. There is no question that the job of the administrative director in particular is lonely and misunderstood when it concerns unpopular decisions affecting the staff. However, if the director involves the staff in the decision-making process rather than making decisions by administrative fiat, the staff will at least be impressed with the difficulty of the issues that must be considered when making such decisions. Involvement will help cement the feeling that staff members also have a stake in the operation of the nursing home, and therefore will work for the good of all concerned.

By assignment of the governing body, the administrative director is responsible for developing a liaison with the outside community. Bringing the community into the nursing home has a twofold benefit: maintaining contact with the outside world for the residents and nurturing an understanding of a skilled nursing facility's purpose and activities by society in general. A volunteer program is the key to community involvement in the nursing home, and the administration should ensure that an active volunteer program is being pursued with formal recognition given to all volunteers. Offering the use of the nursing home premises for organizational meetings and the assistance of the residents in completing civic projects, inviting local dignitaries and officials to participate in special programs such as volunteer recognition or professional seminars, and requesting politicians to address the resident group at election time should be part of the nursing home community contact program.

As representatives of one segment of the local health care delivery structure, the administrative director and other nursing home personnel must become active in organizations dealing with community health care issues. Participation in civic organizations whose goals are the betterment of the entire community and in professionally related organizations where knowledge of long-term care and the problems of the aged, particularly the ill aged, is desirable should all be part of an administrative director's plan for community involvement. Needless to say, all staff members are ambassadors for the skilled nursing facility, and as such they must be familiar with the facility's goals, programs, and problems to enable them to represent the nursing home accurately and positively to all those who are uninformed.

SUMMARY

Whether the nursing home is large or small, freestanding, or attached to the hospital; under voluntary, proprietary, or government sponsorship; located in an urban, suburban, or rural setting; the triad of patient, family, and staff constitutes the nucleus of the therapeutic community. Personnel need to be aware of the changing nature of the chronically ill patient population and to be sensitive to the goals of family members, or patient placements will be unstable and therapeutic programs will suffer. Administration must strive for a continuing collaboration of the three constituencies, with educated and interested staff delivering personalized care to patients and cultivating the concerned involvement of family members.

NOTES

1.   U.S. Department of Health, Education and Welfare, Social Security
Administration, "Skilled Nursing Facilities: Standards for Certification
and Participation in Medicare and Medicaid Programs," *Federal Register*
39, no. 12 (January 17, 1974).
2.   U.S. Department of Health, Education and Welfare, Public Health
Service, *Minimum Requirements of Construction and Equipment for Hospitals and Medical Facilities* (Washington, D.C., 1978).
3.   American National Standards Institute, *Making Buildings and Facilities Accessible to and Usable by the Physically Handicapped* (New York, 1961).
4.   National Fire Protection Agency, *Life Safety Code*, No. 101 (Boston, 1967). Subsequent editions not currently applicable to nursing homes.
5.   U.S. Department of Health, Education and Welfare, "Rehabilitation Act of 1973, Section 504," *Federal Register* 42, no. 86 (May 4, 1977), pp. 22676–22697.
6.   Ibid.

Personnel

INTRODUCTION

There is a direct correlation between personnel who are technically and emotionally supportive and the quality of patient care. The importance of staff as part of the therapeutic community in a long-term-care facility cannot be overemphasized. Ratios of staff members to patients are less meaningful than the ability, interest, and concern of the staff in the care of the chronic ill aged.

Projections for the future foresee that nurses, physicians, social workers, and the like will have the benefit of specific instruction in geriatrics and gerontology during their professional training. Administrators, too, will be better educated, and it is hoped that qualified graduate students will enter the long-term-care field out of choice, not for job security. However, changes in the value system in this country regarding service to one's fellow humans and the current notion of personal service as demeaning may affect the availability of nursing attendants—those who engage in the largest portion of direct day-to-day care of nursing home patients. The recruitment of nurses and other professionals should become easier, while conversely, the recruitment of nonprofessionals should become more difficult.

Like other health care institutions, nursing homes usually employ many married women. As a result, vacation schedules of staff can be related to their families' schedules rather than to the nursing home's operational needs. Similarly, an emergency involving a child can pose a conflict for the working mother who, at the moment, may be caring for a critically ill patient. The increasing emphasis on women's equality may or may not effect a change in such problem areas.

It should be remembered that some patients, both male and female, may relate better to men than to women. A male physical therapist or physical therapy assistant may instill confidence in and encourage some patients who are fearful of falling during ambulation or gait training. Some patients may be inspired to participate more fully in the activity program that is led by a male activity director. This is a matter of a resident's individual preference, but in any case, employment decisions should be made on a sex-blind basis, in concurrence with federal Equal Opportunity Law.

STAFFING PATTERN

In a skilled nursing facility, the number of staff members, particularly clinical staff members, largely depends on the care needs of the patient population. Ideally, however, there should be at least a one-to-one ratio of personnel to residents. Nursing, of course, has the largest number of employees and will probably represent well over 50 percent of the entire staff complement. Workers in dietary, housekeeping and laundry, administration, and maintenance represent the next largest components in the order noted. Other staff members may include physicians, activity personnel, social workers, physical and occupational therapists, record coordinators, and educators.

One administrative staff member should be assigned the responsibility of functioning as director of personnel. Depending on the facility's size, these duties may be delegated to the assistant administrator or the administrative director, or a full-time director of personnel may be employed. The personnel director should report directly to the administrative director and develop rapport with each department head and supervisor.

This position should include responsibility for the entire recruitment process, including interviewing prospective candidates in conjunction with department heads, continuously communicating with department heads regarding their staffing needs and problems, maintaining up-to-date personnel files, counseling employees when appropriate, terminating staff with the assistance of department heads, reviewing and amending personnel policies, interpreting personnel policies, scheduling and recording minutes of personnel committee meetings, and remaining current on applicable labor laws and state code regulations regarding health care workers and personnel administration. Obviously, a candidate for this position must be versed in personnel management, should have some supervisory experience, and should have a proven ability to relate well to both professional and nonprofessional people. If the facility is unionized, experience in unions would be helpful if not mandatory.

Some personnel executives have had training in psychological testing. Such expertise could be useful in evaluating job candidates' ability to function effectively with the physically and mentally ill nursing home residents.

RECRUITMENT

To work effectively with long-term-care patients, potential personnel need more than technical skills. They must be able to become involved with and relate to sick, often depressed old people, many of whom suffer from varying degrees of behavioral disabilities and who bring with them into the nursing facility all their prejudices concerning minority groups. Thus all staff must be made aware of this potential problem so that they do not respond in anger to disparaging remarks made by prejudiced residents.

In contrast to the general hospital, where staff members are frequently trained to be able to rotate through various departments, patient care staff in the nursing home should be assigned to units where they will function most effectively. For example, some nursing personnel cannot handle working with intellectually impaired residents but do very well with the severely physically handicapped, while others can relate well to the brain damaged.

Some reasons for nursing home staff turnover may help guide recruitment and interview programs. Turnover has been ascribed to sex, age, marital status, education, salaries, geographic location, sponsorship of facility, the depressing nature of the work, the lack of commitment of personnel, and the generalized negative attitude of American society toward nursing homes, which can lower staff morale.

It has been demonstrated that the significant factor influencing nursing home personnel to remain on the job is liking their coworkers, followed by liking the patients and fulfilling a personal need.[1] Thus, during the interview process, the candidate's ability and desire to work with the chronic ill aged as well as to blend with other staff should be examined.

Transportation is another important concern, especially for evening and night workers. Thus proximity to the facility might be a determining factor in selecting employees. The interviewer should explore the candidate's reasons for seeking work, for example, whether this is to be a second job, whether the job is needed on a temporary basis for a special purpose such as childrens' college tuition or an important purchase, or whether it is to be a permanent position because the individual truly wishes to work. Has the candidate selected this kind of job because of a liking for old people (another major factor for nursing home job satisfaction), for humanitarian reasons, or because he or she is unqualified for other than a service position?

Discrimination based on age, sex, race, marital status, religion, national origin, or handicap ought not influence the selection of employees on an ethical basis. Federal mandates relating to funding also prohibit such discrimination with respect to civil rights and, more currently, on the basis of handicap. Indeed, the interviewer may not ask if the person is handicapped or inquire about the severity of a handicap, but only if the interviewee is able to perform the tasks required. The decision about whether he or she can perform the job well or safely is left to the job applicant rather than to the employer. Thus the interviewer must thoroughly review the performance requirements of the position with the candidate in case it is later determined that the applicant cannot carry out the duties of the job adequately. When selecting new personnel, the interviewer must always bear in mind the special responsibility of the nursing care facility to its ill aged residents.

It is preferable to recruit employees via other personnel. The personal integrity of the individual recommended by a staff member is generally assured, and such selection methods probably tend to attract people who will fit into the group satisfactorily. Furthermore, the staff member will want a friend's or acquaintance's employment experience to be successful. Care should be taken in hiring spouses and siblings, as an unsuccessful episode with one may cause the loss of both. In a unionized facility, of course, recruitment is circumscribed according to the union contract or contracts.

For locating employees in more specialized areas such as physical therapy, activities, and social service, contacting local professional associations may be useful, although it may be necessary to place classified advertisements in newspapers and journals. Vocational offices in professional schools may be a good source when a qualified person without experience is an acceptable candidate.

An in-depth screening is well worth the time involved. The interviewer should consider both potential and present qualifications of the candidate. Hiring the wrong person is detrimental to patient care and to staff morale, and it is financially costly in terms of time and energy wasted in training, completion of forms, payroll data, and so on.

For whoever handles personnel, the difficulty of evaluating the quality of professional staff by lay persons needs to be emphasized. When interviewing prospective directors of nursing, the medical director's assistance is advisable. Administrative staff can evaluate the administrative capabilities of nursing directors—for example, how they supervise, delegate, plan, and communicate—but they cannot adequately judge nursing skills. The medical director can also be helpful in appraising the abilities of other professionals such as physical therapists. Even so, a person's professional capability probably cannot be determined until after the decision to hire has been made, when the person can be observed on the job.

For the record, the applicant's background should be checked. The licensure of professional staff should be validated, and previous job experiences of all candidates should be explored via a written request to the previous employer. However, references are not gospel: they are only as good as the person who writes them and in no way should they replace a thorough interview.

PART-TIME VERSUS FULL-TIME EMPLOYMENT

Continuity of care is particularly important in the care of the long-term patient. This is crucial among intellectually impaired residents who are not able to describe symptoms or aches or pains to the treating staff. Therefore the clinical staff must be aware of changes in residents' appetites, in their facial appearances, in their abilities to ambulate, in their sleep patterns, in their elimination patterns, and so forth. Part-time and/or per diem personnel will be unable to engage in this type of ongoing individual patient evaluation.

Occasionally, however, a candidate with impressive personal or professional credentials will seek part-time employment. The interviewer will have to exercise discriminating judgment in determining the potential value of hiring such a person on a part-time basis with the hope that the candidate will become full-time in the near future. Management should be flexible enough to make exceptions when especially qualified candidates present themselves.

On the other hand, there are advantages to employing part-time persons. Frequently, such employees can work only when their spouses are home to care for the children, and thus important weekend coverage may be secured. Likewise, part-time personnel are particularly helpful to fill the gaps during the summer vacation schedule. Students in nursing and nutrition, for example, are good choices for summer and other part-time posts, and such experience will afford them an exposure to the geriatric patient and the long-term-care setting. A successful work experience will ensure the availability of future nursing home staff or at least future professionals with some knowledge and sympathy for the care of the ill aged. If the organization is unionized, the ability to hire part-time personnel and students must be verified.

PRIVATE DUTY PERSONNEL

Private duty attendants or nurses should be utilized sparingly. Although they are employed by the resident or his sponsor, the nursing home should verify their current licensure and be satisfied with the individuals selected and the reputation of the agencies from which they were hired, if applicable.

Companies that contract for private duty personnel may operate differently. They may function as a listing service, in which case the private duty nurse or attendant is paid directly by the client and the registry fee is paid either by the client or the employee. Alternatively, the agency may charge the client an all-inclusive fee that covers its percentage, insurance costs, and bonding of the employee, and then the company pays the employee. In any case, it is essential that the nursing home determine that private duty personnel are covered by malpractice insurance—either by the agency or, as is common with nurses, by individual policies. The facility's own malpractice insurance should cover institutional liability if a suit is brought as a result of an action by a private duty nurse or attendant.

Private duty personnel must be given an orientation to the philosophy and program of the skilled nursing facility, with particular emphasis on rehabilitation and the promotion of maximal patient functioning. A complete orientation is especially important for nurses, as their professional training may not have included geriatrics. Furthermore, nurses who work exclusively in private duty may be removed from learning experiences. They sometimes have no meaningful supervision, in-service education, or intellectual stimulation from their peers or other professionals. When they begin an assignment, they should be asked to sign a statement that they agree to abide by all the nursing home's administrative and patient care policies and to be responsible to the director of nursing or a designee. Personnel who do not abide by this agreement should be terminated. All private duty personnel work under the direction of the charge nurse of the unit; however, the amount of supervision varies according to the position—i.e., registered nurse, licensed practical nurse, or attendant—as well as an assessment of the individual's capabilities.

It is particularly important for special duty staff to relate to the families of residents constructively. Contact with physicians and outside consultants should be conducted in the spirit of professionalism and cooperation; facility personnel should never be bypassed. Communication and an effective working relationship between private duty personnel and their nursing home supervisors are essential to providing continuity of care, since special duty nurses and attendants usually are assigned to a nursing home patient for only one tour of duty per day or a maximum of twelve hours per day, after which the patient returns to regular floor staff care. Furthermore, this arrangement may be maintained for a long period due to the lengthy stay of nursing home patients.

PERSONNEL POLICIES
Orientation and Training

First and foremost, new personnel must be exposed to the philosophy of the nursing home and to the needs of skilled care patients, their families, and the other staff members. The importance of working as a team and communicating with all staff members—professional and nonprofessional—must be stressed. People who are accustomed to working only in a hierarchical setting where nurses relate only to nurses and not to aides and porters will need specific surveillance to determine their ability to function in an open social system.

It is vital that employees be given a clear picture of their jobs, through thorough verbal explanations and clearly written job descriptions. Indeed, for future reference, it may be important to document that staff members have read and understood their job descriptions. Staff also must be told and shown on the organizational chart how they relate to the rest of the organization, who supervises them, and to whom they present grievances. Every new employee is entitled to receive a thorough orientation to the facility and its programs and to his position, with special emphasis on patients' rights, infection control, safety, and emergency plans. He or she must be shown the interrelationships among departments and services and how they affect patient care. For example, the housekeeping schedule must take into account what the nurses need to do for the patients and the scope of the activities program on a particular day.

For every employee, standards of performance need to be set and schedules made that include projected completion dates. Such dicta need to be modified according to the responsibility of the position. For example, target dates for maids and porters will be short range, while target dates will be much longer for the executive housekeeper.

Personal qualities that need to be stressed are dependability, punctuality, and reliability, which are so important in a health care setting where helpless people depend on staff. Absolute honesty and ease of communication are indispensable to patient welfare. Open lines of communication must begin with the administration. The example set by administration and department heads will be replicated, and a democratic environment where all levels of staff enter into the decision-making process will create a positive atmosphere for the residents. If all staff members cannot participate actively in decision making, it is essential that they be made aware of the reasons for specific actions.

Sensitizing staff to what it is like to live in an institution where meals are served at a particular hour, where food is mass produced, and where staff members often are standing above and looking down on residents in wheelchairs should be part of the orientation and ongoing education program. Emphasis must be placed on the feelings of dependence, of needing help, and of waiting for assistance in all personal acts, including the use of the lavatory. Finally, difficulties in seeing, hearing, speaking, or ambulating must be reiterated, demonstrated, and if possible, experienced by staff.

Compensation

If possible, salaries, wages, and supplemental benefits for staff members should be commensurate with community standards in other health care facilities. Overtime pay is mandatory according to federal wage and hour regulations for all who work over forty hours per week except for executive, administrative, or professional employees, who, as salaried personnel, generally are not affected by overtime legislation. An employee is considered professional if the work to be done requires knowledge acquired by a lengthy course or specialized intellectual study, or if a primary task is to impart knowledge via teaching. Also, professional work necessitates consistent responsibility and judgment and is predominantly intellectual, varied, and not standardized. Further, at least 80 percent of the time spent working must relate to these criteria, and compensation must be a regular specified sum per week.

Other individual state wage and hour laws should be researched before the completion of personnel policies. Generally, the more stringent laws or portions thereof will prevail.

Uniforms

The use of uniforms in long-term-care facilities is under increasing discussion. With the current thrust toward deinstitutionalization, questions regarding uniforms for staff—including professional staff—have been resolved in a variety of ways. Following the trend in psychiatric institutions, some facilities do not require uniforms. Proponents of this position believe that increased personalization and communication and a more therapeutic milieu prevails among residents, staff members, and families when uniforms are not worn. Critics state that patients and families become confused and uncomfortable when they are unable to identify staff members by their dress. Others question the sanitary aspects of patient contact with staff members who wear street clothes. Some also are concerned with a loss of patients' rights if uniforms are not the practice, insisting that it becomes even more difficult for residents and families to identify and complain about staff members if they wear street garb. Some facilities exhibit the other extreme and have everyone dress in some type of uniform, smock, or coat, ascribing this approach as a desire to appear professional. A middle-of-the-road approach might suggest uniforms for treating staff and street attire for other personnel.

Uniforms are required in some departments and when the facility does not provide them, existing federal and state labor laws should be examined. Generally, the employer is not responsible for uniform reimbursement if the employee earns more than the minimum wage and if the differential between the minimum wage and the person's salary is equal to or greater than the purchase price and cost of laundering the uniform.

All personnel should wear legible name pins that note their position or department for easy identification by residents and family members.

Performance Appraisal and Staff Development

Personnel are entitled to periodic performance appraisals by supervisors or department heads after a specified probationary period—say, three months—and then annually or as necessary. A written form should be devised that is tailored to the needs of the long-term-care facility and to the varying comprehension abilities of staff members so that those completing the evaluation and those reading it have the same understanding of its contents. After the employee has had an opportunity to study the appraisal, constructive responses and suggestions should be encouraged by previously trained supervisory personnel concerning the department or service and the operation of the entire institution.

A beneficial environment is created when a nursing home has an active career ladder policy of staff development. When nurses' aides are encouraged and assisted in becoming licensed practical nurses, when practical nurses are helped to become registered professional nurses, when activity staff members are recruited into the nursing home and helped to attend school, all staff members feel a sense of pride. Even if individual staff members are not able to advance, the fact that their peers can improve their status helps develop a positive climate and a sense of stability among personnel.

Attendance

Sometimes specific personnel policies can be inaugurated that may prove particularly beneficial in a service facility where regular staff attendance is so crucial to the entire operation. Where one or two paid sick days per month are provided, it can be anticipated that most staff members will use them and thus that sick days will become almost a routine part of the schedule. However, some organizations have found that if workers are permitted to accumulate their unused sick days to be collected in the form of a monetary bonus, they will use fewer sick days and employee attendance will be stabilized. While this practice may not save money, attendance will probably improve, benefiting patient care and general staff morale. This policy may help minimize the inappropriate use of sick time and the resultant heavier load left to staff members who are on duty. Of course, staff members may not be permitted to come to work when they are ill but only when they are fit.

Staff Meetings

Regular meetings of all staff members of an inpatient facility are almost impossible when the facility is open day and night for 365 days a year. It is critical, however, to develop a mechanism for ongoing communication. Sometimes staff meetings can be arranged to cover day staff and another shift by requesting the evening nursing staff to arrive fifteen minutes earlier or the night nursing staff to leave fifteen minutes later. Even so, one nursing shift would still be excluded.

Therefore the facility should pursue the development of a personnel committee composed of representatives from all departments and all tours of duty. For further discussion of the personnel committee, refer to Chapter 16.

PERSONNEL RELATIONSHIPS WITHIN AND OUTSIDE THE FACILITY

Within the nursing home, ongoing communication among all staff members is highly desirable. It is essential for nurses to relate to aides and for administrative staff to relate, for example, to unskilled housekeeping and kitchen personnel. A climate of warmth and caring in the staff will assist greatly in the development of a therapeutic community.

Communication must be in the best interests of the residents and their families. In the hospital, families relate to physicians and save their questions for them. In the nursing home, due to the extended stay of residents and the absence of physicians, families get to know staff members and often direct their questions to nurses, social workers, aides, or whoever is available. Conflicting reports by different staff members to families can be damaging to the well-being of the residents and/or family members. Thus all staff members must be trained to differentiate between friendliness to residents and families and behavior that violates patient privacy and is both unprofessional and counterproductive to the well-being of the individuals involved.

When families single out certain staff members for presents, gratuities, or special favors, the integrity of the entire operation is threatened because of the unspoken assumption that special attention is being sought. The value of a staff fund benefiting all employees, supervised by the personnel committee, should be continually reinforced as the appropriate manner for families and/or patients to express their appreciation.

Personnel should be encouraged to participate in professional activities outside the nursing home to enhance their knowledge and expertise. They might be reimbursed for memberships in appropriate professional organizations on the basis of one organization per annum. The administration should approve and foster staff activity in community affairs such as membership on boards of community health and welfare agencies.

To foster a sense of pride and express appreciation for work well done, recognition ought to be given to staff members based on length of service. Awards could be presented upon the completion of one year's employment and five years' employment, and at five-year intervals thereafter. A staff awards program honoring the recipients and acknowledging the efforts of all staff members could be an annual festive event attended by staff, residents, and families.

In addition, individual initiative to further education may be recognized by the granting of modest amounts of money as scholarships. This fund could come under the supervision of the personnel committee, which would organize and sponsor fund-raising events specifically for this purpose. Staff members who are currently attending or who have been accepted for a professionally related educational program would be candidates for a scholarship, and the committee would then distribute the fund as it deemed fit. Staff members working together for the benefit of one another can do much to enhance the feeling of staff unity.

Finally, an annual staff party, with spouses invited, can further staff harmony by cementing a feeling of friendship among the staff community through sharing non-work-related happy occasions. When arranging this kind of party, the personnel committee must remember that there will always be some employees on duty no matter when the party is scheduled. Thus the best possible location may be the facility itself, so that working staff may also attend. Alternatively, the party may be scheduled at a different time from year to year so that it is not always held when one particular shift is on duty.

RECORDS

All policies affecting personnel should be organized into a written handbook that is distributed and explained to all new employees. The personnel committee should review it annually and amend it as needed.

The application for employment (Exhibit 2-1) is designed to conform with specific government guidelines as well as to elicit data that have proved to be deciding factors in employee turnover. The absence of questions regarding sex, marital status, number of children, and specific age is very important. Indeed, even the question of whom to notify in case of emergency must now be answered voluntarily. The alien registration number is requested due to the influx of immigrants who are working in the United States illegally and is, in fact, an administrative responsibility. The availability of transportation is included because lack of transportation can be an important reason for staff turnover. And, finally, whether the applicant is willing to work the proper share of weekends and holidays should be clarified prior to employment.

FIGURE 2-1
Staff Party

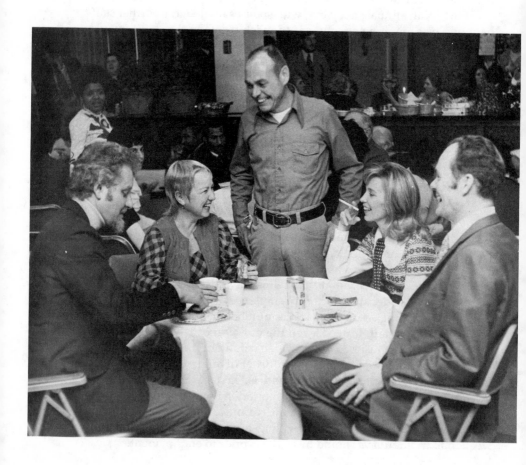

EXHIBIT 2-1
Application for Employment

XYZ Nursing Home

APPLICATION FOR EMPLOYMENT

This nursing home admits and treats patients, selects staff, and recruits volunteers without regard to race, color, creed, sex, national origin, sponsor, or handicap.

Name _____ _____
      Last   First   Middle   Today's date

Address _____
          Street   City   State   Zip code

Social Security no. _____ Telephone no. _____

Are you between the ages of 18 and 65? ___Yes ___No If no, state age ____	If not a citizen of the U.S., do you have the legal right to remain permanently in the U.S.? ___Yes ___No
Do you have any physical, mental, or medical impairments that would interfere with your ability to perform the job for which you are applying? ___Yes ___No If yes, please explain:	Alien registration no. _____
	Date of last physical examination _____
	Family physician _____
	Foreign languages spoken _____
Position desired	Shift desired (in order of preference) _____

Training for this position other than formal education _____

Other specialized training or experience _____

Present employment	Reason for desiring change

What prompted you to apply here for employment? _____

Are you related to anyone presently in our employ (other than your spouse)? Whom and how? _____

Type of transportation to and from work _____

Is there any reason you could not work your share of weekends and holidays? If so, what? _____

Nurses and Technicians:

_____   _____   _____
  Permit no.   State   Expiration date

_____   _____   _____
  License no.   State   Expiration date

Would you volunteer the name of someone to notify in case of emergency?

_____   _____   _____
      Name   Address   Telephone no.

If employed, I agree to abide by the policies and practices of the nursing home and to carry out my duties to the best of my ability. Also, I understand that I must have a physical examination upon employment and annually thereafter.

                        Signature _____

EXHIBIT 2-1 (cont.)

EDUCATION

Name and Location of Schools or Colleges	Major Subject	Degree & Date	Attendance From	To

FORMER EMPLOYERS AND EXPERIENCE (Most Recent First)

Name and Address	Job Description	Period From To	Salary	Reason for Leaving

PERSONAL REFERENCES (Not Relatives)

Name	Address	Phone No.	Business

(Applicant, please do not write in space below)

Interviewed by _____ Date _____

Position _____ Remarks _____

_____

Date to start work _____Starting salary _____

_____

RELEASE INTERVIEW AND RATING

Last day worked_____ Left without notice__ Resigned__ Released__ On leave__

Better job _____	Relocation _____	Incompetence
Family _____	General	Misconduct _____
Illness _____	Dissatisfaction _____	Insufficient pay _____
Death _____	Retirement _____	Other _____

(Superior, Average, Poor)

Overall job performance_____ Job knowledge_____

Cooperation with others_____ Initiative; leadership_____

Ability to grasp new ideas_____ Dependability_____

Appearance_____ Character; integrity_____

Further information on termination: _____

_____

_____

Interviewed by_____Date_____Rehire:____Yes____No____

The employee reference inquiry (Exhibit 2–2) should be mailed to the last employer on record directly after the interview.

The employee performance appraisal (Exhibit 2–3) should be characterized by clear and concise language. So that the same form can be used for all personnel, some questions should be specifically geared to administrative, executive, and professional staff.

The personnel checklist (Exhibit 2–4) should form the history of the employee, providing easily available data for all initial and ongoing employee records.

A warning notice must be completed and presented to an employee to sign whenever his or her performance is unacceptable. Any refusal to sign should be noted. This form testifies to the employee's awareness of unacceptable behavior or work and provides written documentation for the personnel file.

A letter to new personnel may be distributed with other written handbooks, forms, and information to new employees, welcoming them to the staff and briefly explaining the purpose and importance of the other handouts. By its content, this form demonstrates an important aspect of the orientation procedure: the distribution of required information to all new employees.

The notice of termination explains why an employee is leaving the job—resignation, discharge, layoff, or retirement. This form provides a good means of fully documenting the circumstances surrounding an employee's termination.

The curriculum vitae form, outlining educational and professional experiences, accomplishments, and association memberships, should be completed by all administrative, executive, and professional staff upon employment.

UNIONS

Given the choice, most nursing home administrators would not seek unionization for their employees. Historically, health care workers, particularly nonlicensed personnel, were not paid the equivalent of similar workers in other fields and thus were likely candidates for union-organizing drives. Although wages and benefits of hospital and nursing home workers have become more competitive with other industries in recent years, union drives proliferate, and an increasing number of facilities have become unionized.

Unionization is not to be considered a catastrophe, but it can curtail the administration's freedom of action and independence.

EXHIBIT 2-2
Employee Reference Inquiry

XYZ Nursing Home

EMPLOYEE REFERENCE INQUIRY

Date _____

To: _____

_____

_____

_____

Re: _____

S.S. no. _____

We would be most grateful if you would give us your forthright opinion of your experience with the above-named person, who has applied for a position as _____.

Since we work with frail and disabled older people, the past record and personal characteristics of our personnel are of primary concern.

If preferred, telephone me regarding this request. Please be assured that all information will be held in complete confidence. Thank you.

Director of Personnel

I hereby release from all liability the company or person named above, and authorize them to release all information regarding my employment with them.

Applicant's Signature _____   Date _____

- -

Applicant employed from _____ to _____ in position of _____

Please indicate Above Average, Acceptable, or Poor

Overall job performance	_____	Ability to grasp new ideas	_____
Character;integrity	_____	Initiative;leadership	_____
Appearance	_____	Job knowledge	_____
Neatness;orderliness	_____	Cooperation with others	_____
Dependability	_____	Punctuality	_____

Reason for Separation: Family____Transportation____Illness____Better job____

Incompetence____Relocation____Misconduct____Insufficient pay____

Other (explain) _____ Would you reemploy? Yes ____ No ____

Would you recommend the applicant for the position applied for? Yes____ No____

Other remarks:_____

_____

Signature and Title _____

EXHIBIT 2-3
Employee Performance Appraisal

EMPLOYEE PERFORMANCE APPRAISAL

Name _____ Position _____ Date _____

___3-month review   ___Periodic   ___Annual   ___Termination

	Above Average	Acceptable	Poor	Comments
Ability to relate to patients				
Ability to be impartial				
Ability to relate to families				
Ability to relate to staff				
Relationship with supervisor/dept. head				
Quality of work				
Quantity of work				
Adaptability to changing situations				
Ability to express oneself orally and in writing				
Ability to learn				
Ability to introduce and act on new ideas				
Job knowledge				
Judgment				
Dependability				
Punctuality				
Cooperation and willingness to work weekends, holidays, emergencies				
Neatness;orderliness				
Appearance				
Ability to use equipment				

EXHIBIT 2-3 (cont.)

(Answer the following questions for administrative,
executive, and professional personnel only:)

	Above Average	Acceptable	Poor	Comments
Does not discuss personal problems with subordinates				
Is effective in leadership role				
Can be impartial with subordinates				

	Above Average	Acceptable	Poor	Comments
Overall appraisal				

Appraised by _____ Date _____
                  (signature of supervisor)

Acknowledged by _____ Date _____
                  (signature of staff member)

EXHIBIT 2-4
Personnel Checklist

PERSONNEL CHECKLIST

Name _____   Today's date _____

Home telephone no. _____   Date of employment _____

Department/position _____

References mailed (to whom and date) _____

_____

_____

References telephoned (must be documented by completing a reference inquiry

form) _____

_____

Initial health examination returned (date)_____Tine test____Chest x-ray____

Annual health examinations (dates) _____ _____ _____ _____ _____

_____ _____ _____ _____ _____ _____ _____ _____ _____

Recognition of Patients' Rights received ___   Personnel handbook received ___

Emergency handbook received   ___   Safety checklist received   ___

Infection control leaflet received   ___ _____ ___

I have read a copy of my job description and the above orientation material.
I understand my duties, responsibilities, and the overall policies of the
nursing home.

                              _____
                              Signature of employee

                              _____
                              Date

Performance evaluations (dates): 3-month _____

Annually: _____ _____ _____ _____ _____ _____ _____

_____ _____ _____ _____ _____ _____ _____ _____

Although many improvements have been made through the years, large, depersonalized institutions where administration is far removed from workers can create a situation in which employees with grievances may turn to union organizers. In addition, the changing value system in our society, the deemphasis on sacrifice and duty to one's fellow humans, and the notion of personal service as demeaning make some nursing home workers ideal candidates for unionization.

Authorities on union activity in long-term-care facilities insist that unrest and dissatisfaction within the institution rather than outside propaganda cause the union to begin its drive. It is generally agreed that poor administration is the greatest asset to the union that is intent on organizing nursing home personnel. Furthermore, since employees tend to be either disgruntled or satisfied with their immediate supervisor, they vote in favor or against the union on the basis of their relationship with their supervisor rather than their relationship with the entire nursing home.

Whoever is in charge of personnel administration should have a clear picture of the status of personnel. Studies should be done to determine the amount and reasons for turnover. In-depth interviews with resigning staff should identify areas needing improvement. If turnover is attributable to institutional deficits, such deficits should be remedied.

Sometimes grievance procedures need to be redefined so that employees can bring their problems to someone outside their department and/or to administration. Or personnel may need counseling for personal problems, and this kind of support may improve the working climate. Staff members may want to feel a greater involvement and a sense of being needed in the operation of the nursing home.

Union Organization[2]

The union organizer does a thorough research job prior to instituting an organizing drive, beginning with a study of the facility's physical layout, including entrances, parking areas, and adjacent properties. The survey elicits information about the locker rooms, the location of the time clocks, the shift schedules, and the cafeteria or coffee shops. The organizer assembles data on the total number of employees and the number in each department together with their home addresses, ages, sex, ethnic characteristics, and salaries. The names of members of the governing body and their company affiliations and other activities will be summarized. The organizer may pay particular attention to soft spots in the organization—to weak or inept supervisors or to departments with poor morale.

Throughout this preliminary study, employees sympathetic to the union will be identified and developed into a working committee. This committee will be given information about the union and its history, with emphasis on its successes and its methods of organizing. The organizer encourages this committee to join all staff activities in the nursing home with a goal of broadening its base and becoming involved in all personnel-related problems. The committee advises the organizer on the best approach to the personnel in that particular nursing home.

The next step in the organizing process is the distribution of handbills that focus on previous successes in similar institutions or promises regarding wages or fringe benefits that the union can attain. Alternatively, the handbills may discuss purported unfair personnel practices—such as discrimination—or unfair disciplinary actions and may include reprints of newspaper editorials and statements by well-known people in the community favoring the union.

At the same time that handbills are being circulated, union authorization cards to be signed by employees are distributed in the nursing home by the in-house committee and outside the facility by the union organizers. The aim is to obtain recognition of the union by receiving the signatures of a majority of employees. Solicitation of personnel is conducted wherever it is needed, and people are approached in their own homes if the union organizer deems it necessary.

Nursing home administrators may forbid the union to solicit or sign up personnel any place in the facility during working hours and may forbid the distribution of union handbills during working and nonworking time on the nursing home premises. However, the facility may not forbid its employees to solicit for the union or to hand out union handbills during their own time in working or nonworking areas.

The union, quite properly, may request an election if 30 percent of the bargaining unit personnel have signed authorization cards. Should this occur, the administration would do well to contact a labor lawyer to act as liaison between management and the union. Labor consultants also advise that immediately after the facility has determined its position on unionization, this position must be communicated to all department heads, supervisors, and all employees carefully, thoroughly, and forcefully.

Both voluntary not-for-profit and proprietary nursing homes are subject to the amended 1974 version of the National Labor Relations Act. Labor unions may seek recognition as representing the majority of personnel in a specific bargaining unit of the nursing home. However, if the nursing home's administrative director does not really believe that the union represents a majority of the personnel, the nursing home is not required to recognize or deal with the union until it has received certification from the National Labor Relations Board (NLRB).

The National Labor Relations Board has found service and maintenance, clerical, licensed practical nurses, registered nurses, and security guard units the most likely groups to participate in collective bargaining. Before acknowledging the correct representation of the unit by the particular union, the NLRB analyzes a number of issues to determine whether there is a community of interests within the unit concerning wages, hours of work, job tasks, fringe benefits, supervision and general administration, overall working conditions, and the degree to which the work of each unit is interrelated. Professional employees may decide for themselves if they wish to be included in the unit, although professionals in some areas are represented by their own association for the purpose of contract negotiations.

At the conclusion of the representation hearing, the NLRB will decide whether the union qualifies, whether it represents an appropriate bargaining unit, whether the bargaining unit has been authorized by the 30 percent of its members completing union membership cards, and whether there are barriers to an election. In due course, the NLRB's regional office will determine whether all the criteria have been fulfilled and subsequently will schedule an election.

Both the nursing home and the union will be asked to appoint observers to identify personnel who present themselves to vote. Where appropriate, the observers and the NLRB agent may challenge an individual's eligibility to vote. For example, an individual desiring to vote may be a supervisor or may have resigned from the staff. Voting is by secret ballot and a majority of valid ballots (*not* a majority of the personnel in the unit) is needed to certify the labor union.

In accordance with the outcome of the election, once the administration recognizes the union, the National Labor Relations Act stipulates that the employer and the union meet to bargain over the terms and conditions of employment for the unit under discussion.

In a nursing home, the Federal Mediation and Conciliation Service (FMCS) must have due notice concerning original contract negotiation or renegotiation—thirty days for the former and sixty days for the latter. Also, a union must give due appropriate notice to the FMCS before striking or picketing a nursing home. Emergency dispute procedures are delegated to the director of the FMCS for problems related to initial contract negotiations as well as for contract renegotiations. The director is authorized to follow a defined procedure, including the appointment of a board of inquiry in case the health service of a community is seriously threatened by a strike or a lockout.

For effective collective bargaining, someone experienced in labor relations should be given the authority to speak for the nursing home. The administrator and appropriate supervisors should advise the facility's negotiator on the practical implications of every point under discussion. Although only one person should speak for management, the final decision on issues must be made by the nursing home's administration and the governing body. The negotiator appointed by the nursing home must be familiar with union contracts and wage scales in other nearby facilities. He must be completely informed about current nursing home wages and benefits and all nursing home personnel policies. In addition, he should know the number of employees involved, the hours worked including overtime, and the backgrounds, length of service, and problems of present personnel.

At the first meeting, the union negotiator generally presents the union's program, assisted by a committee of employees from the nursing home. At the second meeting, the union demands are explained; at the third, the negotiator presents counterproposals for the nursing home.

In some areas of the country, groups of long-term-care facilities have banded together for collective bargaining either with one union or with several unions. The advantages to association collective bargaining are uniformity and standardization, fewer strikes, better acceptance of increased costs by fiscal intermediaries, and better-informed negotiators. The principle disadvantage is the impact strikes would have on such a large group of nursing homes.

Once the negotiation has been completed, the nursing home must learn to live with the union. The National Labor Relations Act delineates what practices on the part of management and the union are considered unfair. The union contract delineates management's prerogatives to discipline and terminate employees. A system of progressive disciplinary actions including counseling—verbal and written—warning notices, suspensions, final warnings, and termination is mandatory in order to be able to function with outside arbitrators. All these steps must be clearly and carefully documented for the record.

While it is generally true that unions are not welcomed into nursing homes, unionization does not preclude effective patient care. It is obvious that the supervisor or department head is the key to the development of a successful working relationship with unionized personnel. The employment of someone experienced in the development of workable labor relations with particular emphasis on avoiding unfair labor practices cannot be stressed enough, as this person will have to learn to deal with the union representative and staff on a daily basis. Second, the supervisor must be able to defend disciplinary action by an affirmative response to questions concerning whether an employee broke a rule or committed the act with which he or she was charged, whether the employee's act, in fact, deserved correction or punishment, and whether the corrective punishment was appropriate for the act.

It is in the best interests of all residents, families, and staff members to develop productive and cooperative labor-management relations with collective bargaining representatives. Service cutbacks, strikes, and walkouts present a serious threat to ill aged patients, and every effort must be made to avert such situations. If an impasse occurs and if work stoppages are inevitable, however, a well-thought-out emergency strike plan should be developed and thoroughly tested prior to the emergency.

SUMMARY

Nursing home personnel may be male or female, young or old, full- or part-time, professionally trained or basically unskilled, American or foreign born, unionized or nonunionized. Such variables may or may not influence the ability of personnel to learn the technical aspects of their jobs. However, it is clear that the care of the frail, elderly nursing home population is less dependent on the technical knowledge of staff than on their compassion for others. Supervising personnel must be alert to employees who are technically proficient, but deficient in human relations skills. In other words, knowing the technique of gait training a disabled patient is worthless if the staff member is unable to encourage the patient to leave his chair. Thus, those who are gifted in interpersonal relationships may prove to be the more satisfactory staff members, for these people can always be given additional skill training, while teaching an insensitive person to be compassionate is another matter altogether.

NOTES

1. D. Miller, J. Barry, and V. Ready, "Staff Turnover in Long Term Care Institutions: Why and Why Not?" *Second North American Symposium on Long Term Care Administration Proceedings* (Washington, D.C.: American College of Nursing Home Administrators, 1976), p. 134.
2. The reference for the bulk of the discussion about unions and health care is Norman Metzger and Dennis D. Pointer, *Labor Relations and Personnel Management in Long-Term Health Care Facilities* (Washington, D.C.: American Health Care Association, 1975).

Medicine

and Allied Health Professionals

INTRODUCTION

Medical care is the key to all other clinical services provided by the skilled nursing facility. Nursing, rehabilitative services, social work, and the like can perform only to the level of leadership provided by the medical team.

By federal mandate effective in 1975, skilled nursing facilities participating in Medicare and Medicaid programs are obligated to employ medical directors. This legislation came about as a result of a void in the medical care of the ill aged in nursing homes. Former Senator Frank Moss of Utah and other critics of the quality of nursing home medical care realized that many physicians were disinterested and, indeed, repelled by the chronic ill aged or by their own inability to diagnose, prescribe, and effect a cure for the illnesses of such patients. Too many "disease-oriented" physicians tended to avoid their nursing home patients and, in effect, neglected them or offered irregular or perfunctory attention.

The long-term-care facility, unlike the acute hospital, is not in a position to discipline attending physicians for their inattention. The physician needs the hospital as a workshop. If peers in the hospital or the medical records administrator finds a physician's work to be deficient, admitting privileges may be denied and his practice* will be directly affected. The loss of admitting privileges in the nursing home presents no similar threat to the physician. Indeed, some physicians welcome this method of relieving themselves of the responsibility for elderly patients.

*Masculine pronouns are used throughout this chapter, and in other chapters, for purposes of succinctness and are intended to refer to both males and females.

The apparent disinterest of the medical community in caring for the chronically ill aged in long-term-care facilities is changing as medical schools increasingly include geriatric medicine in their curricula. Some schools have integrated it voluntarily; others must do so to be eligible for federal funding. As medical schools become involved in long-term care, clerkships, internships, and residencies in the field will become more common and will eventually improve the quality of nursing home medical care. When medical students are exposed to the problems of the ill aged and have positive experiences in working in long-term-care settings, they will carry their experiences with them in whatever settings they choose for their future careers.

MEDICAL DIRECTION ALTERNATIVES

Medical societies and planners recognize that not enough physicians are currently available to serve as medical directors in the 8000 skilled nursing facilities in this country. To fill the gap, medical leaders have formulated a community-wide method known as the medical staff equivalent. In this system, a county or district medical society can join with the area's long-term-care facilities to develop committees that will monitor nursing home medical care.

The medical staff equivalent model comprises four working committees: executive, medical audit, procedural review, and utilization review. These committees include both physicians and long-term-care personnel. It is suggested that physicians selected to participate in medical staff equivalent programs be well respected in their community to afford them "clout" with their medical peers.

The executive committee, composed of a two-to-one ratio of physicians to long-term-care administrators, coordinates general medical policies and specific medical activities of the facilities under its jurisdiction. It serves as the final determinant in all decisions recommended by the three other committees and is responsible for disciplinary actions involving physicians and nursing homes.

Only physicians may serve on the medical audit committee, which reviews all clinical records in order to ascertain that the description of the patient's illness and physical condition are congruent.

An equal number of physicians and nursing home representatives constitute the procedural review committee, whose purpose is to scrutinize all treatment given to each patient to determine that all possible community resources are being used.

Finally, the utilization review committee, entirely composed of physicians, is concerned with the proper use of beds and the level of practice of attending physicians.

In lieu of the medical staff equivalent, medical direction agents or organizations are also being used. Indeed, in some instances nursing homes contract with hospitals to provide medical direction. Such a practice should be explored when other alternatives fail.

Duties of the Medical Director

The nursing facility's medical director may be on the staff of the facility or may be retained on a consulting basis. Serving as liaison between the administration and the governing body and the entire professional staff of the skilled nursing facility, the medical director is the leader of the interdisciplinary team. Via an ongoing assessment of the nature of the patient population, he is in a position to recommend and implement patient care policies to meet the changing needs of the residents. Furthermore, the medical director should interpret to the administration and to the governing body the significance of government regulations as they affect patient care and services.

The medical director should participate in policy making and long-range planning and should supervise the development of guidelines and rules and regulations for attending physicians, consultants, dentists, and allied health professionals. He should establish standards of medical practice and should supervise or coordinate medical care by maintaining contact with the attending physicians to discuss their patients' medical and management problems. He should be available to provide emergency medical coverage in the absence of the attending physician or his designee.

The direction of the personnel health program is part of the medical director's responsibility. Also, he should assist in planning and participate in the education program related to improved patient services. He should conduct clinical rounds and should supervise all clinical research activities.

The medical director serves on the patient care policy, infection control, pharmacy, safety, interdisciplinary, and budget and capital expenditures committees. If he is an employee of the nursing home, the medical director may not be a member of the utilization review committee but can serve as a valuable resource person. As a consultant, however, he may serve on the utilization review committee. He should advise and make recommendations to administration with respect to the adequacy of medical equipment and supplies and the maintenance of a safe and hygienic environment. He should review and analyze all patient incidents and accidents to determine whether they resulted from medical or environmental problems.

Finally, the medical director serves as the arbiter for solving problems of a medical-administrative and medical-legal nature. In a sense, he is the buffer between attending physicians, patients, families, administration, and the governing body.

In terms of patient care, it is interesting to highlight those times when the medical director is asked to intervene in the absence of the attending physician. He is called by the nursing staff to provide direction for a patient with an unstable medical condition—physical, behavioral, pharmacological, etc.—and to develop a thorough nursing care plan for a newly admitted patient whose condition presents a particular challenge to the staff. When the attending physician or his alternate fails to make a thirty-day visit for whatever reason—illness, vacation, etc.—the medical director is asked to renew orders and write progress notes. Unlike the hospital, where interns or residents are always on the premises to pronounce death, the nursing home does not have physicians in attendance around the clock. Often the attending physician is not available to perform this duty, so the medical director is asked to pronounce the patient dead and sign the necessary papers. If doctors do not return to the nursing home to complete their written chart work, when residents are discharged unexpectedly or expire, the medical director is asked to write the discharge summaries. Although the patient's physician usually performs the admission physical, he rarely will complete annual physicals and the medical director may be requested to do so. In addition to emergency situations when time is critical, the medical director's services are essential to fill the gap left by uninterested physicians.

Performing all these tasks and educational endeavors takes considerable time. Therefore it is suggested that the position of medical director in a 100-bed facility be at least half-time. What kinds of physicians with what kinds of training will seek such posts? Probably younger physicians beginning their professional careers or older physicians who wish to taper off their work schedules. With the increasing number of women in medical schools, it is conceivable that if some of these physicians have children and choose to devote more time to their care, they may welcome the opportunity to find part-time positions.

While the patients' physicians cannot be permitted to ignore the nursing home's rules, which are generally based on federal and state legislation, the medical director cannot be considered the chief of the attending physicians. Rather than direct them, he gives them guidance and advice and coordinates their efforts. Attending physicians strive for autonomy, and the medical director for conformity to patient care policies. Thus the relationship has to be a negotiated one, characterized by tact, diplomacy, and a professional mutual understanding. The medical director actually represents administration and has a mission to see that quality care is delivered. On the other hand, the attending doctors have a primary allegiance to the practice of medicine, which may subvert the effective functioning of the nursing home treatment team.

The aggressiveness with which the medical director deals with the attending staff may be tempered by the administrator's wish not to offend those who refer patients to the facility. Administrators with this point of view probably have not studied the admission process. In the main, patients are referred to the nursing home by lay people, frequently families of former or present residents or by social workers in health and welfare agencies.

ATTENDING MEDICAL STAFF

While the medical director is the coordinator of the professional staff and liaison to the attending physicians, members of the medical staff engage in direct patient care. The term "medical staff" may be interpreted to include all physicians who attend patients in the facility.

The skilled nursing facility may have an open or closed medical staff. In an open medical staff, any physician with a state license to practice medicine is entitled to admit patients to the nursing home in accordance with the facility's admission criteria. Physicians in an open staff arrangement are basically on call and allocate no regularly scheduled time to see their patients.

By and large, nursing homes tend to have an open staff arrangement, with the individual's personal physician able to follow him from hospital or home to the nursing home, thus affording a sense of continuity to the dislocated, ill elderly person. Of course, many patients are in skilled nursing homes removed from their home community, in which case their family physician cannot continue to care for them.

In an open medical staff, the medical director should develop written guidelines (which should then be approved by the governing body) to delineate the attending physicians' responsibilities. The medical director may also schedule medical staff meetings and plan other activities that are usually identified with an organized medical staff. The physicians may or may not participate in such activities on a voluntary basis.

A closed medical staff is an organized medical staff. The governing body appoints physicians on the recommendation of the medical staff's credentials committee. In nursing homes with closed medical staffs, only members of the staff may admit and treat patients. As few as three physicians (or two physicians and one dentist) may constitute a closed medical staff, according to the Joint Commission on Accreditation of Hospitals.[1] Community physicians are frequently invited to continue to visit their patients or, in some instances, are given courtesy privileges. But in fact, the organized medical staff of the facility has the ultimate responsibility for patient care. (See Figure 3-1.)

FIGURE 3-1
Suggested Organizational Structure of the
Medical Staff in a Skilled Nursing Facility

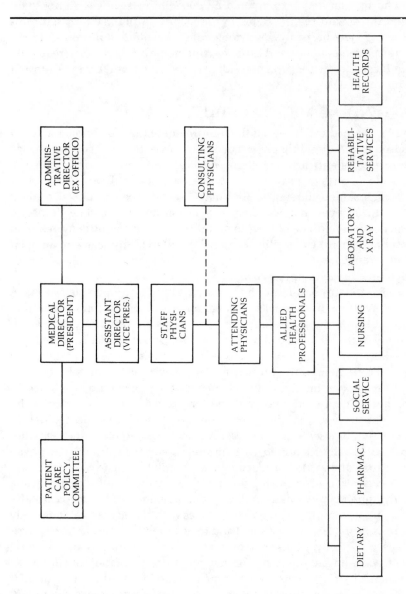

One of the advantages of an organized medical staff is that the physicians often attend their patients according to a prearranged schedule, allowing for better communication with the nursing home staff and greater continuity of care. When professional staff members know when to expect the attending physician, they will hold their telephone calls and prepare themselves and the patients for the medical visit.

Physicians selected to serve on the medical staff must meet certain qualifications. All candidates should be physicians of good character who have graduated from an approved school of medicine and are currently licensed to practice in the state in which the skilled nursing facility is located. It would be useful if nursing home staff physicians were also on the staff of hospitals with which the nursing home maintains transfer agreements. House staff physicians could include interns or residents participating in an approved training program within the skilled nursing facility, or residents working as house staff away from their own educational institution.

The appointment of physicians must follow a procedure outlined in the bylaws of the medical staff. Nominations should originate from the president of the medical staff and should be made in the form of a written application accompanied by a signed statement that the nominee agrees to abide by the medical staff's bylaws and rules and regulations. The application is referred to the administrative director for transmission to the entire medical staff for study and consideration. With the approval of the president of the medical staff, and accompanied by recommendations of the medical staff, the application should be offered to the governing body for action. The administrative director should relay the governing body's decision to the candidate in the form of a letter.

The governing body should appoint and reappoint members of the medical staff annually, subject to the medical staff's approval. In no case should the governing body be permitted to take action on any application or reappointment, or to alter the status of a member of the medical staff, without prior consultation with and subsequent approval by the medical staff.

The medical staff should develop bylaws, outlining the organization of the medical staff, its activities, and the responsibilities of its members, and it also should formulate rules and regulations that describe behavior and procedural requirements for the proper conduct of its work. A valuable guide in their development is the *Monograph Medical Staff By-Laws* published by the Joint Commission on Accreditation of Hospitals.[2]

The rules and regulations form a part of the bylaws; however, the amendment process differs for each. Amending bylaws can occur only when notice of same is given at a regular meeting of the medical staff, after which the matter is referred to a special committee that reports at the next regular meeting. The approval of bylaw amendments requires a two-thirds majority vote of the membership of medical staff present. In both instances, amendments become effective only after approval by the governing body. When adopted and approved, bylaws should be equally binding on the governing body and the medical staff.

The bylaws should describe the qualifications and duties of the officers of the medical staff. The president of the medical staff, who also serves as medical director, should be appointed by the governing body for a three-year term of office to allow him time to develop and organize the medical staff. In addition to his duties as medical director, the president would call and preside at all meetings of the medical staff, keep accurate and complete minutes of meetings, and attend to all correspondence.

Other officers would include the vice-president, who would be charged with acting on behalf of the president in his absence. If the medical staff is of sufficient size, a secretary and treasurer with appropriate functions should be appointed.

As prescribed in the bylaws, an organized medical staff has certain standing committees—executive, credentials, professional activities, and special—to facilitate its business. Members of these standing committees would be the president, vice-president, and additional members appointed by the president.

The executive committee's chief responsibility is to act on behalf of the entire medical staff under such limitations as may be imposed by the entire staff. This entails representing the staff at the joint conference committee (a committee composed of representatives of the governing body, medical staff, and administration), the patient care policy committee, and the utilization review committee. At each regular meeting of the medical staff, a report of all actions taken by the executive committee since the previous meeting should be given.

The credentials committee should be concerned with the examination of the credentials of all applicants for medical staff privileges and, for the purpose of advice to the entire medical staff, recommendations on appointments to, changes in privileges of, or removal from the medical staff. In addition, the credentials committee should review the applications and make similar recommendations regarding dentists, podiatrists, and other allied health professionals.

Peer review is carried out under the auspices of the professional activities committee, which conducts a regular review of medical records and other evidence of professional activity in the skilled nursing facility. Its findings are reported to the medical staff and the governing body.

The special committee of the medical staff would be called to act on the staff's special activities. One of its designated duties should be to study and make recommendations on suggested amendments to the bylaws.

The entire medical staff should meet at least annually before the end of the fiscal year, and more regularly if mandated in the bylaws, at which time committees should present reports of their activities; recommendations should be made on reappointments, committee appointments, and executive positions; and new business should be discussed. Special meetings, when only the business for which the meeting has been called is considered, may be convened by the president or two members of the staff, provided that sufficient advance notice is given to the entire staff. All members of the medical staff should be expected to attend every meeting; 50 percent of the total membership should constitute a quorum.

Medical care in the nursing home may also be provided by a panel of physicians, such as provided by the Health Insurance Plan in the greater New York area. With the anticipated growth in health maintenance organizations, together with the difficulty in attracting physicians to the long-term-care setting, it is likely that medical care in the nursing home increasingly will be provided by contract with a group or panel of physicians.

SCOPE OF RESPONSIBILITY

Whether facilities have an open medical staff, a closed medical staff, or another arrangement to provide medical care to their residents, the responsibilities of the attending physicians and medical director should be clearly defined. Job descriptions should be available for physicians who are on staff. A contract should be executed for the medical director, setting forth the responsibilities of each party, the terms of the agreement, conditions for termination, and financial arrangements.

Although the nursing home does not make special arrangements with patients' private attending physicians, it has a legal responsibility to ensure the provision of competent medical care to its residents. Physician licensure may be verified via confirmation in the state medical society directory. Attending physicians should be required to confirm in writing that they agree to provide medical care for the patient during his stay in the skilled nursing facility and designate the name, address, and telephone number of an alternate physician who may be called in his absence. Such a statement should be placed on the patient's chart for quick reference. Attending physicians should develop weekend, night, and off-duty patterns of coverage and provide same to the nursing home.

Attending physicians are responsible to the patient, the patient's family and/or sponsor, and the governing body for the quality of medical care practiced in accordance with standards established by the skilled nursing facility and for their ethical and professional practices. The principles of medical ethics as outlined by the American Medical Association serve as a guide for the professional conduct of attending physicians.

Each attending physician is responsible for giving guidance, direction, and supervision to all medical, paramedical, nursing, and other staff members involved in his patient's care. Physicians are required to abide by all policies of the facility as defined in the administrative, patient care, pharmacy, and infection control policies and, if provided, in the medical staff rules and regulations.

To inform physicians of their responsibililities according to state and federal law and nursing home policy, all physicians should receive specially developed guidelines that enumerate those items as well as duties and procedures affecting attending physicians and their relationship with allied health professionals, third-party payers, and the services of the nursing home. Such a manual, prepared by each facility according to its policies, would be useful for an organized medical staff as well as for an open staff since it synthesizes the physician's role. Changes or additions in federal or state regulations and/or nursing home policies may be relayed via an issue of a medical memo, a newsletter designed for attending physicians and allied health professionals and mailed to their respective offices.

DUTIES AND PROCEDURES

Patients should be admitted to the skilled nursing facility only on the recommendation of licensed physicians. However, if the patient's family physician does not plan on following him into the nursing home, the patient, his family, and/or sponsor can be assisted by the social service department in appointing an appropriate attending physician. The social worker is in a position to suggest physicians that he believes would be suitable and would relate well to both the patient and the family.

Ideally, the referring physician should continue to care for his patient upon admission to the nursing home. At the time of admission, the physician should provide the nursing home with certain information about the patient: a complete diagnostic statement and admitting diagnosis; a medical summary of all previous laboratory work and x-ray data; a transcript of the patient's hospital record, which includes a history, a summary of recent physical examinations, and a discharge summary; an outline of current medications, diet, and treatment; and a description of the patient's functional status. The last item should be stressed, for it is the real crux of nursing home care. As opposed to the hospital, which is oriented to diagnosis and treatment within a limited period, the nursing home must "live" with the patient—must develop and provide a program based on the patient's behavioral and functional as well as medical needs.

Patients admitted to the nursing home from another health care facility should have this information noted on the transfer form. However, because hospitals frequently do not have a total picture of the patient, the transfer information may be incomplete.

The admission of patients who have been living at home poses problems in securing this data. In such cases, the referring and/or attending physician should be contacted and reminded to provide the necessary documentation either prior to or on the day of the patient's arrival.

Unless a history and physical examination have been performed within five days prior to the patient's admission and the details of such investigation are documented on the patient's clinical record within forty-eight hours of his admission, the attending physician must appear at the facility to do so. Too often, the physician has visited the patient daily in the hospital and therefore feels no urgency to visit the patient in the nursing home, stating that he has completed an interagency referral form that gives up-to-date information on the patient.

However, the skilled nursing facility needs a complete new set of orders irrespective of the hospital experience. It is perfectly reasonable not to repeat certain diagnostic tests if such procedures have been performed at the hospital within five days and if documented results of these tests are presented to the nursing home. It does not help if the tests were done at the hospital but no records sent to the nursing home. Sometimes the attending physician will not visit the patient but will give telephone orders. In such a situation, the medical director will have to be asked to do the complete initial workup.

The following information must be provided and/or ordered by the doctor:

> history and physical examination
> chest x ray and/or interpretation
> x ray if patient has potentially unstable skeletal pathology
> electrocardiogram and interpretation
> urinalysis
> diagnostic screening profile
> other tests if necessitated by the patient's condition
> consultation if appropriate
> drug and treatment orders
> description of the patient's functional capacity, rehabilitation
>   potential, and prognosis
> orders for restorative services and podiatry when appropriate

orders for dental services

nursing orders with respect to patient management and
safety

permitted level of physical activity, including physician
permission for the patient to go off premises

Finally, the physician should document the patient's knowledge, or lack
of knowledge, about his medical condition. If the patient is intellectually
unable to comprehend, the doctor must keep the family and/or sponsor
informed, and this must be documented in writing. Without effective
medical leadership in the provision of all the above, a lack of direction
exists for the nursing home treatment team caring for the patient.

Frequently, patients are transferred from the hospital with diagnoses of recent fractures. It is wise to have a policy of requiring x-ray
studies following admission to make certain that the bones are setting
properly. For example, the pin used in the surgical procedure may not be
in the right place, but this may not be noticed until the patient begins to
bear weight. At this point, the nursing home may be blamed when in
fact the surgical procedure was at fault. X rays should also be taken
before the physical therapist begins an active rehabilitation program.

Within two weeks after admission, the attending physician, with
the aid of other medical and paramedical disciplines, should direct the
completion of the patient care and discharge plans. The care plan summarizes the patient's problems related to the various nursing home
staffs—medicine, nursing, dietary, social service, activities, rehabilitation, and so on—realistic goals for overcoming those problems, and the
treatment program to achieve those goals. The discharge plan should
identify the patient's potential for returning to the community or for
transfer to a different setting. If discharge is imminent, the staffs must
then identify their various roles in preparing the patient for discharge as
part of the patient care plan.

All patients in a skilled nursing facility should be visited by their
physicians every thirty days, and more frequently if their condition
requires. When the physician makes his scheduled monthly visit, he
should review, in conjunction with the charge nurse, the patient care
plan and the discharge plan, rewrite all orders, and write a progress note.
On the anniversary date of the patient's admission, the physician should
conduct a comprehensive reevaluation of the patient's health status, including a complete physical, electrocardiogram, chest x ray, urinalysis,
and diagnostic screening profile. Certainly, physicians who attend quite
a few patients in the nursing home may want to make their monthly visit
to all of them at one time; however, it is important that an appropriate
amount of time be spent with each resident and that "gang" visits not be
tolerated.

Physicians who attend residents sometimes request or require office visits in place of nursing home visits. In very few instances is this practice medically necessary. Complete diagnostic laboratory and x-ray work can be done less expensively and more conveniently for the patient on the skilled nursing facility premises. Office visits do not afford the attending physician—or for that matter, dentist—the opportunity either to see the resident's whole health record or to communicate with the various services at the facility. Where physicians insist on this practice, the family should be asked to provide transportation, and a full written report of the office visit should accompany the patient on his return to the nursing home.

Medical supervision can be evidenced only by signed written orders, progress notes, and discharge notes on the patient's medical record. Telephone orders may be accepted and initialed by the nurse, with the doctor countersigning the order within forty-eight hours. Since the doctor is often not available to countersign, the medical director will have to do so.

It is recommended that patients whose attending physician is a psychiatrist be seen by an internist or family practitioner on admission, for an annual workup, and if a specific need arises. As a courtesy, physicians who are relatives of patients may be permitted to write orders on the chart, although such orders must be countersigned by the attending physician.

If unclear in the choice of diagnostic and/or treatment programs, physicians should be encouraged to seek consultative advice. Although patients and families may select consultants of their own choice, the nursing home should be prepared to suggest a number of local reputable specialists from whom they may choose. The charge nurse should always give reports of consultations to the attending physician promptly for consideration of recommended action and/or approval of treatment or drugs ordered.

The nursing home must take special precautions in conjunction with the physician for the safe management of agitated and confused residents who may be a danger to themselves and/or to others, or who may wander off the premises. Families and/or sponsors and physicians should be notified by the medical director or director of nursing of the risk involved and the preventive measures being taken. The use of physical restraints as one form of patient management should be suggested to the family. If after advice and counsel with nursing home personnel and the attending physician, the family expresses a strong desire to forgo the use of restraints, they should be asked to state such desires in writing for the nursing home records. The written request should include a statement to absolve the nursing home and all attending professionals of all related liabilities.

FIGURE 3-2
Physician Writing Monthly Orders

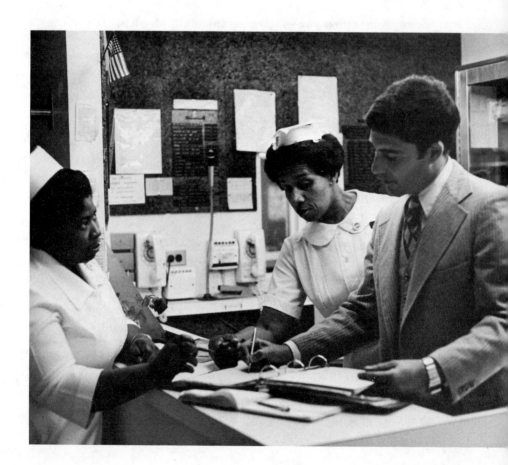

In the event of a change in patient status, the charge nurse should contact the attending physician, who must respond promptly and whose responsibility it is to notify the patient's family and/or sponsor. Except in a medical emergency, a patient should not be transferred, discharged, nor be the recipient of radical change in treatment without notification of and consultation with the patient and/or his family or sponsor. Further, the physician must inform the family of the need for special care, services, or equipment, of the transfer of the patient to another health care facility, or of the patient's expiration. Except in the case of death, the nursing home will assume those duties only when specifically requested to do so by the physician. As the physician must come to the nursing home to pronounce death, it is suggested that he immediately notify the family and/or sponsor of the death.

It is preferable to transfer patients as infrequently as possible from the skilled nursing facility, as the move may be traumatic for them. Every effort should be made and alternatives exhausted to maintain the patient in the nursing facility during an acute illness. Often this entails much persuasion of the attending physician, who—for his own convenience or because he does not understand the capability of the nursing home staff—would like to have the patient in the hospital, where he can more readily attend him. The attending physician should be assured that the nursing home can provide all but the most complicated diagnostic services and can closely monitor the patient's condition. Furthermore, hospitalization for the ill aged can be a frightening and costly experience. As hospital staff members are not trained specifically to care for confused, disoriented, and sometimes noisy and abusive geriatric patients, they are frequently impatient with and misunderstand the patients' problems and needs. The support that friendly and caring faces in the nursing home can give the patient during a crisis may be more beneficial than sophisticated hospital procedures.

When a patient is discharged, the attending physician must write a complete discharge diagnosis on the medical record. All too often, however, he will not return to the nursing home, so the task devolves to the medical director.

Upon the death of a patient, the physician must respond to the nurse's call within a reasonable period and appear on the premises to make the pronouncement of death, sign the death certificate and other necessary papers, and write a complete discharge diagnosis on the chart. If a patient dies when neither the attending physician nor the medical director is available to sign the death certificate and the covering physician refuses to comply because he had not previously seen the patient, the covering physician should be requested to sign a statement that the patient has expired and that he is arranging for pronouncement elsewhere, usually at the medical examiner's office.

The skilled nursing facility should encourage physicians to request postmortem examinations on their patients to aid in the accurate determination of the "cause of death" for public health statistics and for medical-legal reasons, to have as complete information as possible about each patient for future research and teaching activities, to see the effects of disease processes that cannot be fully evaluated by the limited diagnostic procedures and tests performed during life, to plan appropriate precautionary measures to be taken by exposed nursing home personnel and family because of contagious disease, to help the deceased's family learn about hereditary conditions, and to help evaluate the efficacy of medical and surgical treatment that was carried out during the patient's life. All these factors are directly related to the improvement of subsequent care of the institutionalized ill aged.

Written permission to perform an autopsy must be obtained from the patient's next of kin. The nursing home may facilitate this process for attending physicians by having available authorization forms. Although arrangements for performing the autopsy are the physician's responsibility, the nursing home should cooperate to the fullest. The medical director should request a report of the postmortem examination.

ALLIED HEALTH PROFESSIONALS

To provide comprehensive care for its residents, the skilled nursing facility should arrange for the services of allied health professionals—dentists, podiatrists, and optometrists—in addition to medical doctors. Although residents and/or their families may select the dentist of their choice, the skilled nursing facility should have a contract with at least one member of each of the allied health professions to ensure that patients will receive the care they require.

Consultations and services rendered by allied health professional staff are under the supervision of and require an order by the patient's attending physician or the medical staff in facilities that have an organized medical staff. Allied health professionals are expected to exercise independent judgment within their areas of competence, with the ultimate responsibility for patient care shared by the attending physician. They participate directly in patient management and are expected to write orders and progress notes within the scope of their licensures. As part of their consultant role to the nursing home, allied health professionals offer the staff guidance and conduct clinical sessions related to patient care.

When recruiting and interviewing dentists, podiatrists, and optometrists, the administration should emphasize the needs of the particular patient population, particularly some patients' disturbed behavior and inability to follow directions. Some patients may impede the dentist by refusing to open their mouths or by biting him. The podiatrist may need assistance while using sharp instruments on agitated residents. And the optometrist may not receive reliable responses in his examination and vision testing. Feet that do not hurt, dentures that fit, and glasses that improve vision can do much to assist the resident physically, socially, and emotionally. Thus grea care should be exercised in the selection of allied health professionals to perform these essential ongoing services.

Administrators must be aware that young professionals with small practices may be anxious to work in the nursing home. It will take a fair amount of time for them to develop a modus operandi in the nursing home—to understand the residents, to become familiar with the staff, and so forth. At some point after one or two years, if their interest is not geriatrically oriented and if their practices have grown sufficiently, they will resign and the administrator will once again be faced with recruitment problems. Therefore it is highly desirable to select professionals whose interests transcend the financial reward. For example, dentists who work alone in their offices often seek the professional stimulation and conviviality afforded by working in an institutional setting, and thus they are better candidates for work in nursing homes.

From another vantage point, the specialist who literally makes rounds in institutions and scarcely has time to get to know the patients should be avoided. Individualization in patient relationships is important to the dignity of the resident; an assembly-line medical service should be discouraged.

Each candidate for appointment at the skilled nursing facility should be asked to submit a curriculum vitae to the administrative director. In a facility with an organized medical staff, the candidate's credentials would then be referred to the credentials committee for recommendations and subsequent action by the medical staff. A facility with an open medical staff would seek the approval of the patient care policy committee before executing a contract.

Dentists, podiatrists, and all practitioners who are accustomed to private office practice need to be oriented to working in an institutional setting. Most physicians and some allied health professionals are hospital affiliated, but many work alone and need to understand that in a nursing home the attending physician and the staff are involved with their patients. Residents are often not responsible for decision making. Rather, families or sponsors are involved and must be contacted, for example, for approval before ordering new dentures. Sponsors may refuse such permission on the basis of cost and the limited life expectancy of the patient. Other constraints may include the illness—frequently both mental and physical—of nursing home residents, the institutional bureaucracy with limitations on the service imposed by finances, or limited administrative orientation to the particular discipline.

The nursing home can often justify office visits to allied health professionals such as dentists who may not have sufficient equipment for any procedure more complicated than routine care in the nursing home dental office. Furthermore, resident wishes to visit a practitioner's office should be honored provided that medical clearance has been obtained. Such office visits constitute a continuation of the premorbid, noninstitutional way of life and thus may help preserve the resident's dignity.

In the majority of cases, when office visits are not practical, examination and/or treatment rooms or the resident's bedroom should be used. The transportation of the patient to the examining room and the scheduling of appointments will need to be organized with the cooperation of nursing staff in assigning an auxiliary staff member or volunteer to assist the practitioner. Alternatively, the practitioner may be asked to bring his own office assistant to help.

Dentistry

Malnutrition is a continuing and real concern among the aged ill. Since poor dentition is very often the cause of an elderly person's inability to eat properly, proper functioning of natural teeth and/or dentures is imperative.

Additionally, the condition of a person's teeth may affect his feelings of self-respect and personal dignity. Missing teeth or lack of dentures can be embarrassing to a person who always took proper care of his teeth. Residents who feel they are unattractive due to poor or no dentition may not want to participate in activities with other residents or receive visitors due to their embarrassment. They may never want to smile, which is demoralizing for them, their families, and the patients and staff around them.

A written agreement should be maintained with one or more duly licensed dentists, signifying his consent to advise and participate in an active oral hygiene program, to visit the facility regularly to examine patients upon the written request of the attending physician, to provide prophylactic and therapeutic care within the scope of the patient's ability to endure such treatment, and to write orders on the dental sheets in the patient's medical record.

The advisory dentist must be available to provide emergency care for all residents, including those whose personal dentist may not be available. In addition, the skilled nursing facility should include as part of its transfer agreement with a community hospital the provision that patients may be sent to the hospital for emergency dental care when the advisory dentist is unavailable or when more elaborate equipment is required than is available at the nursing home.

The advisory dentist should assist the skilled nursing facility in identifying routine care that can be performed on the premises, such as examinations and evaluations, dental hygiene, taking measurements needed for fabricating new dentures, and denture adjustments. Emergency fillings and extractions can usually be carried out at the nursing home setting. Other treatments requiring a visit to the dentist's office and/or hospital should be clarified with the dentist.

All residents admitted to a skilled nursing facility must have a record of their current dental status entered on their medical record within ninety days of admission. Subsequently, all patients should have annual reevaluations of their dental needs, and any necessary work should be completed. These surveys may be done by the patients' own dentists or by the facility's advisory dentist.

Optometry

Visual deficiencies or problems can undermine the day-to-day functioning of nursing home residents. If reading or even television viewing was once an important leisure-time activity, the loss of such outlets can be devastating to a resident's general well-being. With medical orders, an optometrist may be asked to examine and analyze the functioning of the residents' eyes and to prescribe preventive or corrective measures for maximum vision and comfort, including eyeglasses but excluding drugs or medicines, which can be provided only by ophthalmologists.

When feasible, such examinations could be scheduled at appropriate intervals for groups of residents at the nursing home. Once such an ongoing relationship is established, a workable system for the rapid repair and replacement of broken eyeglasses is more likely to ensue. Otherwise, residents may have to await family visits for the work to be accomplished.

Podiatry

Foot problems can be painful and tiring and may curtail the rehabilitation of nursing home patients. Movement is essential for the ill aged—physically to prevent muscle contractions and psychologically to prevent depression. Thus it is important for residents to have access to podiatric care on a regular basis so that they may continue to remain active.

As patients should receive ongoing treatment from the podiatrist, it is recommended that, along with the initial physician's order, the podiatrist should complete an evaluation for the physician's approval, noting the recommended visitation schedule. This order would remain in effect for a year. At the time of the annual physical examination, podiatric care would be reordered. This format precludes a PRN (*pro re nata*, "as is necessary") order, and yet the patient can receive regular podiatric care between physician visits.

FIGURE 3-3
Dental Survey

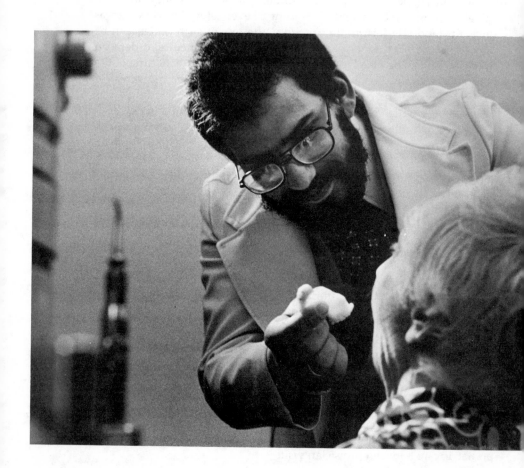

FIGURE 3-4
Podiatry Treatment

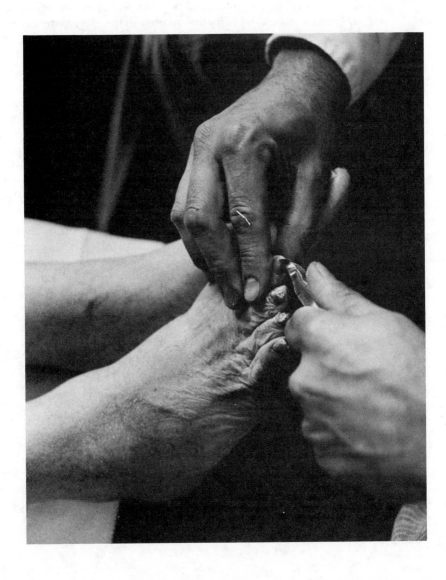

DIAGNOSTIC SERVICES

Within the skilled nursing facility, certain diagnostic procedures should be available to aid in the prompt treatment of residents and to preclude unnecessary transfers to the hospital for such services. For example, a patient who has recently fallen may require an x ray to check for a fracture. An in-house x ray is less disruptive to the patient and less costly than a round-trip ambulance ride.

All laboratory, x-ray, and electrocardiogram studies require a physician's order. The results should be promptly placed on the chart; abnormal results should be verbally reported to the physician immediately.

Laboratory procedures that should be conducted on the premises are complete blood count, routine urinalysis, and stool examination for occult blood. Other biochemical, hematologic, agglutination, serologic, bacteriologic, and pathological studies should be performed by a licensed laboratory with which the nursing home has a contract. To simplify test ordering and the accompanying bookkeeping when dealing with an outside laboratory on a contract basis, it is advantageous to arrange that a standard series of tests be conducted under a specific title or number, rather than having to order multiple individual tests for admission and for annual laboratory workups. Customizing laboratory procedures to the needs of the nursing home will ensure better service.

The skilled nursing home should provide for electrocardiography and have facilities for radiology. Individual x-ray films should not be removed from the premises but made available to attending physicians for bona fide study and used for in-house educational purposes.

The employment of technicians to conduct diagnostic work should vary according to the size of the institution. A facility with more than 100 beds may require a full-time laboratory and x-ray technician who is properly qualified and licensed by the state to take x rays. Certain skill is required of such a person when he works with the geriatric patient population. It may not be easy to draw blood, take an x ray, or perform an electrocardiogram on an agitated or confused patient who is unable to follow directions. In addition to having technical abilities, he must exhibit the other qualities inherent in nursing home personnel.

PHARMACY

Skilled nursing facilities with more than 150 beds may justify the development of an institutional pharmacy. To have a pharmacy on the premises, the nursing home must be licensed by the appropriate state agency as an institutional dispenser.

However, several variables must be considered in planning for an institutional pharmacy, not the least of which is the cost efficiency of its maintenance, both to the nursing home and to the residents. Savings can most often be achieved by ordering drugs and supplies in bulk quantities; hence the nursing home must demonstrate the need for a large stock of drugs according to the number of prescriptions filled. The nursing home must have sufficient operating capital to allow a large amount to be tied up in the pharmacy inventory as well as to have funds available to replenish that inventory.

Other considerations in determining the costs of establishing a pharmacy would be the need for a registered pharmacist on a full-time and/or part-time basis, and decisions concerning whether the pharmacy should be open seven days per week. Finally, the facility itself must have a sufficiently large and safe area to house the pharmacy.

Once all the overhead expenses are evaluated and it is decided how much it will cost to maintain a pharmacy on the premises, a study must be done to determine the markup required on prescriptions to meet the overhead expenses. The amount to be charged for prescriptions must be competitive with prevailing area prices and should be commensurate with the Medicare and Medicaid reimbursement schedules.

The operation of an institutional pharmacy would be advantageous in emphasizing the use of generic drugs rather than brand names, which should effect dollar savings to patients and their sponsors. Physicians would be requested to order the generic equivalents stocked by the house pharmacy in accordance with their formulary. This system would be especially viable in the case of an organized medical staff, whose members would be instructed to order by generic name.

An institutional pharmacy on the premises would ensure the immediate availability of all patient records under the nursing home's supervision. When a community pharmacy services the skilled nursing facility, the patients' profiles and billing records are maintained by the pharmacist in his store files, which is an inconvenience to the nursing home, for when a family or sponsor questions a drug bill, most often they will refer to the nursing home rather than the pharmacy for explanation.

Unit Dose

Nursing facilities, whether large or small, with or without an institutional pharmacy, must weigh the advantages and disadvantages of supplying medications in unit doses. The main constraint to unit dose is its cost, which, when considered for the patient who receives that medication for an exceptionally long period, becomes an important reservation. Further, the amount of space required to store unit-dose pharmaceuticals is significant and must be taken into account, especially on the nursing units.

Of course, having an institutional pharmacy may alleviate these constraints and make the use of unit doses more feasible. If the drug is prescribed frequently enough, the nursing home can order it in large quantities, which would lower the cost per dose. Second, with an institutional pharmacy, space on the nursing unit would not be a problem as the pharmacy would send up medications on a daily basis, so entire prescriptions would not have to be kept on the unit.

The advantages of using unit doses lies in nursing administrative efficiency—pouring medication, controlling drugs, and reducing chance of error. Also, waste would diminish. For example, if a patient did not take the medication at the appointed time, or if medication orders were changed, the particular drug could be saved as long as the individual wrapper was not opened.

A compromise to all these considerations might be to use unit doses for controlled substances that must be closely inventoried three times per day. It would be easier and more efficient to have numbered packets than to have to count all the pills in a bottle, which sometimes results in damaging or losing the tiny pills.

Community Pharmacy

Smaller facilities would contract the services of a community pharmacy to provide drugs and some medical and surgical supplies. The contract (Exhibit 3–1) should be specific as to price structure and the pharmacy obligations to patients and to the nursing home, emphasizing prompt and emergency response.

Before selecting a community pharmacy, the administrator and the director of nursing should interview a number of interested pharmacies to determine their capabilities for providing the needed twenty-four-hour service and the range of pharmaceuticals ordered by attending medical staff, as well as their ability to handle the necessary health and financial records.

The designated dispensing pharmacist should plan a schedule of routine visits to the nursing home at least three days a week to check individual patient medicine boxes to ascertain that each patient has a sufficient supply of prescribed medicines, to review the doctor's order book for new orders, and to check the supply of the emergency medications box. If there is a change in medication or if new medications are ordered between the pharmacist's visits, the charge nurse should call the order into the pharmacy.

EXHIBIT 3-1
Pharmaceutical Service Contract

XYZ Nursing Home

PHARMACEUTICAL SERVICE CONTRACT

In accordance with the state health code, Medicare and Medicaid regulations, and other pertinent state and federal regulations, I agree to provide drugs and medical and surgical supplies to XYZ Nursing Home with the following conditions:

Price Structure

a. Markup to the patient will be based on the cost of the prescription plus $____ (which is the Medicaid markup).
b. Cost of the prescription will be determined by the wholesale price as base starting cost.
c. Cost will be determined by the number of pills, regardless of how many are contained in a bottle.
d. Quantity dispensed will be determined by the physician.

Pharmacy Service to Patients

a. A profile will be kept for each individual patient and will contain:

1. Diagnosis
2. Prescription number
3. Date filled or refilled
4. Name of drug, quantity, dosage
5. Price charged to patient
6. Doctor
7. Any drug interactions or drug allergies

b. Billing system procedures will be the following:

1. Patients will be billed monthly.
2. They will receive a statement with the prescription number, date received, name of drug, amount received, and cost. There should be no question in the patient's mind as to what he is receiving.
3. For Medicare patients, the nursing home will be billed. Medicaid (except when included in daily rate) and private patients will be billed directly.

Pharmacy Services to the Nursing Home

a. An inventory of patients' needs will be maintained a minimum of three times per week or more if necessary, with the nursing home to receive delivery the same day.
b. Nursing home delivery will be available if needed seven days per week.
c. Twenty-four-hour emergency service is assured.
d. The pharmacy will participate in in-service education programs and cooperate with nursing staff and physicians for efficient service operation.
e. A copy of the Druggist Red Book will be provided to the nursing home to verify questions regarding the price of drugs.

EXHIBIT 3-1 (cont.)

f. A copy of prescriptions delivered to the nursing home will be
    left at every delivery for proof of delivery and drug control,
    in that if there is ever a question by the nursing home or the
    patient, the proof of delivery will verify the presence of the
    prescription.

g. Each month, an accounting will be rendered to the nursing home
    of all business to the nursing home, private patients, and
    Medicare and Medicaid patients.

h. Drugs used from the emergency drug box will be charged to the
    patient or his sponsor.

i. The pharmacist will attend quarterly pharmacy committee meetings
    and will participate in periodic patient care policy and
    utilization review committee meetings.

j. The pharmacist will review drug storage and administrative areas
    regularly for proper records and neatness.

k. The pharmacist will assist in amending and adhering to pharma-
    ceutical, patient care and administrative policies, and state
    and federal regulations.

l. The pharmacist will cooperate with the pharmacy consultant to
    provide an opportunity for him and the administrative staff of
    the nursing home to review all records pertaining to patients
    and institutional accounts.

m. The pharmacist will provide a monthly and an annual report on
    pharmacy activities and all appropriate statistical data.

n. The pharmacist will remain informed of all pertinent state and
    federal regulations, and ascertain that the nursing home
    personnel are informed of same and that the nursing home
    policies reflect changing requirements.

Pursuant to federal and state laws, I agree there will be no
discrimination against anyone because of race, color, national origin,
creed, sex, sponsor, or handicap.

This agreement can be cancelled by either party with thirty (30)
days' written notice.

_____   _____
Administrative director   Pharmacist

_____   _____
Date   Name of pharmacy

                                      _____
                                      Date

The pharmacist must communicate with the business office to establish the billing status of each patient—Medicare, Medicaid, or private. Prescriptions for Medicare and Medicaid patients may be billed to the nursing home. In some states, Medicaid sponsors are billed directly by the pharmacist. It is strongly recommended that private families or sponsors be billed directly by the community pharmacy to keep families from suspecting that drug costs have been inflated. Should the community pharmacy bill the nursing home and the nursing home in turn bill the families or sponsors for drugs, questions will arise as to whether the skilled nursing facility is overcharging for medications. It is also suggested that the nursing home receive a monthly accounting of pharmacy business with patients so that inquiries from patients and/or sponsors regarding pharmacy bills may be responded to promptly.

Irrespective of who bills for drugs, it is a good idea for a nursing home to use the allowable Medicaid reimbursement cost as the charges for drugs paid by private patients or other third-party sponsors, thereby allowing for easy reference should any questions arise as to approriateness of charges. Although the community pharmacy may not receive as much profit by using the Medicaid figure for all drugs, it is assured of considerable business on a continuing basis and therefore should be satisfied with a smaller profit margin.

When the skilled nursing facility does not have its own pharmacy, some sponsors may request the opportunity to purchase drugs for their patients from discount drug houses, from their own pharmacy, or from some relative or friend who may own a pharmacy. This request should be denied, as it will lead to problems such as not having drugs when needed as physicians change orders, not having properly completed records and labels, the absence of the drug profile in a central place, and the possibility of drugs being handled by a third party if they are not sent from the pharmacy directly to the facility.

Consultant Pharmacist

Facilities that use a community pharmacy for procuring medications should also appoint a separate consultant pharmacist to assist in reviewing and monitoring the facility's pharmacy program. Hiring a consultant pharmacist is recommended to avoid a conflict of interest in having the vendor pharmacist advise the nursing home about its pharmaceutical services.

The consultant pharmacist's responsibilities are to supervise the pharmacy program of the nursing home: record keeping; labeling; storage, administration, and safe handling of drugs; and monitoring the community pharmacy by reviewing patient and institutional accounts. Each patient's drug profile should be reviewed monthly, and any unusual situations should be brought to the attention of the medical and administrative directors. The consultant pharmacist must attend all meetings of the pharmacy committee, where he should present a written report of his review of the pharmacy services of the nursing home. He must keep the nursing home apprised of changes in federal and state regulations concerning the procurement, distribution, and use of drugs, and he must review the nursing home pharmacy policies and procedures annually and suggest amendments, when needed, to ensure their compliance with all applicable statutes. Finally, the consultant pharmacist should attend meetings of the infection control committee and should present a minimum of two in-service programs per year.

PHARMACY POLICIES

Copies of pharmacy policies should be available at all nursing stations and appropriate offices. Procedures affecting the policies should be included in the appropriate manuals, especially the nursing manual. Certain practices would apply whether the nursing home has an institutional pharmacy or utilizes a community pharmacy. Its policies must reflect all applicable federal and state regulations.

In general, only medications listed in the *U.S. Pharmacopeia*, the *National Formulary, Accepted Dental Remedies, New Drugs, U.S. Homeopathic Pharmacopeia*, or listings approved by the pharmacy committee should be used at the skilled nursing facility. A current drug reference book and a list of drug interactions should be provided at each nursing station.

The nursing home should not accept drugs that a patient was using prior to admission. Such drugs have been handled by someone in addition to the dispensing pharmacist—e.g., the patient or his family—so there is no assurance that the drugs in the bottles are what the labels indicate. If drugs are sent directly to the nursing home from the pharmacy, however, the accuracy of the labeling is assured.

Absolutely no medications, even over-the-counter drugs, should be administered to a patient without a physician's order. Medications should never be given to a visitor unless ordered by a staff physician.

Ordering

The patient's attending physician must order medications in writing unless an unusual circumstance justifies a verbal order, in which case the verbal order must be given to a qualified nurse and countersigned by the doctor within forty-eight hours. Unlike the hospital, where a patient's physician visits daily and therefore can easily countersign orders, the physician may not come to the nursing home for weeks at a time. Getting verbal orders countersigned can pose a great problem to nursing staff. The order sheet can be mailed or taken to the doctor's office for his signature, but doing so is often time consuming. This is an instance where the medical director would be asked to intervene on an emergency basis.

Legally, controlled substances such as narcotics and sedatives cannot be ordered verbally. Physicians must meet state and local regulations governing the ordering of controlled substances, such as the use of a special prescription form. Again, due to the absence of physicians in the nursing home, abiding by such requirements may cause some difficulty, so the services of the medical director may be used to conform with pertinent laws.

Experimental Drugs

The use of experimental or research drugs should be permitted only under certain conditions. The drugs should be supplied by a recognized research institution. Acknowledgment of and approval of usage in writing must be received from the patient and/or his family, the attending physician, and the dispensing pharmacist. Literature about the specific drug must be available to the dispensing pharmacist and the nursing staff to make them aware of side effects and contraindications.

Labels and Records

Each prescription label must state the patient's full name; the physician's name; prescription number; name and strength of drug; date of issue; expiration date (if time-dated medication); name, address, and telephone number of the pharmacy; directions for administering the drug, as well as other legally required information in the case of controlled substances. Any medication container with a blurred or missing label must be discarded unless the pharmacist can verify the information.

When medications are delivered to the institution from the community pharmacy, the charge nurse should check them against written orders, and, if they are correct, sign the attached slip, giving one copy to the pharmacist and retaining a copy for nursing home records. The receipt of all controlled substances must be noted in a bound log book, and they must be inventoried on each nursing shift.

Storage

Medications must not be stored in patients' rooms, but rather at the nursing station in a locked compartment, with controlled drugs in their originally delivered container, placed under double-lock protection. Each patient should have his own container for medications, properly labeled with name and room number. Transferring between containers is prohibited. Locked refrigeration must be provided for drugs requiring it, and drugs for external use must be stored separately from internal medications to minimize the possibility of any confusion. Only authorized personnel should have access to medications.

Even such staples as aspirins and antacids should not be kept by residents in their rooms. This restriction may seem to curtail patients' rights, but nurses and the medical staff must know exactly what medications patients have taken.

Stop-Order Policy

Because of the long-term residencies of nursing home patients, it is appropriate to institute a stop-order policy. Unless specified otherwise in the facility's policies, there would be a thirty-day stop-order policy on all drugs, which conforms with the length of time for which any physician's order is valid in a skilled nursing facility. Therefore the charge nurse should regularly check the physician's orders and progress notes to verify how long a medication is to be continued. When a specific time is not designated in the order, the attending physician should be notified of an automatic stop-order prior to the administration of the last dose. In all cases, doctor's orders supersede the stop-order policy.

Release of Medications

The release of medications to residents who are leaving the premises for an extended period or to residents who are to be permanently discharged should be permitted only with the attending physician's approval. If the attending physician cannot be reached, the medical director may be asked to provide approval. Whenever drugs are being released to a patient or his family, the responsible family member must complete and sign a drug release form.

For residents who will be returning to the nursing home, the pharmacist should be requested to make up a prescription with the proper labeling for the specific time period involved. The nurse must *not* remove the required number of pills from an existing bottle to give to the patient or family with directions for administration since doing so would be construed as the dispensing of drugs. If the pharmacist does not have advance notice to prepare a "take-out" prescription, or if the patient is being discharged permanently, the nurse should give the patient or his family the entire remaining amount of current prescriptions in their original containers. However, the pharmacist must verify the contents of the medication container upon the patient's return. Controlled substances cannot be released from the nursing home to the patient or his family in this manner. Such a problem would rarely occur, of course, if the nursing home were to have a pharmacy on the premises, because drugs then would be issued and administered daily rather than on an extended basis.

Emergency Drug Box

An emergency drug box can be maintained, but it must be reviewed annually by the pharmacy committee, which specifies its contents. It may be useful to conduct a longitudinal study to assist the pharmacy committee in determining what drugs should be maintained for emergency situations. Again, however, such emergency medications require a physician's order. In an emergency, if a physician orders a drug that may not be delivered for some time—even an hour may be critical—the nurse can suggest a substitute from the emergency drug box.

One emergency medication box should be available in the facility and must be locked at all times. The contents should be limited to medications that would be essential in a crisis when time is of the essence; hence, they should be in injectable form only. The box may include the following:

> various sizes of syringes
> tourniquet
> cardiac emergency medications
> Dilantin for seizures
> diuretics for pulmonary edema
> antibiotics for acute infections
> antiemetics to halt vomiting
> corticosteroids as anti-inflammatory agents
> dextrose for hypoglycemia
> coagulants
> medications for respiratory distress, fainting, and low blood
> pressure

The emergency drug box must be carefully controlled and maintained. Attached to the box itself should be a list of the entire contents and the expiration date of all time-limited medications to make sure that they are replaced on schedule. In the absence of an in-house pharmacy, the drugs should be provided on consignment only by the dispensing pharmacist. Thus, a record must be kept of drug administration for the pharmacist's billing. When a medication is removed from the emergency drug box, the nurse administering it should immediately inform the pharmacist so that it may be replaced with the next delivery.

Disposal

The preferred method for drug disposal—with the exception of controlled drugs, which must be surrendered to the Bureau of Narcotics and

Dangerous Drugs—is by incineration or water disposal. The destruction of routine canceled and unused drugs should be witnessed by two licensed nurses and entered in a notebook, indicating the date, drug, and quantity. To avoid wastefulness, medications for patients discharged to a hospital should not be destroyed until the nursing home is officially informed that the patient will not be returning to the facility or when the patient returns to the nursing home and new orders are written indicating a change or discontinuation of the medication.

FINANCIAL ARRANGEMENTS

Unless the daily rate of the nursing home is an all-inclusive rate covering all or part of these services, charges for attending physicians, consulting physicians, dentists, podiatrists, optometrists, pharmaceuticals, and diagnostic studies are the responsibility of the patient and/or his sponsor. These providers bill the patient or sponsor directly.

Attending physicians have certain obligations to their patients whose costs are covered by third-party payers. For a Medicare beneficiary, it is absolutely necessary that the attending physician sign certification forms immediately upon the patient's admission, and recertification forms periodically thereafter. If this requirement is not met, Medicare benefits will automatically be denied the patient, regardless of his medical condition. However, compliance with the signing of Medicare certification and recertification forms does not necessarily imply that the patient will receive covered benefits. In some states, it is also mandatory that attending physicians sign certification and periodic recertification forms for their Medicaid patients if they are to continue to receive Medicaid benefits in the nursing home.

RECORDS

The monthly physicians' orders and progress notes are noted on a form (Exhibit 3-2) designed especially for use in a nursing home. It emphasizes areas that are important in terms of patient activity and the necessity for skilled observation of unstable medical conditions that qualify the patient to remain in the nursing home.

The medical director's guidelines integrating the orders of the attending physician with the nursing care program according to the patient's functional status should be separately stated in writing.

The confirmation-by-attending-physician form, indicating agreement to care for the patient and designating an alternate, must be completed upon admission of the patient and reviewed by the attending physician annually. This information should always be available on the chart in case the attending physician is unavailable and the alternate must be contacted.

EXHIBIT 3-2
Monthly Physicians' Orders and Progress Notes

MONTHLY PHYSICIANS' ORDERS AND PROGRESS NOTES

Date _____

Physician's name _____ Phone _____ Patient's name _____

PROGRESS NOTE: _____

_____

_____

PHYSICIAN'S PLAN OF TREATMENT AND CARE

Diet Plan and Orders

___ Regular salt restricted (2.5 g)
___ Puree
___ Chopped
___ Special diet--type
___ Supplemental feedings
___ Levine tube
___ Routine tube feeding regimen

Nursing Care

___ Enema PRN
___ Douche type
___ Digital rectal exam PRN
___ Foley catheter
___ Change Foley every month
___ Catheter irrigations PRN
___ Toilet-training program
___ Weekly weight
___ Decubitus or wound care
___ Debridement PRN
___ Dressings
___ Irrigations
___ Positioning

___ Skilled observation for unstable
    medical condition (please specify
    what should be observed) _____
    _____
    _____
    _____

Rehabilitation and Restorative Nursing

___ Retraining in ADL (activities of
    daily living)
___ Physical therapy (complete prescript'n)
___ Occupational therapy (" ")
___ Speech therapy (complete prescription)
___ Supportive nursing psychotherapy
___ Supplemental nursing rehabilitation

Activity and Restrictions

___ OOB (out of bed) ad lib
___ OOB with assistance
___ OOB with no assistance
___ Locomotion aids (specify below)
___ Off-premises permission, no escort
___ Off-premises permission with escort
___ Restraints PRN (complete prescription)
___ Siderails
___ Recreation activities contraindicated

Paramedical Modalities

___ Podiatry PRN (complete prescription)
___ Dentistry PRN
___ Optometry PRN

Diagnostic Tests

___ Fractional urines daily
___ Urinalysis 2x monthly
___ Other _____
    _____
    _____

MEDICATIONS AND ADDITIONAL ORDERS

_____

_____

_____

_____

_____

Physician's signature _____ Date _____

The designation-of-dentist form is completed upon admission of the patient. It clarifies immediately whether the patient has his own dentist or is to be seen by the facility's advisory dentist.

The dental order form may include the initial evaluation by the dentist, treatment rendered, and ongoing progress notes.

The podiatrist evaluation and prescription form (Exhibit 3-3) serves two purposes: (1) it documents the podiatrist's evaluation of the patient's need for podiatry services, and (2) it is the physician's signed orders indicating his agreement to the treatment plan suggested.

Certification and recertification forms are completed by the attending physician and document the reason for the patient's need for skilled nursing care. They conform with requirements for utilization review and are a requirement in order for Medicare and Medicaid patients to receive benefits.

The diagnostic requistion form simplifies the procedure for ordering diagnostic tests. Requests for all tests may be made on this one duplicate-copy form. The carbon may be kept on the patient's chart as a reminder until test results are received.

The outpatient consultation record (Exhibit 3-4) should accompany the patient to the doctor's office so the consultant may complete it immediately for return with the patient. Certain data needed by the consultant for his records are provided by the charge nurse on the form.

The history-and-physical-examination form (Exhibit 3-5) must include current medical status and past history. It is planned to cover every aspect of the individual from head to toe, and it includes goals for the patient and a discharge plan. Additionally, the physician notes on this form if the patient has been informed of his medical condition, and if not, the medical reasons why.

The restraint prescription form (Exhibit 3-6) is as specific as possible to preclude PRN orders. It includes the type of restraint, when it should be worn, procedure during release of restraints, and a statement that the physician recognizes that the restraints are ordered in an effort to control an agitated and/or unsafe patient.

FACILITIES AND EQUIPMENT

The nursing home should have available certain medical facilities for the use of physicians, dentists, and technicians. A properly maintained examining room should always be accessible to physicians. It should include an examining table, blood pressure unit, electrocardiogram machine, scale, sink with foot pedals, examining light, otoscope and ophthalmoscope, and cabinets with appropriate supplies.

EXHIBIT 3-3
Podiatrist Evaluation and Prescription Form

PODIATRIC EVALUATION AND PRESCRIPTION FORM

Name _____ Date _____

Specified Need for Prescription (to be obtained from medical records):

_____ Diabetes mellitus   _____ Chronic thrombophlebitis

_____ Arteriosclerosis obliterans   _____ Peripheral neuropathies

_____ Buerger's disease   _____ Vascular insufficiencies

_____ Dystrophic toenails

Podiatric Evaluation:

_____ Diminished or absent dorsalis pedis pulse

_____ Diminished or absent posterior tibial pulse

_____ Onychomycosis (fungus of nails)

_____ Dystrophic nails

_____ Keratosis such as corn or callus (excrescences)

_____ Skin changes _____

Suggested amount of podiatric care:

_____ Every 4 weeks _____ Every 6 weeks _____ Every 8 weeks _____ None

Comments:

_____ D.P.M.
                    Podiatrist

I concur with the above notes, and with the suggested intervals of podiatric
care. In the event the podiatrist notes a condition requiring further
attention, I give my permission for initial treatment and request a follow-up
report from the head nurse.

_____ M.D.
                    Physician
Comments:

EXHIBIT 3-4
Outpatient Consultation Record

OUTPATIENT CONSULTATION RECORD

XYZ Nursing Home

Date _____

Patient's name _____Birthdate _____

Responsible relative _____

Medicaid number _____ Medicare number _____

Referring physician _____

Consulting physician _____

Diagnosis _____

Service to be rendered _____

Summary of condition _____

PLEASE COMPLETE AND RETURN WITH PATIENT

Results of Examination:

Prescribed Drugs and/or Treatment:

Next appointment date _____

Physician's signature _____ Date _____

EXHIBIT 3-5
History and Physical

HISTORY AND PHYSICAL

Physician _____ Date _____

I. Present illness _____
_____
_____

II. Past medical history _____
_____
_____
_____

III. Past surgical history (dates--include injuries, fractures, operations)
_____
_____
_____

Physical Examination

Blood Pressure _____ Temperature _____ Pulse _____

          Respiration _____ Weight _____

Nutritional status _____

Mental status _____

Skin _____

Eyes _____

Ears _____

Nose _____

Mouth _____

Pharynx _____

Neck _____

Patient's name _____ Sex ____ Age ____ Birthdate _____

EXHIBIT 3-5 (cont.)

Heart _____

Lungs _____

Breasts _____

Abdomen _____

_____

Musculoskeletal _____

_____

Genitalia _____

   Rectal _____

   Pelvic _____

Neurological _____

_____

Pertinent Lab Findings: _____

_____

Functional Status:

Physical _____

_____

Behavioral _____

_____

Complete Diagnoses: _____

_____

_____

Goals: _____

_____

Discharge Plan: _____

_____

The above patient has (has not) been informed of his current medical status.

If not, state medical contraindications for same _____

_____

Physician's signature _____ Date _____

See monthly order sheet for plan of treatment and care.

EXHIBIT 3-6
Restraint Prescription

RESTRAINT PRESCRIPTION

Type:

During Day	During Night
_____ Belt	_____ Belt
_____ Vest	_____ Vest
_____ Hand/wrist	_____ Hand/wrist

Indication:

_____ When in chair	_____ When Levine tube is in situ
_____ When in bed	_____ During parenteral administration of fluids
_____ When agitated	
_____ When on the toilet	_____ If patient has had recent and/or recurrent falling episodes

Siderails:

_____ No siderails needed

_____ Yes (check below)

_____ When in bed

_____ Bedtime only

Procedure: Release every 2 hours in order to perform any or all of the following:

_____ Ambulate	_____ Take to meals
_____ Take to the toilet	_____ Reposition
_____ Perform daily care and grooming	_____ Take to activities
_____ Prevent irritation and circulatory impairment	

Comments:

I am aware that this patient has fallen one or more times and/or is difficult to manage because of agitation. I believe the above measures will help provide a safe/secure environment for this patient.

Physician's signature _____ Date _____

Patient's name _____

The dentist should have available a designated area with the following equipment: hydraulic dental chair, light, drill, buffing and grinding machine, ultrasonic denture cleaner, instrument tray on wheels, automatic timer, work shelf, and cabinets for supplies. The dental area must be large enough to accommodate the dental chair and a wheelchair for patients who can be examined only in a wheelchair. The lighting, x-ray, and other equipment must then have arms sufficiently long and flexible to be used when the patient is in a wheelchair. The advisory dentist should inform the nursing home what instruments and supplies need to be routinely maintained, or he may prefer to bring those items when visiting.

The x-ray room should be equipped with an x-ray unit with fluoroscope, x-ray view box, and x-ray filing cabinets. The dark room, adjacent to the x-ray room, should have x-ray cassettes, film cabinet, developing tank, light, timer, hangers, and cabinets.

For the limited laboratory studies that are to be done on the premises, the laboratory should have a microscope and light, centrifuge, refrigerator, sterilizer, blender, sink, cabinets, and necessary supplies.

In addition, the nursing home should provide a conference room where physicians and other staff members can talk privately with patients and families.

SUMMARY

Although state and federal regulations designate to the administrator the responsibility for providing medical and allied health services in the nursing home, the administrator has neither the training nor the clinical expertise to evaluate the quality of these services and must depend on the counsel of the medical director. Physicians, dentists, and other professionals cannot function in a vacuum. They will be attracted to the nursing home if they derive professional satisfaction and stimulation therein. The medical director provides an operating structure, as well as the opportunity for peer review and professional audit.

NOTES

1.   Joint Commission on Accreditation of Hospitals, *Accreditation Manual for Long Term Care Facilities*, 2nd ed. (Chicago, 1975).
2.   Joint Commission on Accreditation of Hospitals, *Monograph Medical Staff By-Laws* (Chicago, 1978).

Nursing

INTRODUCTION

The nursing department in the skilled nursing facility must be planned with an understanding of the nature of the patient population to be served. The average age of the patients can be expected to be about eighty years, with the ratio of female to male patients three or four to one.

The predominant patient disability relates to cerebral arteriosclerosis with organic brain syndrome of varying degrees plus other organ involvement and vascular disease, such as in heart, kidney, and peripheral arterial disease. Typical of the geriatric patient is the concurrent involvement of multiple organ systems, such as chronic pulmonary edema, arthropathies, urologic disease, and neoplasms of various organs.

Providing comprehensive nursing for these complicated patient care problems requires more than the expeditious execution of medical directions. It requires even more than high standards of nursing in conjunction with compassion and understanding for the patients and their families. To encourage the rehabilitation of these patients and to promote maximal physical, social, and emotional functioning, nursing must be integrated with other professional services so that patients may benefit from a total coordinated care program involving nursing, and physical and social rehabilitation.

GERIATRIC NURSING IN A LONG-TERM-CARE FACILITY

In contrast to the daily medical supervision available in the general hospital, less frequent medical visits have placed the director of nursing at the hub of virtually all patient activities. He must relate patient and family activities to the operating management and vice versa. Thus the nursing service is responsible for translating operational policies to all nursing and paranursing professional services.

In contrast to the usual patient stay of ten to fourteen days in an acute hospital, the average patient placement in a skilled nursing facility is considerably longer. Consequently, the nursing staff must be deeply committed to the psychological and social rehabilitation of the patient population in several areas: the personal psychological status of the patient and interpersonal patient relationships involving other patients, visiting families, and staff. Indeed, studies of friendship among nursing home patients have shown that the severely physically handicapped list members of the nursing department as friends;[1] nursing staff members truly represent significant others in the lives of such patients.

In the absence of immediate access to medical leadership, physical diagnosis is an important tool in the nursing armamentarium. However, because of the frequency and degree of organic brain disease in the patient population, valid symptomatic complaints may be lacking. Therefore objective evidences of patient disability in terms of change in patient behavior require the nursing skills of sound observation, smell, hearing, feeling, and judgment. In a long-term-care setting, the nurse should be able to diagnose clinical shock, acute and small stroke phenomena, congestive heart failure, dehydration, Cheyne-Stokes and Stokes-Adams syndrome, certain cardiac arrhythmias, diabetic acidosis and insulin shock, and bone fractures.

A knowledge of the clinical use and toxicology of commonly used drugs can be particularly important in the skilled nursing facility because of the general absence of physicians. Knowledge of the clinical behavior of the various insulins and hypoglycemic oral medications and of the various tranquilizers, depressants, and opiates, with their frequent paradoxical behavior and other toxic manifestations, along with a working knowledge of digitalis and its derivatives, with and without the presence of intensive oral and parenteral diuretics, can be important tools for nursing assessment. Familiarity with the various antibiotics and their clinical, toxic, and related allergic phenomena is also important, as is understanding the relative advantages and disadvantages of intravenous administration of water and electrolytes versus administration of clysis in the agitated, noncooperative patient who does or does not have chronic cardiac disease.

In the chronically ill aged, body movement is the cornerstone of physical rehabilitation and physical reconditioning. It can prevent debilitating disease and disabilities. Maintaining the relationship of body movement to psychosocial rehabilitation, physical therapy, occupational therapy, and recreational therapy, and the therapeutic use of the institution's physical environment should be distinctly a nursing function related to the prevention of decubiti, motor hypotonia, and loss of range of motion, and to the rehabilitation of a chair- or bedridden patient into a functional, social, and reasonably intact individual.

With organic brain disease, the feeding, bathing, and dressing of the elderly may require special skills. The importance of good nursing techniques in bowel and bladder function can be appreciated only when breaks in those techniques literally threaten the patient's existence. Bladder training associated with the use of either intermittent catheterization or the use of an indwelling Foley catheter can be either a life-saving procedure or a life-threatening experience, requiring an understanding of the anatomy, pathology, bacteriology, and pharmacology of the urologic tract. Bowel training for the prevention or treatment of fecal impactions should be a fundamental nursing technique of particular importance in a patient population whose fluid intake may be low— particularly with the frequent use of diuretics—and whose physical activity is often limited.

Recognizing the unsophisticated development of geriatric nursing techniques and the very limited exposure of nursing students to the needs of the chronically ill aged, the nursing department must develop education, training, and retraining programs for registered nurses, licensed practical nurses, nursing aides, and orderlies. Nursing personnel in the long-term-care facility need to learn how to relate to their elderly charges—to touch their patients whose visual and auditory acuity may be impaired, to understand that elderly residents must be permitted to function at a slower pace, and to be patient with slower responses and movements.

The director of nursing must pursue techniques for more effective liaison with other paramedical professions involved in the total care of the chronically ill aged. Ongoing clinical research relative to the use of new and adapted nursing techniques and the improvement of conventional tools of nursing care is an essential part of the entire nursing program and serves as a stimulus to continuing staff efforts in the long-term-care setting.

STAFFING PATTERN

Primary factors in establishing a proposed staffing pattern include the facility's philosophy and structure, the nature of both the resident population and the staff, and the involvement of the family members. Whether the physical configuration of the entire building—including the exterior recreation areas and the individual nursing units—is compact or spread out definitely influences the number of staff members needed. For example, where nursing stations are far from many private bedrooms, obviously it will take more time for each patient to be observed than if the nursing station is in the center of a double corridor unit composed primarily of double or multiple rooms.

Of course, the facility's philosophy regarding patient care affects the staffing pattern. Some institutions are bedroom oriented, as in acute hospitals, where patients are usually confined to their beds or chairs in their own rooms. Other facilities use the entire structure, including the exterior and interior environment, as a stimulus to the physical and social rehabilitation of the resident population. Obviously, a smaller staff is needed if patients remain in their beds or rooms throughout the day than if they are encouraged to go outdoors and to attend recreational activities during the course of the day. For example, it is less time-consuming to assist a patient to use the lavatory if he is in his bedroom than if he is in the garden and thus has to be transported in and out of the building.

The care needs of the patient population may vary from facility to facility depending on the institution's admission policies; for example, some skilled nursing facilities may not admit comatose patients because they require a high intensity of care and more nursing staff. The level of resident disabilities may also vary from time to time so that the number of staff needed in January, for example, may be insufficient in June.

Likewise, the staffing practice may affect the number of staff members needed. If the skilled nursing facility has a policy of hiring registered professional nurses and nursing aides exclusively and does not employ licensed practical nurses, the total number of professional staff members may be smaller because of the greater skill of the registered nurses, while the total number of nursing aides may need to be larger to compensate for the absence of practical nurses.

The level of training of individual staff members, both professional and nonprofessional, will also influence the overall size of the staff. If many of the nurses are recent graduates of a collegiate program, more nurses will be required until the new graduates have had sufficient clinical experience. Likewise, the tenure of the staff affects the staffing plan. A relatively stable and experienced group of nursing personnel can do more than inexperienced staff in a facility that has a high turnover rate.

Sometimes family members appreciate and benefit from the opportunity to participate in the care of their relative. If a wife feels guilty about having placed her husband in a nursing home even though it was physically impossible for her to care for him at home, this guilt may be somewhat assuaged if she can, say, feed him one meal per day. Feeding a patient is very difficult and time-consuming, so this practice can be helpful to both staff and spouse.

It is said that where nursing home residents have a full, varied, and active day, they will have less occasion to call the nursing staff. Further, it is postulated that when residents are secure and trusting in the genuine concern and conscientiousness of the nursing staff, they will be less apt to use the call bells at night, as bells sometimes are used to ascertain the availability of help and not because help is needed.

FIGURE 4-1
Family Member Feeding Patient

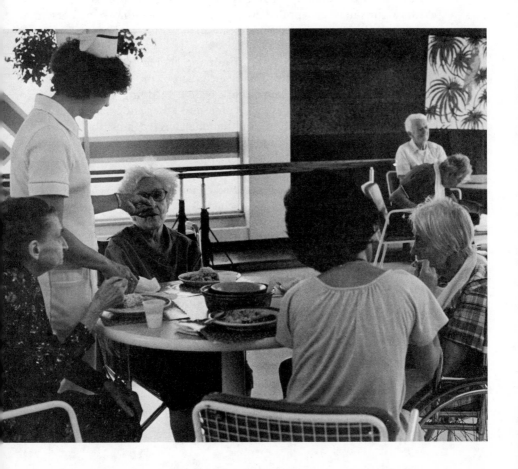

Thus the staffing complement is not something a computer can dictate. Many factors influence the staffing pattern, and the individual charged with the responsibility of scheduling must have a good sense of the needs of the care givers and care receivers at particular times.

The performance of the director of nursing and the supervisors will suffer if they are not completely familiar with the residents' problems and needs. The management of the nursing home must not permit executive nursing staff to be deskbound, as leaders must be informed to be able to lead. There can be no dissociation between administrative and bedside nursing.

Master Staffing Plan

A useful way to measure the amount of care needed by each resident is to assign a numerical value based on set criteria to each resident according to the amount of nursing care required. Once the average number of nursing care hours required per patient on a single unit is determined, this figure may be applied to determining the number of personnel needed to provide direct patient care, that is, care exclusive of supervision and education.

Once a year, the director of nursing should complete the master staffing plan, a twelve-month advance plan of the nursing department schedule of hours and personnel needed. In doing so, he takes into account holidays, sick time, vacations, and other anticipated exigencies that will affect the schedule, and then matches it against the anticipated amount of nursing care hours required in direct patient care. This schedule also indicates the total number of persons necessary to fill the head nurse, supervisor, and director of nursing positions on an annual basis.

The master staffing plan is used as the basis for the current department schedule. A three-month schedule is highly desirable, affording employees the opportunity to plan their free time, particularly weekend duty, well in advance. Unless the nature of the patient population changes dramatically, following the staffing requirements indicated in the master staffing plan should guarantee adequate coverage.

A 100-bed skilled nursing facility with three nursing units needs a director of nursing, four to five supervisors—one of whom covers for the director of nursing on his free days—and four head nurses. The fifth supervisor will be able to fill in as head nurse for the extra day or two needed. Although full-time staff members are more desirable than part-time staff, one part-time supervisor and one part-time head nurse, who in emergencies would be willing to expand their work week, do offer a certain amount of flexibility to the carefully staffed nursing home.

Additional flexibility is possible when the head nurse works during the evening rather than during the day. When a highly qualified nurse can work only evenings and his ability exceeds that of the day nurse, he should be selected for the position of head nurse. There is a special advantage for a skilled nursing facility with an open medical staff to have the head nurse on duty after 3 or 4 P.M., when many attending physicians come in to visit their patients. Too often, the evening charge nurse is not sufficiently cognizant of the around-the-clock picture of the patient and fails to obtain adequate information from the doctor. The head nurse is in a better position to question and make demands on the attending physician.

For the hypothetical 100-bed facility, about eleven licensed practical nurses would permit coverage of all units, allowing for one extra practical nurse assigned to the concentrated care unit and one to the unit for the intellectually impaired during weekdays for optimal care. One practical nurse would also supervise the central storage in the absence of a full-time purchasing agent. During periods of especially heavy nursing loads, such as during a flu epidemic or when several patients are experiencing acute exacerbations and problems, additional staffing should be provided.

Eighteen aides and orderlies are suggested for the concentrated care unit, ten for the unit for those who can engage in some self care, and twenty-two for the unit for confused patients. More orderlies will be needed during the daytime to help with bathing and dressing, but orderlies must be available during the evening to help prepare patients for bed, and during the night to lift heavy patients. Often, male patients will prefer to be handled by male orderlies.

Administrative Assistant

A well-oriented administrative assistant to the nursing department, not a clerk, could be taught to complete much of the paperwork so that the entire nursing staff—those providing direct patient care and those in a supervisory role—will have maximum time to care for patients. The administrative assistant would make out the routine weekly schedules following the pattern set by the master staffing plan.

Working under the direction of the director of nursing, the assistant would ensure that all clinical chart material is current, complete, and accurate, and would assist in the utilization review process with respect to records required on individual residents. On a continuing basis, he would review, in conjunction with staff nurses, the documentation on all clinical records of inpatients.

A candidate for this position should have some knowledge of personnel relations and clerical skills; previous exposure to a health care setting would be useful. Most of all, he must be cognizant of the needs of the staff and demands of the different nursing units. He should be familiar with government standards and regulations, particularly with respect to staffing requirements and records documentation.

Director of Nursing

Administratively responsible to the administrative director and professionally responsible to the medical director, the director of nursing supervises and administers the entire nursing service, including but not limited to nursing personnel, orientation and education, drug management, clinical nursing techniques, nursing records, nursing supplies, and the coordination of nursing with the other disciplines. Maintaining quality care and conforming to physician's orders and nursing home policies are primary responsibilities of the director of nursing. He interprets the role of nursing to the administration and to the medical community. Since participation in family counseling as it affects both the patient's and family's adaptation to the nursing home is crucial for a successful patient placement, the director of nursing must interpret this process to the nursing staff. He should attend family counseling sessions with the medical director and social work consultant. On a continuing basis, he should develop, revise, and/or adapt techniques for nursing in a long-term-care setting and undertake research for the improvement of patient care.

As one of the top executives in the nursing home, the director of nursing must have the tact, patience, and understanding to deal effectively with the staff he supervises, other nursing home staff, the outside professional and lay communities, patients, and families. He must be skilled in identifying problem areas and utilizing initiative and judgment to solve those problems and make frequent decisions.

Professionally, this registered nurse should have advanced preparation in administrative nursing techniques, supervisory experience, and rehabilitation and/or geriatric nursing experience. He must be familiar with the policies of the skilled nursing facility, current standards of geriatric nursing, and all applicable government regulations.

Although the director of nursing should be a full-time employee, his working hours may vary so that he can supervise all nursing shifts properly. On a regular basis, he should overlap one or two hours into a nursing shift other than the day shift.

Nursing Supervisor

The nursing supervisor reports to the director of nursing and is responsible for all nursing units on his shift. The full-time day supervisor acts as director of nursing in the director's absence. On a regular basis, the supervisor provides and coordinates nursing care for patients, cooperating with other departments to meet all the patients' needs. He makes rounds every day with the head or charge nurse to observe each patient, determining the need for additional or modified care.

Supervisors oversee the maintenance of all nursing records on their shifts, including accident or incident reports on patients, staff, and visitors, the proper completion of administrative records, and the availability of all supplies and equipment. They are responsible for staff knowledge of and conformance with all sanitary regulations regarding supplies and equipment, aseptic techniques, and nursing procedures. Supervisors instruct all nursing personnel on new procedures and treatments to allow for the most efficient use of nursing time. At the end of his shift, a supervisor completes a written report on the condition of unstable patients, and any changes that occurred during the shift.

In addition to being registered nurses, supervisors should demonstrate both leadership and administrative ability and have a knowledge of geriatric nursing standards. They must be capable of maintaining good working relationships with the nursing staff, department heads, and subordinates. Familiarity with the organization of the nursing home, its policies, and the requirements of government regulatory agencies is essential.

Head Nurse

The main duty of the head nurse, who is directly responsible to the supervisor on his shift, is to oversee the functioning of an assigned unit for a twenty-four-hour period, that is, to direct treatments and procedures to be done during the entire twenty-four hours and supervising personnel assigned to his unit. The head nurse should visit each patient on his unit several times a day and know the routine of all those patients. He should be able to recognize and interpret symptoms and report all pertinent information with clarity and skill to physicians. It is important for the head nurse to maintain open lines of communication with attending physicians and to assure that all patients are visited by their doctors.

The head nurse is responsible for the quality of all nursing records on the unit and for thinning charts, completing admission or monthly nursing assessments or summaries, and writing ongoing clinical notes. He should routinely inventory supplies and equipment on the unit and reorder them when indicated. The cleanliness of the unit with respect to those areas falling under the purview of nursing—bedside tables, patients' closets, drawers, cabinets, and the like—is the head nurse's responsibility. He should ensure that medications are properly stored, and should remove the discontinued medications from the medication room monthly.

The position of head nurse should be held by a registered nurse who enjoys and has training in caring for the ill aged. Good organizational ability and leadership are prerequisites for this job, as the head nurse truly directs the operation of his unit. Encounters with family members and friends are constant and require tact and understanding and sensitivity to the nurse's role in the confidential relationship between patient and doctor. He must be able to respond calmly in emergency situations. A knowledge of nursing home policies and procedures and applicable government regulations is mandatory.

Charge Nurse

The charge nurse works under the direction of the head nurse on the unit or the supervisor on duty for that shift and renders nursing care to the patients on his unit for his shift only. Responsibilities include knowing the condition of all patients on the unit, carrying out all physician orders, and accurately noting orders on the chart or Kardex (discussed later in this chapter). When new medications are ordered, the charge nurse notifies the pharmacist and removes discontinued medication from the patient's tray. He ensures the proper record keeping for all controlled substances.

In conjunction with the head nurse, the charge nurse determines patient care assignments for each nursing attendant on his unit. He sets up and maintains all treatment trays and notifies the head nurse when supplies are low. In addition, he completes accident reports for patients and staff and notifies the supervisor of such accidents.

The charge nurse may be either a licensed practical nurse or a registered nurse with a knowledge of geriatric nursing as well as general nursing theory and practice. He must be able to work under supervision and also must direct the nursing attendants under his charge. Familiarity with the organization of the nursing home, its policies and procedures, and requirements of government agencies are within the scope of the charge nurse's responsibilities.

Nursing Attendants

Nursing attendants work under the direct supervision of the unit charge nurse. Both female aides and male orderlies should be employed by the nursing home. They perform all nursing tasks that do not require professional training, including bathing, feeding, dressing, toileting, transferring, and transporting patients from one area of the facility to another. In addition, they perform certain housekeeping tasks such as making beds and cleaning bedside units. The attendants' main responsibility is to carry out assigned duties in a manner conducive to patient safety and comfort, and in conformance with established nursing home routine.

Persons seeking attendants' positions must have a genuine interest in caring for institutionalized ill aged. They must be willing to perform repetitive, sometimes unpleasant, tasks and be able to recognize changes in patients' conditions to report to the charge nurse. An understanding of the principles of asepsis and sterile techniques to avoid infecting patients or themselves or contaminating equipment and supplies is mandatory in this position, for it places the attendant in constant direct contact with patients. Attendants should be familiar with the functioning of each department and with the general regulations of the nursing home.

In some states, nursing attendants who have undergone a special training program are permitted to administer medications. Obviously, the practice of using medication aides has occurred in areas where licensed nurses are in short supply. As a general principle, only qualified nurses should be performing such skilled services in a skilled nursing care facility.

Private Duty Nurses and Attendants

Private duty nurses and attendants always work under the supervision of the nursing home nursing staff. Frequently, they are less well trained in rehabilitation nursing than regular staff, and their efforts may be counterproductive if they treat their charges like infants instead of helping them become more independent. When possible, it is preferable to assign regular staff for special duty. This, of course, is possible only for limited periods.

"Feeders"

Some nursing administrators advocate the employment of "feeders," who generally are students who assist in feeding residents the evening meal. Such a program may or may not be successful because the feeders will not know much about the patients if they see them only an hour a day. If, however, they are able to relate to the residents, they may have more patience than full-time staff to devote to the monotonous task of feeding. Naturally, the feeders must be carefully oriented, observed, and evaluated. Sometimes they can work a full tour of duty on weekends, which will help give them a broader view of patient needs.

Night-shift Personnel

Nursing staff members who work evenings and nights have additional and unique responsibilities, as they are virtually the only department on duty. Thus they are more involved with telephone calls, with visitors, and with building emergencies. If the elevator should break down, they must know whom to contact. In the case of fire or other catastrophe, they must be in command until off-duty staff are summoned.

The director of nursing may find it necessary to suggest to the administrator the need for a transportation service for the evening and night shift change, for some women may be fearful of traveling unescorted and public transportation may not be operative.

The director of nursing, supervisors, and head nurses should make every effort to incorporate all three nursing shifts into planning and decision making within the department. Too often, the evening and night workers feel removed from the rest of the staff, which may lead to disinterest in their work and subsequent poor job performance. The director of nursing must be sure to meet with all nursing staff members regularly. Perhaps adjusting his schedule by an hour or two either way would guarantee regular communication with evening and night staff.

PATIENT CARE PROCEDURES

The unique aspects of nursing in a nursing home begin even before the admission of the patient, when the social worker counsels with the director of nursing about which unit would be most appropriate for the patient. Indeed, whenever possible the director of nursing should accompany the social worker on a hospital or home preadmission visit to assess the patient's medical and psychosocial needs and to plan for an appropriate placement. If a double room is contemplated, the director of nursing can be particularly helpful in making suggestions for possible roommates. At admission, the nursing assessment must be sufficiently intensive to compensate for the absence of interns to do complete physicals and for the possibility that the attending physician may not appear for one or two days.

Members of the nursing staff play a major role in helping the patient adapt to congregate living. If the new patient is disruptive or in conflict with a roommate, nurses often determine when to act and what to do. They will be faced with decisions about how to deal with one resident who is disrupting an entire unit. If, for example, a resident is transferred to the hospital and a new patient admitted and seated in the former patient's place in the dining area, nurses must decide what to do if the former patient returns to the nursing home and claims his old spot in the dining room. Nurses may have to intercede to make peace in the selection of television programs or the selection of seating at an activity.

Personal Care

The nursing staff in the long-term-care institution will become involved in all aspects of patient clothing, from daytime wear to night clothes, and from summer garments to winter coats and hats, even to suggesting the use of sneakers rather than shoes for some unsteady residents. Information from the hospital may mislead nursing home staff by incorrectly describing the patient as able to dress himself when in fact he continuously remained in a gown and bathrobe in the hospital. Head nurses will find themselves responsible for asking for clothing replacements and for making suggestions about the preferable type of clothing for individual residents, particularly for the severely physically disabled, who need simplified closures like Velcro, and the mentally impaired, who may destroy certain types of garments.

Personal care procedures such as bathing differ in the nursing home setting. Bed baths are de rigueur in the hospital, but nursing home patients are showered while seated in mobile shower chairs. In some instances, tub bathing is preferable and may be facilitated with the use of a hydraulic patient lift.

The procedure for the ordinary enema differs from the hospital practice of giving enemas in bed. In the nursing home, results are best when enemas are administered with the patient seated on the toilet. To preclude fecal impactions among intellectually impaired residents, rectal examinations are a more frequent occurrence and may be done by trained nursing attendants.

Catheter Care

Certain nursing procedures require creative adaptation and special care in the long-term-care facility. Nurses use indwelling catheters for hospital patients for brief periods, while nursing home patients may be catheterized for extended periods, necessitating careful management to prevent urinary tract infections and urinary retention. Urinary tract infections can be life-threatening to elderly debilitated residents, who may become comatose or severely agitated from the ensuing urinary retention. It is helpful if nurses are trained to insert urethral catheters on an emergency basis during an episode of acute urinary retention. Patients who have infections may need a special bladder irrigation program.

Special Care Requirements of the Intellectually Impaired

Nursing observation takes on an added dimension in the nursing home, where a substantial percentage of the patients are intellectually impaired and cannot express valid verbal symptoms when they feel nauseous or when they are constipated. All staff members—in particular, licensed practical nurses who have continuous patient contact—must be sensitized to smell, to touch, and to observe.

Routine nursing tasks involving this same group of residents often become complicated, for example, when the patient who requires colostomy care pulls out his bag and eats fecal material. Or, a bowel and bladder training program for a confused resident may work only some days in contrast to the same program for an alert person, who is able to cooperate on a regular basis.

FIGURE 4-2
Mobile Shower Chair

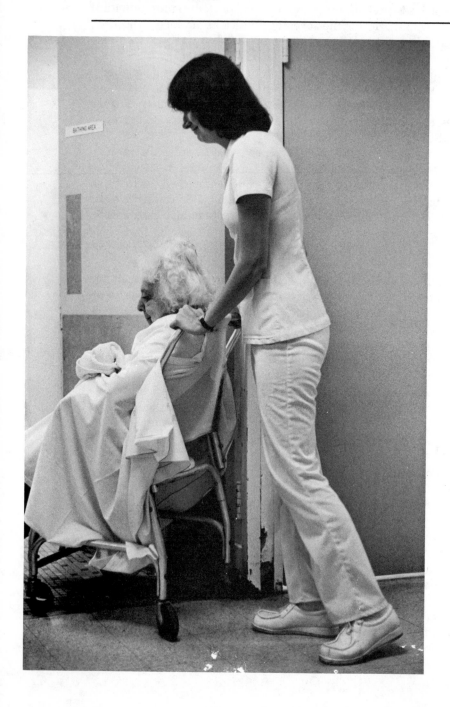

Checking vital signs of agitated residents may be aided by the use of electronic thermometers. After inserting the conventional mercury thermometer, the nursing attendant must remain with the patient until the temperature has been recorded. Since the electronic thermometer affords instantaneous recording of temperature, this equipment saves staff time, is safer and more accurate, and reduces the possibility of breakage.

Supportive Nursing Psychotherapy

Supportive nursing psychotherapy certainly is not indigenous to nursing home nursing, but its relative importance to the entire care program in this milieu is immeasurable. Depression in newly admitted patients is almost universal; it is manifested by apathy, weight loss, and diminished locomotion. Some residents engage in passive and active suicidal acts, refusing to eat, to take medications, to ambulate, to get out of bed, and the like. Further, patients with severe depression; with a suicidal history; with low self-esteem; with ego loss resulting from paralysis, colostomy, or disfiguring illness; and with fears, anxieties, and panic can all benefit from concentrated emotional support from the staff. While in the hospital, the psychiatrist will be contacted for help; in the nursing home, it is really up to the nurses to support these patients on a continuing basis, using all their skills to relate to residents in meaningful ways.

Diagnostic Tests

Nursing home nurses should be able to draw blood if a laboratory technician is not on staff. They must be familiar with abnormal laboratory findings, for it is their responsibility to inform the attending doctor of possible abnormalities in the results, which are telephoned and/or mailed to the institution rather than to the physician. Nurses also need to be familiar with what tests should be ordered. For example, if a patient is jaundiced and vomiting, liver studies are in order. Likewise, long-term-care nurses should be sufficiently familiar with diseases like osteoporosis to know when x rays should be ordered.

Preparing a brain-damaged patient for a barium enema in order to do a gastrointestinal x-ray series mandates skillful nursing assistance. The x-ray technician simply cannot handle this procedure alone: the patient may defecate before the x ray or refuse to remain on the x-ray table.

Feeding Patients

Nursing staff members cannot help but become intimately concerned with the intricacies of community dining. In the selection of tablemates, the organization of personalities vies in importance with the organization of residents in wheelchairs, which crowd a table. When two residents at a table for four may not use salt and sugar, what is the correct

FIGURE 4-3
Electronic Thermometer

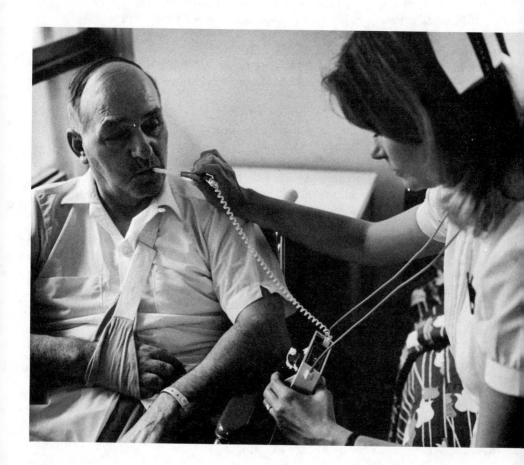

course of action—to remove all salt and sugar, to monitor, or to trust? Is it more important to encourage residents to eat unaided no matter how repellent this may be to tablemates, or should such patients be asked to eat alone?

Decisions have to be made regarding which department should be responsible for supervising meal service on the nursing units. Since much more is required than merely distributing the meals, nursing staff members who truly know the residents and have evaluated exactly what needs to be done for each at mealtime are better qualified for this task than are dietary personnel. This is particularly true in the case of brain-impaired nonambulatory residents, whose eating patterns require careful observation to preclude sustained long-term weight loss, which may be related to the interpersonal climate of the patient and attendant at feeding time.

Nurses also must become intimately involved in the feeding process. One problem is that the patient may not actually swallow his food. He may refuse the food outright or may accept it, roll it around in his mouth, and finally spit it out; all this is very time-consuming and taxing. When spoon feeding proves totally unacceptable, nurses may suggest the need for nasogastric tube feeding to the attending physician.

Nasogastric tube feeding is a procedure routinely associated with the hospital newborn nursery. In the nursing home, it is of special value to the ill aged because of the difficulty of administering intravenous therapy, which offers only the limited nutritional value of sugar and water. Special training must be offered in the technique of insertion and monitoring nasogastric tube feeding to preclude the possibility of aspiration pneumonia. Nurses must ascertain that the tube is in the correct place and must know what to do if the patient vomits or experiences diarrhea.

There are instances, however, when physicians will order intravenous therapy, so the nurses, in the absence of interns or the hospital IV team, must be able to handle this procedure. Hypodermoclysis—fluid with enzymes, actually a clysis with nutrients—is especially useful for comatose patients. Nurses must be able to handle intravenous administration of water, electrolytes, and antibiotics and must be capable of doing a cutdown, making a small incision into the skin to insert intravenous therapy.

Supplemental Nursing Rehabilitation

Instituting supplemental nursing rehabilitation before physical therapy is ordered and after it is terminated provides for the interface between nursing and the restorative services and for true continuity of care. Supplemental nursing rehabilitation is more intensive than the customary

FIGURE 4-4
Monitoring Patient on Intravenous Therapy
and Nasogastric Tube Feeding

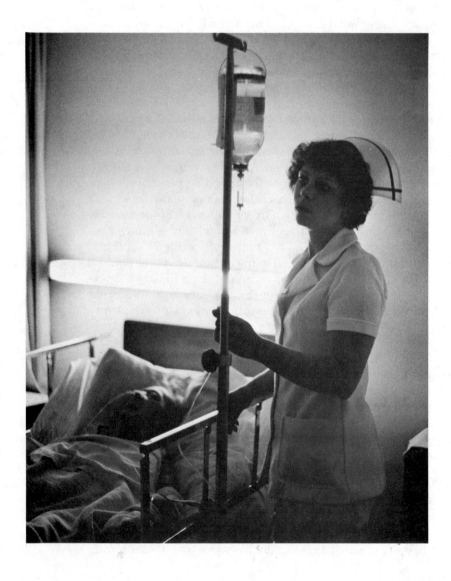

rehabilitation program conducted by the nursing staff. When the physical therapist judges and the attending physician concurs that the patient is ready to graduate to supplemental nursing rehabilitation, the physical therapist alerts and counsels the nursing staff. To provide continuity, a specific nursing attendant in each unit should be designated as the individual responsible for regularly walking and exercising the residents under the supervision of the professional nurses. This will encourage other nurses' aides to ambulate residents and should provide a beneficial, competitive spirit among the aides.

Patient Protection

The question of patient protective or safety devices is fraught with physical, social, and ethical considerations. It is common to hear discussions about the overuse of chemical restraints for nursing home patients. However, studies have shown that the medications most frequently used by ill aged nursing home patients are laxatives and analgesics, with tranquilizers ranking third or fourth on the list. For the very agitated patient, drug therapy is essential but need not continue ad infinitum. Proper management will identify correct dosages for the changing requirements of chemical restraints. Continuous observation is mandatory, as drugs can be hazardous by causing residents to be unsteady on their feet and to fall.

Physical restraints are even more offensive to family members than are tranquilizing drugs. The vision of an aged relative virtually tied to one spot may so disturb the family that they insist that no protective devices be used. The nursing home should concur only if the family or sponsor will affirm in writing that the nursing home will be held blameless if the resident falls.

Families need education regarding the advantages and the safety provided by restraints for the effective management of agitated patients. Using the term "protective devices" may be more acceptable to families and, indeed, aptly describes the purpose of restraints.[2] However, some agitated patients respond poorly to restraints and act out even more. It is important to remember that restraints promote safety when patients exhibit injurious behavior so they will not endanger themselves, other patients, or personnel, and that they prevent patients from removing dressings, contaminating wounds, or removing hypodermoclysis.

If restraints are used, a regular program of careful observation to see that the resident is correctly positioned, plus regularly scheduled periods of ambulation or freedom from restraints, is the responsibility of the unit charge nurse. Locked restraints are not permissible, and restraints can be applied only with medical orders for specified periods.

FIGURE 4-5
Nurse Checking Patient with Restraints

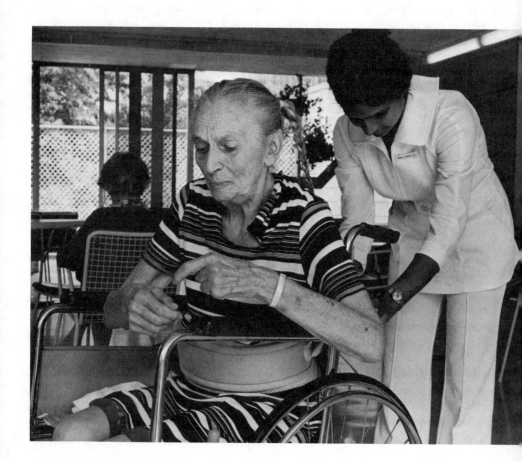

Decubiti Management

The management of decubiti (bedsores) is a major nursing problem. Too often, patients are admitted who present severe decubiti, although it is not documented on the interagency referral form. Frequent position changes to relieve pressure around the clock, not just during the daytime, are indicated.

Contrary to the popular notion, decubiti are not always the result of poor nursing care. With some severely debilitated patients, pressure sores may be inevitable despite the most intense nursing program. Depression and resultant immobilization may contribute to decubiti. Proper cleansing, exposure to the air, frequent change of position, the use of water mattresses, good nutrition, and most important, continuous nursing observation are the cornerstones of an effective decubiti treatment program. The nursing staff must learn to think of the whole patient. While concentrating on a fractured hip, they must not neglect decubiti and weight loss.

Nursing staff should be able to determine when flotation therapy is needed as a treatment modality to relieve pressure or as a preventive measure when nurses anticipate pressure problems due to prolonged immobilization following orthopedic surgery. Water mattresses should be available in each nursing unit as routine equipment. If a rental fee is charged for this therapy, doctors, at family (sponsor) direction, might not order the equipment for financial reasons. However, treatment plans should be based on patient need, not finances, and nurses in consultation with the medical director should be the final arbiters of such decisions.

Off-premises Considerations and Concerns

Hospital-trained nurses need to be educated in the psychological and physical value of the outdoors for long-term patient care. However, they must also be alerted to the problem of patient disappearance. In the hospital, patients are customarily in night clothes and would be easily identified if they attempted to leave the building. In the nursing home, however, residents are fully clothed and could be confused with visitors when they leave the building.

Special precautions must continuously be taken to prevent a confused patient from wandering off the premises—including the regular accounting of patients when administering drugs, checks at mealtime, and routine bedchecks. Fire exits cannot be locked but may have alarms on them. Gates in the parking area must be kept latched at all times. Elevators, doors, and exits should be carefully observed by all staff, especially during visiting hours.

All patients should wear wristbands and have their pictures taken upon admission. Photographs of newly admitted patients are taken to permit ease of descriptions in case they disappear. Patients are more apt to wander before they become accustomed to the nursing home and before all staff have had time to become familiar with their appearance. A series of photographs also serves as a pictorial history of patient progress.

Although residents may have medical and family permission for off-premises outings, the nurse will have to determine whether the resident is well enough to leave the facility each time. Nurses must follow through by learning how patients function while out of the institution.

Family Relationships

Nursing home nurses continuously deal with families of patients. In the hospital, families question physicians about patients' conditions. In the nursing home, nurses and even aides are interrogated by families, and they must exercise caution about overstepping their authority by offering information. If too many people give direct reports to families, confusion may ensue. Often a nurse's aide will not be aware of the full picture or its ramifications. Serious problems can arise when, for example, a patient dies in the presence of family but cannot be considered dead until the attending physician has arrived to pronounce death. This may take some hours, and the family may be outraged at not being able to go ahead with funeral arrangements. Less serious, but ever present, are questions by family members concerning the use of the catheter or of protective devices. Of particular interest are questions and concerns of families and visitors about other unrelated residents and their problems. Nurses must be careful to protect personal rights and privacy of other residents.

Families truly become a part of the therapeutic community, and thus they require sensitive treatment. Although families sometimes treat nurses as paid servants, the nurses really are acting in place of families in caring for their ill aged relatives. In this endeavor they can be made scapegoats by long-standing patient-family interactive behavior of guilt, anger, and hostility. Staff members may be accused of moving mother too much when, in fact, it is completely necessary for the patient's welfare.

Nurses learn that it is essential to notify some families prior to their visits if their relative has sustained an injury, albeit a very minor one. Some relatives become suspicious and distrustful if they are not informed about each incident. They will feel they must be in continuous attendance to safeguard their relative.

The key to effective nursing management is the development of a workable homeostasis of interpersonal relationships among patient, family, and nursing staff.

Nurse-Physician Interaction

Nurses generally have no part in the medical consultation process, but they may need to function as intermediaries in the nursing home. For example, in the hospital the attending physician will request a consultation and will confer directly with the consultant. In the skilled nursing facility, the attending doctor may ask the nurse to contact the consultant, who may refuse to come to the nursing home for the consultation. This is particularly onerous when a nursing home patient has been hospitalized for surgery and the surgeon insists on seeing the patient after surgery in the hospital or in his office. Or, if the consultant does visit the patient, he may forward his report to the nursing home, giving the nurse the task of relaying the report to the attending physician.

Nurses in the skilled nursing facility must be able to identify bona fide emergencies, as patients are frequently sent to the hospital based on the verbal report of the nurse to the attending physician. While the doctor is charged with the responsibility of notifying the family of the transfer of their relative to the hospital, in effect this task often devolves to the nurse during the evening periods when he also has the burden of completing accompanying interagency referral forms.

Patient Discharge

Patients can be discharged only on the written order of their physicians. Sometimes, however, patient and family insist on discharge against medical advice. This situation is likely to occur at the initial stages of placement before the resident and his family have had the opportunity to adapt to the nursing home.

When patients do leave against medical advice, the patient and/or his sponsor should be asked to sign a release in the presence of a witness, absolving the attending physician and the nursing home from all responsibility for any adverse effects that may result from this action. Otherwise, an angry family may fault the facility should the patient, for example, sustain a stroke directly after leaving the nursing home premises. If no one will consent to sign the release, this should be noted and recorded in the patient's record in the presence of witnesses.

Unsuccessful and premature discharge probably is caused by a combination of episodes. Perhaps the patient purposely reported false incidents to his family in order to coerce them into taking him home. Perhaps the patient truthfully reported incidents that could have been remedied given time and improved communication. If the family member has mixed or unresolved feelings about the appropriateness of the placement, a little pressure from relatives becomes the catalyst for premature and inappropriate discharge. Such episodes are less likely to occur if patient, family, and nursing home work out mutually acceptable and realistic goals for the patient.

Thus the continuing involvement of the social service department with the newly admitted patient and his family is essential to the success of the placement. A mature, trusting family may not respond to obviously inaccurate stories or may request an explanation from the nursing home staff, but an immature, guilt-ridden family may permit suspicions to run rampant and may respond by summarily terminating the placement without conferring with nursing home representatives.

Patient Death

The dying patient deserves to receive empathetic and concerned nursing care. If possible, the same staff members should care for the patient on a continuing basis. Even when constant care is not required, a planned visitation and reassurance program should be implemented. In conversation, the resident should be reassured, and every effort should be made to see that he is not alone. Family members should be given free access at all hours and should be notified promptly when their relative's condition so warrants.

The feelings of other residents associated with the dying of a patient present problems. Should the dying patient be transferred to the concentrated care unit or should he remain in the room to which he has been accustomed? When making these decisions, it is necessary to think about the welfare of the entire community of patients. Their feelings should be explored via group discussions. Their wishes, as well as the wishes of the dying patient, should be considered. It is important to remember that the other residents will relate what is happening to another associate in terms of their own future experience. Thus they have a deep interest in and concern for how the deaths of peers are handled.

As mentioned previously, the attending physician is rarely in attendance if the patient dies on the nursing home premises. In the hospital, the resident staff can pronounce the patient dead. In the nursing home, however, the attending physician must do so and complete the death certificate before the body can be moved.

Most nursing homes do not have morgues, yet it is patently undesirable for the body to remain on the premises for an extended period. At times, the relative or sponsor of the patient is unreachable and an alternate plan will be needed until the family or sponsor can be notified. It is useful to work out an arrangement for a local funeral parlor or parlors to provide a holding service until final burial plans are made. A holding plan is also useful when the individual is to be buried in a different state and an out-of-state funeral parlor requires travel time before picking up the deceased. Autopsies, which are valuable teaching tools, are all too rare, although it is conceded that death certificates of nursing home patients are not known for their accuracy.

Following the death of a nursing home patient, notification must also be given to the fiscal intermediaries: Medicare and Medicaid. Clothing must be collected and made ready for the family. Equipment such as wheelchairs, televisions, and furnishings should be assembled and placed in a safe place until the family collects them.

The Ethics of Treatment Versus Nontreatment

Probably the crucial ethical issue faced by the nursing home, and particularly nursing personnel, relates to nontreatment of reversible conditions. For example, a severe urinary tract infection may cause the patient to become febrile and comatose. Family members and attending physician may request no treatment when the use of antibiotics may arrest the infection. Likewise, if the patient is comatose, he will have to be fed by means of a nasogastric tube, which requires a medical order. If nasogastric tube feeding is not ordered, what is the nursing staff's responsibility? Do they have a right to participate in the decision-making process?

If the nursing staff thinks that the patient is not receiving appropriate treatment, the attending physician and the family must be so informed. The physician and family have the option of transferring their patient to another setting where their wishes will be honored. If the stated philosophy of the skilled nursing facility is clearly and explicitly committed to treatment, this is the only available course of action.

From an administrative point of view, how is it possible to train nursing staff on one side of the hall to do everything to help patients to function at the maximal level when, on the other side of the hall, patients with reversible illnesses are not treated?

Medications

On the average, approximately five or six medications are administered per patient in the nursing home, representing an important aspect of therapeutic treatment. In the absence of physicians, nursing home nurses must be aware of the uses and effects of drugs and what signs or symptoms to observe for untoward reactions.

Some patients may refuse to take drugs, so the nurse must tread the fine line between what he is supposed to proffer and the patients' right to refuse. This becomes most complicated when a resident is not intellectually intact and the nurse must decide whether the patient should be coerced into accepting the medication.

Nurses should follow the approved procedure of the facility when administering medications, keeping in mind several factors. The eight "rights" of a medication system are a good rule of thumb:

1. the right drug
2. the right form of the medication
3. the right dosage
4. the right strength
5. the right expiration date
6. given at the right time
7. given to the right patient
8. given by the right route of administration

While crushing pills and then mixing them with a soft food is a good method for administering medications when patients have difficulty swallowing pills or when the drug cannot be obtained (or is too costly) in liquid form, it can be done only with very careful direction from the pharmacist or physician. As coated pills are meant to be dissolved in the small intestine, removing the coating causes the medication to be digested in the stomach, bringing on the possibility of a toxic reaction.

Extra caution must be taken when wheeling the medication cart through the unit housing the intellectually impaired patients. These agitated and confused patients can be very distracting to the nurse who is trying to pour medications. It might be advisable to pour liquids and prepare crushed medications immediately prior to bringing the medication cart into the unit. However, in no other instance should medications be prepared in advance.

Patients may not always be found in their rooms, or even on the nursing unit, when it is time for them to take medication. If they are attending an activity or are in the garden or receiving physical therapy, the nurse may have to bring the medication to them. However, residents who are able to should be encouraged to present themselves at the nursing station to receive their medications.

The nursing staff has responsibility for control of medications on the premises, particularly if the nursing home does not have an institutional pharmacy but a contract with a community pharmacy for the provision of drugs. Nursing staff members must be completely familiar with the pharmacy policies, especially stop-orders, and the procedure for releasing medications when a patient will be out of the building for a significant period or is discharged. All nurses must be aware of the location of the emergency drug box, its contents, and the procedure for administering drugs contained in it.

When a doctor has ordered a new prescription, the nurse must call it in to the pharmacist. Upon delivery to the nursing home, the nurse must

FIGURE 4-6
Medication Cart

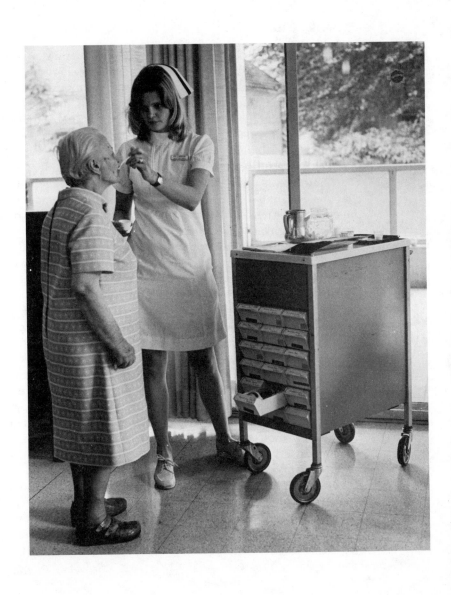

check the medication received against that ordered and record specified information in a bound log book. Mandatory record-keeping requirements also involve the inventorying of all controlled substances by two nurses at the change of shift. The director of nursing should oversee the disposal of unused medications and the surrender of all controlled substances to the Bureau of Narcotics and Dangerous Drugs.

RECORDS

Patients' Charts

The long-term stay of patients coupled with a nursing home's record-keeping requirements produce very thick patients' charts. In the nursing home, every single chart must include material from social service, the dietitian, the activities department, and so on, while only physician-ordered services are noted on hospital charts. The volume of inter-disciplinary data on each patient's chart is advantageous in the respect that a total description of the patient may be found by perusing his chart; in hospitals, records are fragmented among the departments.

These factors present obvious problems in record keeping, since the chart material must be current while also providing a complete picture of the patient. It is necessary to thin patient charts constantly and carefully, leaving enough material on the health record to give a full physical, social, and emotional description of the patient at that time, and to provide a continuum of care. The documentation that is removed from the current chart must be placed in a certain order for easy reference and must be readily available to provide background information and fill in the gaps in the current record. It may be necessary to conduct a semiannual or annual chart review to ensure the accuracy and completeness of long-standing active charts.

Maintaining current material on the chart is also affected by the frequent discharge and readmission of residents to and from the general hospital. Social service histories, dental records, activities plans, nutritional problems, and the like will not often change from discharge to readmission; it is useful to pull that material from the patient's discharge file and place it on the new chart. This can be easily done by noting in the discharge chart what material was taken out for placement on the patient's current record.

Information on patients' health records is confidential and should be available only to authorized people. In most cases this would mean professional staff, although key personnel in a nursing home may be technically nonprofessional people such as the activities director, social worker, or physical therapy assistant who treat patients daily.

The outside cover of the chart should list the patient's name and room number, the physician's name, the patient's status (e.g., Medicare or Medicaid and appropriate numbers), and a notation of the patient's allergies, if any. At the immediate top of the chart should be a copy of the admission record card received from social service and the most recent nursing assessment form. The assessment form (Exhibit 4–1) is completed in conjunction with the patient's utilization review dates, as it provides a total medical, functional, and psychosocial picture of the patient.

As a reminder, it is helpful to keep a copy of the diagnostic requisition form in the front of the chart to be removed when the results of the studies are received.

Nursing Progress Notes

Nursing progress notes should be specific, accurate, and pertinent and must reflect that the patient's care plan is being carried out. Any changes in the patient's condition should be documented with notes written by every shift until the problem is resolved. At the time of a physician's visit, nurses should write notes indicating the reason for the visit and, when a patient has a complaint, including subsequent documentation describing the action taken to resolve the problem. A note should be written by every nursing shift for the first forty-eight hours after a patient's admission and *at least* weekly thereafter, indicating the patient's improvement, deterioration, or maintenance of status quo. Every nursing note should be dated and signed by the recorder with the shift time also indicated.

Except for the months when a nursing assessment is required, a monthly summary should be routine. Its purpose is to give a twenty-four-hour picture of the resident for the thirty-day period. The monthly summary should include notes written on the same date by nurses on the day, evening, and night shifts. This form is unique to long-term-care facilities where patients remain for thirty-day periods.

Diagnostic History

The diagnostic-history form (Exhibit 4–2) provides a continuing record of the patient's medical problems. It comprises the original admission diagnosis, past medical history, and a description of new conditions encountered while in the nursing home. All new diagnoses should be noted; if the physician does not provide a diagnosis, symptoms should be documented. Readmissions with new diagnoses as well as the discharge diagnosis should be included. At the time of the patient's annual physical, the attending physician should be requested to initial this form so as to make it an official record of the patient's status.

EXHIBIT 4-1
Comprehensive Nursing Assessment

COMPREHENSIVE NURSING ASSESSMENT

Patient's name_____

Admission no._____   Admission date_____

Type of Review_____   Date of Review_____

Attending physician_____

DIAGNOSES

1. Admitting note diagnoses:

    _____
    _____

2. Attending physician diagnoses_____
    _____

3. Additional Diagnoses by medical director_____
    _____
    _____

PATIENT DATA

1. Birthdate_____   Age_____

2. Sex_____

3. Marital Status   S   M   W   Sep.   Div.

Answer Yes or No to Following:

                                        Yes   No
1. Does patient wear dentures?   ____   ____

2. Does patient wear partial
    dentures?   ____   ____

3. Does patient have own teeth?   ____   ____

4. Does patient wear hearing
    aid?   ____   ____

5. Does patient wear glasses?   ____   ____
              reading glasses?   ____   ____
              distance glasses?   ____   ____

DAY OF ASSESSMENT MEASUREMENTS

1. Weight   _____

2. Blood pressure   _____

3. Pulse   _____

4. Respiration rate_____

5. Temperature   _____

FUNCTIONAL STATUS
(Check appropriate answers)

1. Mobility

    ____Fully ambulatory
    ____Ambulatory with assistance
    ____Nonambulatory
    ____Uses walker
    ____Uses cane
    ____Able to propel own
        wheelchair
    ____Must be pushed in wheel-
        chair
    ____Confined to bed at all
        times
    ____In bed most of day; placed
        in chair periodically
    ____(# of hours)

2. Transferring

    ____Can transfer alone
    ____Needs some assistance
    ____Must be totally assisted
    ____Bedfast

3. Stairclimbing

    ____Independent
    ____Needs assistance
    ____Unable to do
    ____Not permitted

EXHIBIT 4-1 (cont.)

FUNCTIONAL STATUS (Cont.)

4. Bathing

___Independent
___With supervision
___With assistance
___Must be done by staff

5. Dressing

___Independent
___With supervision
___With assistance
___Must be done by staff

6. Eating

___Independent
___With assistance
___Must be spoon-fed
___Nasogastric tube
___Difficulty swallowing

7. Toileting

___Independent
___With assistance

8. Bowel Function

___Normal
___Frequent impactions
___Incontinent
___Diarrhea
___Rectal bleeding
___Hemorrhoids
___Colostomy

9. Bladder Function

___Normal
___Periodic retention
___Totally incontinent
___Incontinent at times
___Cystostomy
___Frequent genito-urinary
   infections
___Hematuria
___Catheter

10. Grooming

___Independent all areas
___Needs help in some areas
___Needs help all areas
___Requires total care

11. Sensory

___No visual deficits
___Visual deficit moderate
___Visual deficit severe
___No hearing deficit
___Hearing deficit moderate
___Hearing deficit severe
___Hypesthesia
___Hyperesthesia

12. Special Functional Problems

___Gait impairment
___Tracheostomy
___Dyspnoea
___Chest pain
___Contractures

13. Orientation and Brain Function

___Totally oriented
___Oriented at times
___Disoriented to time and place
___Disoriented to place only
___Disoriented to time only
___Alert and intellectually intact
___Occasionally confused, forgetful
___Moderately confused, forgetful
___Severely confused, forgetful
___Can meaningfully communicate
   verbally
___Can communicate only with
   gestures
___Can communicate only at times
___Totally unable to communicate
___Aphasic

14. Behavior

___Appropriate
___Hyperkinetic
___Passive
___Aggressive
___Belligerent
___Combative
___Hostile
___Paranoid
___Confused
___Depressed
___Wanders
___Euphoric
___Lethargic
___Pleasant
___Cooperative
___Unstable
___Agitated
___Hallucinates

EXHIBIT 4-1 (cont.)

```
MEDICAL AND NURSING NEEDS

1.  Medications                      7.  Rehabilitation, including
                                         Restorative Nursing Services
      ___Oral
      ___Rectal                          ___Speech pathology/audiology
      ___Intramuscular                   ___Skilled physical therapy
      ___Intravenous                     ___Skilled occupational therapy
      ___Clyses                          ___Supplemental nursing rehab
      ___Irrigations                     ___Training in transfer
      ___Instillations                   ___Ambulation retraining
      ___Topical                         ___Exercises for prevention of
      ___Ophthalmic                         contractures
      ___yes ___no  Can self-administer  ___Exercises for reduction of
                    medication             contractures
      ___yes ___no  Can be trained to    ___Training in use of brace
                    self-administer       ___Training in use of cane
                    medication           ___Training in use of walker
                                         ___Training in use of prosthetic
2.  Medications                             device
                                         ___Heat applications
    Specific meds    Dose   Frequency    ___Whirlpool
             Route                       ___Training in ADL (activities of
                                            daily living)
                                         ___Bladder-training program
3.  Dressings and Bandages               ___Bowel-training program
                                         ___Oxygen
      ___Unsterile                       ___Inhalation therapy
      ___Sterile                         ___Blind training
      ___Bulky
      ___Ulcer
      ___Protective                  NURSING CARE
      ___Elastic
      ___Site _____       1.  ___Administration of ordered drugs
                                     2.  ___Titration of drugs that tend to
                                             cause untoward effects
4.  Frequency of Dressing/Bandage    3.  ___Frequent positioning
    Applications Per Day             4.  ___Pharyngeal suctioning
                                     5.  ___Tracheostomy care
      ___Once a day                  6.  ___Wound care
      ___More than once a day        7.  ___Decubitus care
      ___Less than once a day        8.  ___Debridement
                                     9.  ___Vital signs:
                                             Once a day
5.  Dietary Needs                            Each shift
                                             Every hour
      ___Low salt                    10. ___Nasogastric tube feedings
      ___Therapeutic diet            11. ___Colostomy care
      ___Supplemental feedings       12. ___Colostomy irrigations
      ___Regular diet                13. ___Digital exam for impaction
      ___Chopped                     14. ___Routine enema program
      ___Puree                       15. ___Catheter care and insertions
                                     16. ___Bladder irrigations
                                     17. ___Fractional urines for sugar and
6.  Ancillary Professional Services          acetone
                                     18. ___Intake and output monitoring
      ___Podiatry                    19. ___Monitoring lab results
      ___Dental                      20. ___Patient preparation for special
      ___Optometry                           diagnostic tests
                                     21. ___Application of restraints
                                     22. ___Water mattress therapy
                                     23. ___Supportive nursing psychotherapy
                                     24. ___yes ___no  Is patient able to
                                             perform or be trained to perform
                                             any of his nursing care or therapy?
```

EXHIBIT 4-1 (cont.)

ACTIVITIES PROGRAM PARTICIPATION

1. ____ Attends with no encouragement
2. ____ Requires moderate encouragement
3. ____ Requires maximum encouragement
4. ____ Refuses to attend
5. ____ Unable to attend

NURSING OBSERVATION

____yes ____no Patient needs daily skilled nursing observations and supervision

Special Observations: Explain: _____

1. ____ Unstable medical condition   _____
2. ____ Shock or bleeding   _____
3. ____ Drug response   _____
4. ____ Unstable psychiatric condition _____
5. ____ Recurrent seizures   _____
6. ____ Symptoms of acute infection   _____

Brief summary of general condition:

_____
_____
_____
_____
_____

Note any acute or specific changes in mental or physical status of patient that
have been resolved prior to date of this review: _____

_____
_____
_____
_____
_____

Present status: Improving___ Stable___ Unstable___ Deteriorating___ Terminal___

_____   _____
Signature of assessing nurse   Date

(THE INFORMATION DOCUMENTED HEREIN MUST BE OBTAINED FROM MATERIAL THAT IS
ACTUALLY DOCUMENTED ON CHART. IF MATERIAL IS NOT DOCUMENTED ON CHART, THERE IS
AN OBVIOUS DEFICIENCY IN THE CHARTED MATERIAL, WHICH SHOULD BE CORRECTED.)

EXHIBIT 4-2
Diagnostic History

DIAGNOSTIC HISTORY
(Note: always asterisk hospital readmissions)

Name _____   Physician _____

Date of original admission _____

Original admission diagnosis _____

_____

_____

_____

Previous Medical Problems (including information from previous nursing home
                           admissions)

   Surgery _____

   _____

   _____

   Resolved medical problems _____

   _____

   _____

   Chronic or unresolved problems _____

   _____

   _____

   Undocumented findings _____

   _____

Additional Diagnoses or Acute Illnesses

Date of Readmission	Date of Onset	Date of Resolution	Condition

Dual Kardex System

In addition to records maintained on the chart, the utilization of a dual Kardex system is recommended to help consolidate other directives and documentation of the patient's care: two Kardexes are kept for each individual patient, allowing four surfaces to be available for information.

One Kardex should contain the medication administration plan, combining notation for transcribing, dispensing, and administering drugs. All medications ordered—PRN, routine, and once-only orders—are noted on one card, which also provides space for recording routine medications administered. The second card in this Kardex records PRN medications administered and notation of vital signs, clinitest, and weights.

Both the nursing care plan and the patient care plan are found in the care plan Kardex. The nursing care plan is a particularly unique adaptation to long-term nursing because it provides a fairly complete description of the patient at a glance. The patient's problems and needs, the plan of approach to meet those needs, implementation of doctor's orders in activities of daily living, nursing treatments (both routine and PRN), and diagnostic work are synthesized on the nursing care plan card. On the patient care plan card, the different disciplines note the patient's problems and needs relative to their specialties, along with their plan of approach to meet those needs and goals.

The dual Kardex system allows for all treating staff to learn the status of any given patient easily and quickly at any given time by including specific material that is not normally found in a Kardex in an acute hospital setting, but is necessary due to the extended duration of the patient's stay. Some data about the patient's status upon admission is recorded, thus precluding the need to review voluminous material from old charts. The Kardex is also particularly useful for change-of-shift reports (see Exhibit 4-3).

The key to the successful use of the dual Kardex system is to have all the material current and accurate; otherwise its effectiveness is compromised. The charge nurse and members of the nursing home treating team must make corrections in the Kardex as new orders are received or as the patient's condition changes. These changes are made easily by using a pencil to mark notes on the care plan.

Physician Reminder Form

A physician reminder form (see Exhibit 4-4) that can be attached to a patient's monthly order sheet is useful in assuring that the physician is informed of and attends to all important matters during a visit. This form is especially necessary because physicians frequently visit in the evening when the head nurse normally is not on duty and the charge nurse may be unaware of the necessity of informing the physician of such matters.

FIGURE 4-7
Use of Dual Kardex System

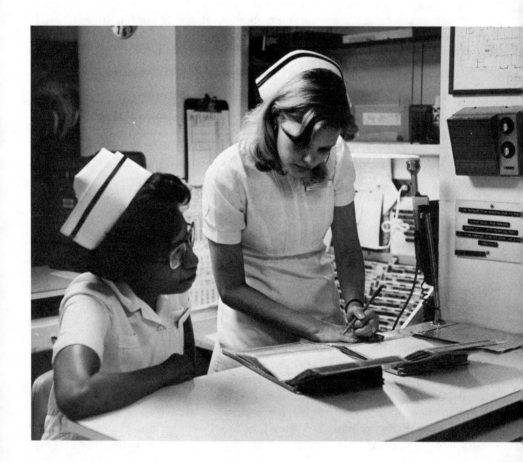

EXHIBIT 4-3
Dual Kardex

ROOM 109 NAME Doe, Jane (1979)	PATIENT CARE PLAN	
DIAGNOSIS s/p CVA c̄ rt. hemiparasis, Diabetes Mellitus	ASHD, seborrheic dermatitis, diab. dermatitis	

DATE	GENERAL NURSING PROBLEMS & NEEDS	PLAN OF APPROACH	RESPONSE
5/24	① Chronic diabetic mellitus requires long term supervision.	① Special care of integument. ② Dietary control. ③ Observation for increased cardiac and renal involvement; increased visual deficits and symptoms of hypoglycemia or diabetic coma.	
	② Recent CVA c̄ rt. hemiparasis has altered her body image which is superimposed upon prior dependent, insecure personality.	① Encourage her to explore and verbalize her feelings. ② Support her c̄ positive acknowledgement of body use and mental capacity.	
	③ Chronic seborrheic dermatitis and diabetic dermatitis.	① Shampoo scalp twice weekly and moisturize skin every day. ② Instruct Miss Doe to keep from scratching lower extremities, especially c̄ finger nails. Keep nails short and clean.	
	④ Long standing ASHD c̄ history of edema of lower extremities.	① Observe for increased weight due to edema and report to Dr. Smith.	(A.F.)

(front view)

EXHIBIT 4-3 (cont.)

ROOM 109 NAME Doe, Jane (1979)	PATIENT CARE PLAN	
DIAGNOSIS S/P CVA c̄ rt. hemiparasis, Diabetes Mellitus,	ASHD, seborrheic dermatitis, diab. dermatitis	
DATE	ANCILLARY PROBLEMS & NEEDS	PLAN OF APPROACH	RESP

DATE	ANCILLARY PROBLEMS & NEEDS	PLAN OF APPROACH	RESP
5/24	DIETARY & NUTRITIONAL 1800 calorie ADA		
	①This lady had lived alone c̄ poor nutritional intake. Caloric intake to be increased after evaluation of present diet tolerance and diabetic status	① Maintain 1800 cal. ADA for 2 weeks. Then reevaluate diet c̄ Dr. Smith for increase of calories (6-7-79).	
	② Pt. likes late evening snack.	② Milk 90 cc. c̄ ½ sandwich @ 9 p.m.	CRN
	REHABILITATION: P.T. - rt. hemiparasis	Goals: Long - amb. c̄ q. cane c̄ supervision	6 mo
	① Range limitation - rt. elbow 15° flexion contracture	Short: Transfer independently 3 mos.	
	② Strength-some general weakness, more on rt. No active motion of R UE, weakness of rt. ankle c̄ pronation of rt. foot.	① Exercise for range ② Exercise for strength. Orthopedic shoe c̄ built in antipronator to be ordered.	
	③ Requires mod. assistance to transfer, and to ambulate in parallel bars and c̄ q. cane.	③ Training in wt. bearing, transfer, balance and gait in parallel bars and c̄ rt. short leg brace and q. cane.	CDF
	SOCIAL & RECREATION		
	Pt. is essentially an isolate and withdrawn at this time. Crewel, her old hobby, is difficult c̄ rt. hand use diminished and visual deficits.	① Start with small group activity to reestablish socialization. ② Introduce weaving loom for familiar activity, using gross muscle movement.	CJ
	SOCIAL & FAMILY SERVICE		
	Miss Doe is last surviving member of her family. Her sister, whom she lived, died 3 mos. ago. They worked as secretaries and spent leisure time at museums and concerts. Family lawyer is caring for finances.	① Help pt. to work through the loss of her sister. ② Help pt. to adjust to community life here. ③ Encourage her participation in cultural programs.	CN.
	BEHAVIORAL		
	Pt. is naturally shy and withdrawn. Since CVA she is frightened and reluctant to move from her bed. She shows increased confusion at night.	① Responds well to 1:1 attention and to a firm but gentle directive. ② Volunteer visiting twice weekly will be encouraged. ③ Keep night light on. Reassure and reorient to surroundings daily.	CA
	SPEECH		
	Dysarthria 2^d to CVA	Allow time for pt. to articulate.	
	PODIATRIC		
	No areas of diabetic ischemia noted.	Have podiatrist attend weekly.	
	DENTAL		
	Upper dentures loose 2^d to wt. loss.	Dental consult for denture relining.	
	VISUAL		
	Visual loss to be evaluated.	Dr. Scott to attend. 5-29-79	
	AUDIAL		
	None		
	RELIGIOUS		
	Methodist	Attends Protestant and Catholic services.	

DEVELOPED IN CONJUNCTION WITH PHYSICIANS PLAN OF CARE   (interior view)

EXHIBIT 4-3 (cont.)

1979	NURSING CARE PLAN	
DATE	**NURSING PROBLEMS AND NEEDS**	**PLAN OF APPROACH**
5/24	I. Recent CVA (4-16-79) c̄ rt. hemiparasis	I. Assist Miss Doe in each area of difficulty
	① Confusion	① Continuous reality orientation and repetition of instructions.
	② Weakness of rt. arm and leg.	② Daily ROM, use of arm sling and short leg brace.
	③ Dysarthria	③ Do not hurry verbal response. Allow time to articulate
	④ Dysphagia	④ Observe for cough c̄ fluid intake. Observe for s/s of aspiration pneumonia.
	⑤ Neurogenic bowel and bladder	⑤ Foley catheter insitu c̄ removal planned in 2 weeks for attempt at bladder training. Enema and laxative program.
	⑥ Diminished vision, especially to the right.	⑥ Stand and place items to pt's left side.
	II. Seborrheic dermatitis of temporal areas of scalp.	II. Use medicated shampoo as directed.
	III. Appetite diminished due to long standing inanition and present depression.	III. Feed slowly, give small portions to start, encourage through praise. Bet. meal nourishments.
	IV. Increased confusion at night.	IV. Keep night light on; reorient pt. to surroundings each night. Check siderails. (A.F.)

ADM. DATE 5-24-79   RELIGION Methodist   BIRTH DATE Jan. 20, 1899   AGE 80

(front view)

DIAGNOSIS 5/p C.V.A. c̄ rt. hemiparasis, Diabetes Mellitus, ASHD, seborrheic dermatitis, diabetic dermatitis

ROOM 109   NAME Doe, Jane   DOCTOR Smith   TEL. NO. 761- 7163

DATE: 5-24-79   DISCHARGE PLAN:

There is no discharge plan at this time. Patient requires full skilled services and rehabilitation program is in progress.

I. D. MEETING - PATIENT EVALUATION				PHYSICIAN'S MONTHLY VISIT			
AND DISCUSSION OF DISCHARGE PLANS				ORDERS AND GOALS REVIEWED AND UPDATED			
DATE	SIGNATURE	DATE	SIGNATURE	DATE	SIGNATURE	DATE	SIGNATURE
5-27-79	R.S.			5-24-79	A.F.		

(back view)

EXHIBIT 4-3 (cont.)

DIET 1800 ADA Need help c̄ feeding self X I & O	ACTIVITY ___ BED REST ___ BATHROOM X OOB IN WHEEL-CHAIR ___ OOB AD LIB	SPECIAL SERVICES X P.T. X DENTAL X BEAUTICIAN X PODIATRIST X NEWSPAPER Large print Times if possible. Also gets large print Readers Digest.	URINE ___ TOILET q2h X FOLEY CATHETER X IRRIGATE N/S qd X F̶ for s/A qid 7-11 - 7-11
NOURISHMENT OR SPEC. FEEDINGS Eggnog - pudding 10am 2pm 90 cc milk & ½ sandwich 9 p.m.	AMBULATION ___ ALONE X ASSIST		SPEECH Dysarthria of CVA causes some slurring
BATH X BATHE PATIENT ___ ASSIST X TUB ___ SHOWER	LOCOMOTION AIDS short leg brace (rt.) quad cane SPECIAL EQUIPMENT sling rt. arm	BOWEL CARE X RECTAL ONCE WEEK X ENEMA q.o.d. prn ___ BEDPAN H.S.	SIDERAILS X WHEN IN BED ___ NIGHT ONLY ___ RELEASE
		SPECIAL PRIVILEGES	ADMISSION T. 99 P. 88 R. 20 B/P 134/60 WEIGHT 94 lbs. SKIN CONDITION scalp shows area of seborrhea, especially in temporal area. Diabetic dermatitis of lower extremities.
MOUTH X UPPER) DENTURES ___ LOWER) ___ PARTIAL PLATE ___ SPECIAL CARE	EYES ___ BLIND X PARTIAL SIGHT R X L ___ X GLASSES 1- gold rim - vision 1- tortoise - reading	ALLERGIES Penicillin	

ORDER DATE	TREATMENTS AND NURSING CARE	TIMES	ORDER DATE	DIAGNOSTIC AND CONSULTATION	DONE	REC'D.
5-24-79	Weigh 3x week	M-W-F	5/24	Chem Screen 25 and CBC	5/26	A.F
5-24-79	Foley inserted #18/5 cc			Urinalysis	"	A.F.
	Change foley q 2 wks.	6-6-79		Chest x-ray	"	R.S.
	Catheter care qd	11 AM		EkG	"	R.S.
			5/26	Opthomology consult c̄ Dr.		
	Check scalp and note condition	qd		Scott on 5-29-79		
	Sebulex shampoo Biw	M&F				
	Keri Lotion to skin especially lower extremities	qd				
	Assist c̄ sling and leg brace when necessary					
	PRN			STANDING LAB WORK		
			5/24	Weekly fasting blood sugar with 2 hr. P.P. q Wed.		

DIAGNOSIS S/p C.V.A. c̄ rt. hemiparesis, Diabetes Mellitus, ASHD, seborrheic dermatitis, diabetic dermatitis

ROOM 109   NAME Doe, Jane   (interior view)   DOCTOR Smith   TEL. NO. 761-7163

EXHIBIT 4-3 (cont.)

1979	P. R. N. MEDICATION ORDERS	#147548-8092	SINGLE ORDERS				
ORDER DATE / EXPIR DATE	MEDICATION, DOSAGE, AND FREQUENCY		DATE	MEDICATION AND DOSAGE	TIME TO BE GIVEN	TIME GIVEN	INIT.
5/24	Milk of Magnesia 30 cc hs prn		5/26	Lasix 40 mgm p.o.	STAT	11am	AF
	Aspirin gr. X q 4h prn for pain						
	or temperature over 100°						
	Regular insulin coverage based on						
	S ċ A − 4⁺ − 15 units subq.						
	S ċ A − 3⁺ − 10 units subq.						
	S ċ A − 2⁺ − 5 units subq.						
	S ċ A − 1⁺ − NO INSULIN						
			INIT	NURSE SIGN	INIT	NURSE SIGN	INIT	NURSE SIGN
			A.F.	Ana Fields	MM.	Marilyn Mills	
			R.S.	Ruth Spencer			
	(front view)		F.M.	Frances May			

AGE **80** RELIGION **Methodist**   DATE ADMITTED **5-24-79**   IF ANOTHER PAGE IS IN USE CHECK HERE IN RED →

DOCTOR **Smith**   PHONE **761-7163** DIAGNOSIS **S/PCVA, ċ rt. hemiparasis, Diabetes Mellitus,**

ROOM **109**   NAME **Doe, Jane**   **ASHD, seborrheic dermatitis, diabetic dermatitis**

EXHIBIT 4-3 (cont.)

MEDICATION ADMINISTRATION RECORD

ALLERGIC TO: Penicillin

ALL ENTRIES MUST BE PRINTED   YEAR 1979   DATES GIVEN May - June

ORDER DATE	EXPIR DATE	MEDICATION, DOSE, FREQUENCY	HR.	5/24	25	26	27	28	29	30	31	6/1	2	3	4	5	6
5/24		NPH Insulin subq. qd 10 u.	7³⁰	MM	MM	MM	MM	MM									
		Digoxin 0.25 mgm p.o. q.o.d.	9A	AF	X	AF	X		X		X		X		X		X
		pulse		88	X	84	X		X		X		X		X		X
	5/26	Lasix 40 mgm p.o. q.d.	9A	AF	AF	←				D/C	5/26						
		K-Lor 1 pkg. in orange juice q.d.	9A	AF	AF	AF	AF										
5/26		Chloral Hydrate 500 mgm po. h.s.	9P		→	RS	RS										
		Lasix 60 mgm p.o. q.d.	9A		→	AF	AF										

(interior view)

AGE 80   RELIGION Methodist   DATE ADMITTED 5-24-79

DOCTOR Smith   PHONE 761-7163   DIAGNOSIS S/PCVA, c̄ rt. hemiparasis, Diabetes Mellitus,
ROOM 109   NAME Doe, Jane   ASHD, seborrheic dermatitis, diabetic dermatitis

IF ANOTHER PAGE IS IN USE
CHECK HERE IN RED →

EXHIBIT 4-3 (cont.)

ROOM 109	NAME Doe, Jane	YR. 1979								TREATMENTS GIVEN		Foley N/S		
DATE	P. R. N. MEDICATION GIVEN		DATE	B.P.	T	P	R	WT.	S & A				
5/24	Milk of Magnesia 30cc @ 9 pm F.M.												
DATE	PRN MEDICATION GIVEN #147794-8092		DATE	B.P.	T	P	R	WT.	S & A				

———— (front view) ————

ROOM 109	NAME Doe, Jane	YR. 1979								TREATMENTS GIVEN		Foley N/S
DATE	P. R. N. MEDICATION GIVEN		DATE	B.P.	T	P	R	WT.	S & A		
5/24	Milk of Magnesia 30cc @ 9 pm. F.M.		5/24	134/60	99	88	20	94	neg. neg. / neg. neg. / neg. neg.	A.F.	
5/25	Regular insulin 5u rt. arm subq. 7 p.m. R.S.		5/25			80			neg. neg. / neg. neg. / 2+ TR / neg. TR	A.F.	
5/26	Regular insulin 10u. left arm subq. 7³⁰ p.m. R.S.		5/26			84		96	neg. neg. / 3+ TR / neg. TR	A.F.	
5/27	ASA gr. X for pain in rt. shoulder 8 p.m. R.S.		5/27			92			neg. neg. / neg. neg. / neg. neg.	A.F.	
	Milk of Magnesia 30 cc 9pm R.S.										

———— (interior view) ————

EXHIBIT 4-4
Attending Physician Reminder

ATTENDING PHYSICIAN REMINDER

Dear Doctor,

Please Sign:

1. ____ Telehpone order dated _____

2. ____ Accident report dated _____

3. ____ Certification

4. ____ Physical therapy prescription

5. ____ Restraint order

6. ____ Adm./annual diagnostic workup

7. ____ Diagnostic history

8. ____ Other: _____

Please Note:

1. ____ Diagnostic reports dated _____

        Type _____

2. ____ Adm./annual physical due

3. ____ Physical therapy evaluation and notes

4. ____ Medical director's note

5. ____ Nurse's note dated _____

6. ____ Consultation dated _____

        Type _____

7. ____ Other: _____

Other Records

The nursing department has certain record-keeping requirements of an administrative nature. Mandated by law are specific records pertaining to controlled medications—narcotics, sedatives, depressants, and stimulants. A bound controlled substances receipt book must include certain information regarding every prescription for a controlled substance that is received at the nursing home. The nurse receiving the order must sign it and note the date, the patient's name, the pharmacy filling the prescription, the drug, the amount ordered, and the amount received.

Each administration of a drug must be noted on an inventory sheet, and the remaining quantity must be accounted for at the turnover of each nursing shift. Both the nurse signing in and the nurse signing out participate in this accounting. These record sheets become a part of the patient's chart when they have been completed.

Cancelled or unused controlled medications should be counted by two nurses, placed in a double-locked container, and routinely inventoried until they are taken to the Bureau of Narcotics and Dangerous Drugs. Just before they are taken, the drugs should be counted and itemized on a specified quadruplicate form, which is signed by the receiving agent and the licensed nurse making the delivery. One copy should be retained by the nursing facility and, along with the receipt of surrender obtained from the agent, placed in a notebook. When the copy with notification of destruction is returned to the facility, all three items are stapled together and placed in the notebook stored in the locked cabinet. Records of controlled substances usually must be retained by the facility for a specified period according to state law.

Completed notification of patient movement slips must be sent to administration, business, social service, and dietary departments at the time of a patient's discharge, death, or room change.

Each nursing station should have a resident off-premises book that records the names of residents who leave the building. Such information can be vital in an emergency situation, when every person in the facility must be accounted for. For each outing, the following should be noted: patient's name, date, time of departure, expected date and time of return, signature and relationship of person accompanying the patient, destination, and signature of the charge nurse indicating awareness of the patient's departure. A record should also be maintained—either incorporated into the off-premises book or kept separately—for the signature of ambulance, Medicab, or taxi drivers who transport the patient to the hospital or outside appointment.

Depending on local laws concerning the retention of copies of death certificates and removal of bodies, the nursing home may want to have other records of that information. If the nursing home can keep a copy of the death certificate, which would list all relevant data including to whom the body was released, that form may suffice. Otherwise, a mortality log should be maintained to record the pertinent data on the death, in addition to the chart material, and the signature of the morti- cian who accepts the body.

A form should be developed detailing important information that needs to be relayed from one nursing shift to the next. Most often, this would be a supervisors' report form, which would highlight admissions and discharges, patients who have received new orders and the content of those orders, and patients in unstable conditions who are to be closely observed during the next twenty-four hours. The supervisors' report, in conjunction with the Kardex, is the main reporting mechanism for com- municating with the oncoming nursing shift.

The nursing supervisors should remit a list of the changing clinical and administrative needs of the nursing department to the director of nursing for the preparation of a monthly report, which is submitted to the administrative director.

The director of nursing should keep on file a list of all licensed nursing personnel. As he is responsible for verifying the licensure of nursing staff, he ought to have a record of all nurses' names, addresses, license numbers, and license expiration dates. This same record must also be kept for nurses working with permits with expiration dates: if the permit expires without being replaced concurrently by a license, the nurse can no longer work. Nurses should always be required to show their new licenses when they receive them.

Reports of patient accidents or incidents should be fully described on an individual form. Corresponding documentation must, of course, be found in the nursing notes. The accident/incident report form does not become a part of the patient's permanent record, however; it is an administrative record to be filed elsewhere. All such reports require the attending physician's signature and must be referred to the medical director for review and comments.

Errors or omissions in administering medications must be put on record. In addition to noting the mistake in the nursing progress notes, a medication incident report should be completed, containing a descrip- tion of the error, verifying notification of the attending physician, and containing his comments and signature. The report should be brought to the attention of the pharmacy committee, as well as the director of nurs- ing and the medical director, for their recommendations.

NURSING DEPARTMENT COMMUNICATIONS

The nursing home must evaluate its needs with respect to the nurses' call system. Unless the patients are intellectually alert, an intercom unit is of no benefit. A closed-circuit television can provide close supervision for patients who are immobile or intellectually impaired.

An audiovisual call system may be installed to summon assistance in each bedroom, lavatory, and shower or tub area. The location of the call button must be within easy reach of the patient or staff member who is attending the patient in that area. The call buzzer should sound continuously at the nursing station until a staff member has responded and turned off the buzzer in the location from which it was sounded. The visual part of the system could be a light over the bedroom door with a color code to indicate lavatory or bedroom, a light over the shower/tub room, and a light at the nursing station. The call system for one unit should be able to be switched over to sound at another unit should all staff members be required to leave the unit in an emergency.

The nursing department should have its own telephone lines to facilitate incoming and outgoing calls. These lines can also be used to receive incoming calls, which are taken on extensions that can be plugged into a jack installed in each room so that residents can take phone calls in private. Outgoing resident phone calls can be made on a conveniently located public telephone, one of which should be wheelchair height. The installation of adaptations for the hard of hearing must be considered for phones used by residents. Some residents will want to have private phones, which should be installed only with family and physician approval.

Each nursing station should have a bulletin board for posting evacuation and emergency plans and relaying information pertinent to that unit, such as the wheelchair cleaning schedule, equipment sterilization schedule, beauty parlor schedule, list of attending physicians and alternates, daily patient assignments, and in-service education program. The entire nursing schedule according to floor assignments should be posted at the main nursing station.

Every nursing station should have a complete list of telephone numbers of professional persons and services available to the facility. This list should include attending physicians, allied health professionals, community hospitals, ambulance services, clinical laboratory, clergy, fire and police departments, the heads of all departments, and professional clinical consultants. As the nursing department is often the only department on duty during the evening and night, it must have a complete list of emergency repair service numbers to use if any type of equipment should break down.

FACILITIES, EQUIPMENT, AND SUPPLIES

The nursing unit must be planned to accommodate necessary work areas and supply space in addition to patient bedrooms, lavatories, and com-

FIGURE 4-8
Patient Using Call Buzzer

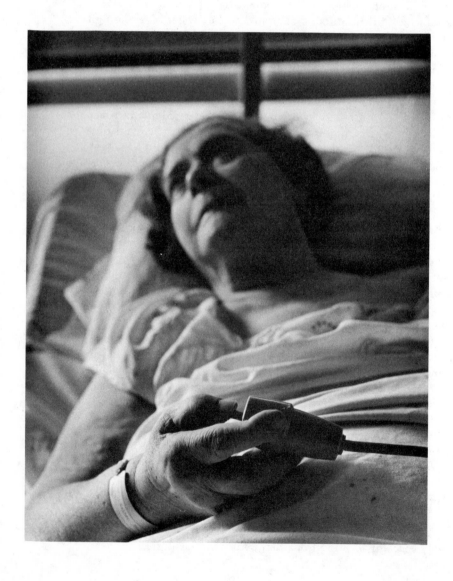

munity and/or dining areas. Lavatories and handwashing areas for staff must be designated throughout the unit. Nursing stations should be of comfortable size to allow the free movement of several people. Space should be allocated to store current patient charts, older chart material of current patients, a sufficient supply of blank forms used on the health record, and a reference shelf that includes the following:

> medical dictionary
> *Physicians' Desk Reference*
> formulary
> policy handbooks for administration, patient care, infection
>   control, and medical service
> nursing procedure manual
> diet manual
> facility emergency plan

Large fluorescent flashlights and extra bulbs should be kept at each nursing station for emergency use during a utility interruption. An instant camera should always be available to record decubiti of newly admitted patients and to record their progress.

In a 100-bed skilled nursing facility, consideration should be given to having two treatment rooms—on the units for the intellectually impaired and for the severely physically handicapped. The treatment room should have complete equipment for an examination: examining table, scale, sink with foot pedals, examining light, and cabinets. The availability of this room would facilitate the carrying out of patient treatments by nursing staff and certainly would be of substantial assistance to physicians in affording privacy and needed equipment and supplies when examining their patients.

All supplies that are clean, disinfected and/or sterilized, and ready for use may be stored in the treatment room or, in its absence, in the clean utility room. The head nurse should stock supplies to last only a limited period—three days at maximum—to provide better control over their use. A physical examination tray—including sphygmomanometer, stethoscope, otoscope, ophthalmoscope, flashlight, gloves, percussion hammer, and tongue blades—should be ready for use at all times. The autoclave or sterilizer and its supplies must be stored in a clean area, as should sterile specimen bottles. If a full-time laboratory technician is employed to collect and prepare all specimens for laboratory testing, the necessary equipment for doing so, including a centrifuge, may be stored in the laboratory; otherwise it may be kept in the nursing unit. The proper setup for passing a nasogastric tube should be available, as should a tray containing sterile vaginal examination equipment.

The head nurse should check the treatment tray daily for restocking.

It should contain the following items:

> small bottle of hydrogen peroxide
> small bottle of tincture of Merthiolate
> small bottle of liquid green soap
> razor and blade
> large jar of one-inch sterile gauze (Iodoform 5 percent) and 5
>   yards of packing
> 6 alcohol sponges
> small plastic case containing safety pins
> roll of adhesive tape
> 2 padded tongue depressors
> 3 sterile packs of cotton balls
> 4 sterile applicators
> several unsterile tongue depressors
> box of adhesive strips (including butterfly closures)
> sterile pack containing four 4 x 4's
> small bottle of tincture of benzoin
> tube of lubricating jelly
> bottle of alcohol
> airway

An emergency cart stored in a clean area should be prepared for use at any time. The cart should contain the following supplies:

> emergency drug box
> complete intravenous setup with a bottle of each type of fluid
> emergency blood work tray
> complete sterile instrument set
>   large and small scissors
>   large hemostat
>   2 small hemostats
>   2 thumb forceps
>   2 probes
>   scalpel and blade
>   four 4 x 4's
>   needleholder
>   suture material
>   airways
>   ambubag for cardiac arrest

Oxygen tanks, affixed to the floor and stored in a ventilated area, must also be available for an emergency. The skilled nursing facility may contemplate having other more specialized equipment on the emergency cart if a physician is likely to be present in an emergency. These items might include a cardiac fibrillator and cardiac board, an emergency tracheostomy tray, and an emergency urology tray containing filaments, followers, and sounds for the urologist's use.

Separate from the treatment room or utility room where clean items are stored should be the dirty utility room, to which all soiled equipment is returned to be cleaned. If required by nursing home practice, the dirty utility room would house the bedpan flusher/sterilizer. A dirty hopper—a sink with a large, open drain with no catches for the disposal of contaminated wastes—would be useful in this room. Disinfectants for cleaning and soaking equipment would be stored here, as would enema equipment and apparatus for gross testing of urine and stool. If the dirty utility room is large enough, a closed container for dirty linen may be kept there.

Clean linen should be stored in a closet designated for that purpose only. A pantry should be planned for each nursing unit, with a refrigerator, stove, toaster, sink, cupboards, and other appliances and utensils as may be needed. Juices, nourishments, and supplements would be kept in the unit pantry areas.

Medication rooms must be provided on each unit, with both single-locked compartments and double-locked cabinets for storing controlled substances. A refrigerator must be available in the medication room for drugs that require refrigeration. Space should be allocated for storing the medication-dispensing cart; the required records for controlled substances also may be kept here.

The nursing department office should be located where it is accessible to patients, staff, and families; it may be either on or off the nursing unit. In addition to adequate desk space, shelves and file cabinets are needed for the many necessary reference books and records. Prospective and past department work schedules and the master staffing plan should be located in the department office. Reference books would include the same items maintained at each nursing station and some additional material, such as geriatric and rehabilitation texts, a medical directory of the state, Conditions of Participation in Medicare, the state hospital code, regulations pertaining to controlled substances, minutes of the nursing policy and procedure committee, and other information that the director of nursing deems necessary.

Additional equipment that should be part of the nursing department inventory on each unit includes electric razors, an electric suction machine, a stretcher, an ultrasonic denture-cleansing device, wheelchairs of various types, and at least three shower chairs with very large, sturdy wheels for ease of movement, durability, and balance. A patient lifter should be available for the severely physically handicapped. Side rails should be attached to all beds. For a 100-bed skilled nursing facility, a minimum of ten water mattresses should be available for flotation therapy.

FIGURE 4-9
Chair Scale

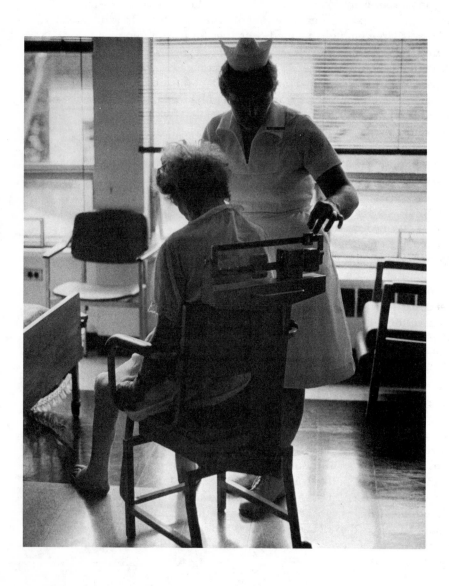

Chair scales should be selected with great care when they are to be used by severely disabled or agitated residents who may lean to one side, thus affecting the scale's accuracy. The beam of the usual chair scale should be sufficiently wide to avoid inaccurate recording. The use of an electronic scale may be advisable, although this apparatus is much more costly. In some instances, ramps may be purchased to fit over the normal doctor's scale, which will permit the patient to be weighed in a wheelchair. In the case of a severely agitated patient, it may be necessary for a staff member to sit or step on the scale while gently holding the patient. It is recommended that there be one scale on each unit to avoid transport, which could affect a scale's accuracy.

Although not necessarily located on the unit, the bulk of nursing department supplies should be inventoried and maintained in a storage room. One nurse should be assigned the duty of maintaining this stock and the responsibility for comparing prices and products for suggestion to the director of nursing. When the inventory falls below a predetermined amount, the supplies nurse should complete a requisition form for the purchasing agent in the business office. With the delivery of supplies, the assigned nurse should check each item to ensure its correctness. Finally, all requests for supplies from the floor nurses should go through the supplies nurse so that he is constantly aware of departmental needs and can exert control over the use of supplies.

SUMMARY

Educational institutions are increasingly emphasizing the special skills needed in geriatric nursing. Some states are requiring nursing aides to pass certifying examinations in order to qualify for nursing home aide positions. Since the elderly ill patient moves from the hospital, to the long-term-care facility, to his own home with home care services, it is imperative that nursing staff in all settings be trained to handle these patients. Then and only then will continuity of patient care be a reality and not a goal.

NOTES

1. D. Miller and S. Beer, "Patterns of Friendship Among Patients in a Nursing Home Setting," *The Gerontologist* 17, no. 3 (1977).
2. "Terminology," Ken Eymann, ed., in *Serving the Aging* (Reno: Eymann Publications, sample copy issue, 1977).

CHAPTER 5

Infection Control

INTRODUCTION

We are all continuously in contact with microorganisms, some of which are pathogenic and some of which are harmless. In response to germs that produce disease, the body rallies its defense system in combat, with usual success. However, when the body's resistance or immunity is low due to already-present illness, disease germs may not be so easily opposed and can cause serious infection. Such is the case in a skilled nursing facility with a patient population that is chronically ill and generally weakened.

Although the principles of infection prevention and control have long been present in the acute-care setting, only in recent years has it been impressed on the long-term-care sector, augmented by the federal government's inclusion of an applicable regulation as a Condition of Participation in Medicare and Medicaid programs. The realization of the increasing debility and disability of nursing home patients has also heightened the awareness of this issue in skilled nursing facilities.

The elderly's susceptibility to infections is aggravated because of the aging body's increasing inability to fight off disease. Cracks in the skin, the natural barrier for keeping out germs, and poor circulation—which prevents the body's defense substances from traveling to the site of infection—increase the vulnerability of the elderly, particularly the ill elderly. Those persons who are nonambulatory present an even higher risk due to their usually weakened condition. Incisions or artificial openings, which do not have the defense mechanisms of natural body openings, pose further complications in warding off disease. All these factors, found in various combinations in the nursing home patient population, compounded by the multitude of chronic organ pathologies, have the effect of lowering the infective dosage—the number of microorganisms necessary to cause infection—for these patients, and thus they are at risk. Indeed, what may be a mild case of flu for a younger healthy person can be a life-threatening experience for the aged ill. A urinary tract infection may be uncomfortable for a young person, but it may prove fatal for a nursing home patient.

Fortunately, the nursing home is not faced with the catastrophic acute infections—such as infectious hepatitis, meningitis, and overwhelming staph—that a hospital is. Hospital patients come in "off the street" often in acute stages of illness, or they may have undergone surgical procedures that increase their susceptibility to infection; hence their exposure to more exotic infections tends to be much higher. Strict isolation is common in a hospital, but not in a nursing home, although the nursing home must be prepared to institute that practice. Most nursing home patients are admitted from the hospital with relatively good assurance that they are free from serious infection (although it is not uncommon for patients to be transferred from the hospital with a fever or a urinary tract infection).

Thus the kinds of infections commonly encountered in the two types of health care settings differ. Upper respiratory infections are frequent in the skilled nursing facility and are easily transmissible, as they are in the general population. Pneumonia, which is also prevalent, can quickly lead to serious complications in a chronically ill person if it is not treated.

The presence of Foley catheters is another ongoing infection control concern in the skilled nursing facility. Long-term Foley catheter management is prevalent; hence the chance for cross-contamination is much greater than in the hospital, where catheters are normally in place for a few days at most. The majority of nosocomial infections (those originating within the institution) in a nursing home with a large proportion of catheterized patients are urinary tract infections attributable to Foley catheters, although it is sometimes questionable whether the infection is new or whether it recurs over extended periods.

Nursing home patients often have eye infections due to the drying of tear ducts that occurs with age. Also, patients confined to bed are good candidates for such infections because, when their heads are to the side, tears secrete outward and dry the eye.

Decubitus ulcers or any trauma to the friable skin of the aged pose a threat of possible infection. Both are constant nursing care problems for the institutionalized ill aged.

INFECTION PREVENTION

The nursing home should establish an infection control committee whose goal is an active prevention program and continuous surveillance so infections may be detected early and dealt with appropriately. In developing this program, several principles should be borne in mind:

separating clean from dirty; avoiding contact with contaminated items, areas, or people; proper sanitizing to prevent the build-up of microbes; and maintaining good health and hygiene habits for all involved. Chapter 16 will discuss the function of the infection control committee further.

An effective infection-prevention program begins with formalized measures for all areas of the nursing home. Since infections are most often caused by a break in technique, it is important that all staff members be aware of the purpose for such procedures.

Germs are omnipresent; hence every object that is handled or every person who comes into the nursing home is considered a possible source of infection. The goal is, therefore, to reduce the number of microorganisms to an acceptable level. This can be accomplished by various physical or chemical methods, depending on the object to be treated.

Sterilization, the most effective method, destroys all forms of microorganisms present, including spores, which are encased in a hard covering and resist other methods. Disinfection kills most living microorganisms, although not usually spores. Sanitizing will lower the microorganism count to an established safe level. Incorporating one of these methods into cleaning equipment, linen, floors, walls, utensils, and so on must be guaranteed to minimize the microbial count.

Autoclaving is convenient and is considered the most effective method of sterilization. The principle of the autoclave is steam under pressure. With the exception of large items and substances that are not penetrable by steam, most objects requiring sterilization may be autoclaved after being properly prepared: thoroughly cleaned, wrapped in autoclave paper, and dated (unless sealed in plastic, sterilization by autoclaving is good for only one month). It is advantageous to provide a temperature-recording device on the autoclave to ascertain that the proper temperature is used at all times.

Objects can be disinfected or sanitized by means of several different methods. Boiling water or various chemical compounds are the agents most frequently used in the nursing home. Which agent to select would depend on the material to be disinfected and the type of organism, if any, suspected to be present. Commercial solutions are available to incorporate into any cleaning routine, but it is important to follow their specific directions closely and to change the wash water frequently.

NURSING HOME POLICIES

Nursing home policies should reflect efforts to contain the incidence of infection. When considering admission policy, the patient care policy committee should specify that no patient who has a contagious disease will be admitted unless the physician certifies that transmissibility is negligible. Admission laboratory work should include a serology test to identify such diseases as typhoid or syphilis. In addition, many states mandate a chest x ray or tine test prior to admission. Residents should receive appropriate immunizations unless the physician's orders forbid them because of medical contraindications. If an inpatient succumbs to an acute infection requiring strict isolation, nursing home policy may be addressed to conditions under which the facility will or will not retain the patient.

Visitor regulations should indicate when visitors are prohibited from seeing a patient, such as when the patient is in strict isolation. Visitors might be discouraged from entering the building if it is feared that an infection that is widespread in the nursing home could be transmitted outside the facility. Such events as flu epidemics in the community might cause the infection control committee to prohibit visitation due to the susceptibility of nursing home residents. Visitors should be requested to inform the nursing home if they or a family member succumbs to a contagious illness in order to determine whether they might be carriers of the infection; if so, they should not be allowed in the facility. Gifts to patients of home canned or jarred food should be discouraged.

If the facility does not have a biological incinerator, arrangements should be made for the incinerated disposal of biological waste. Such arrangements may be effected with a neighboring hospital on a fee basis. Using disposable supplies whenever possible would further reduce the chance of contamination, but it would also increase the amount of waste generated by the facility.

Personnel policies must be directed to infection prevention and control. In conformance with federal law, all new employees must have a physical examination including a tuberculin tine test (followed by a chest x ray if the tine test is positive), a serology test, and a stool examination if required by area law. The importance of sound personal hygiene and health habits should be impressed on all personnel. The administration should consider recommending uniforms for employees who work in high-risk areas and hairnets for dietary personnel. The infection control committee should address policies concerning personnel who have, or who have come into contact with, communicable illnesses or who have open abrasions. Employees should report such instances to their supervisor, who should determine whether they should continue in their routine work or be reassigned to another job category.

The most important aspect of any infection control program is proper instruction about and implementation of handwashing. The orientation and ongoing in-service program should clearly reinforce this principle and highlight the instances when it is critical: between patient treatments, after using the lavatory, after handling soiled equipment and supplies, and so on.

FIGURE 5-1
Administering a Tuberculin Tine Test

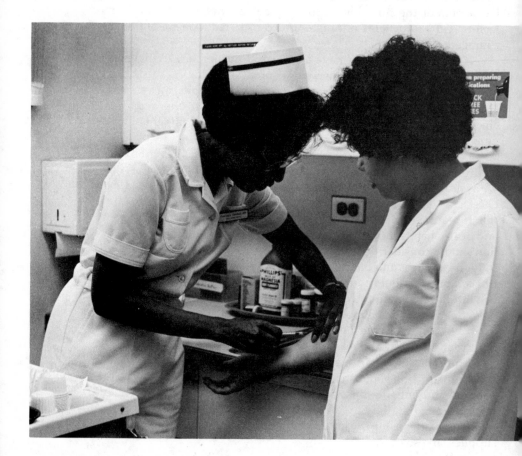

FIGURE 5-2
Handwashing

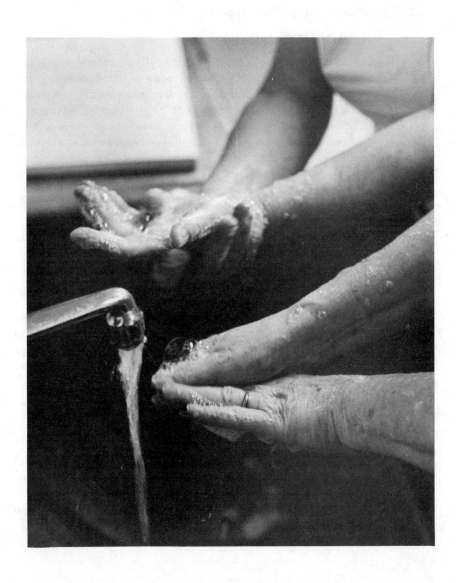

The infection control committee should work with the director of education to develop a useful program for all facility staff. The broad goals of the program should be to provide an understanding of the basic concepts of infection, to provide a general knowledge of the infection hazard inherent in a specific job category, to impress on each employee his personal responsibility in the prevention and control of infection, to reduce the possibility of acquired infection, and to provide ongoing education related to standard infection control techniques. The committee should review even such obvious acts as staff members eating in their offices and the resultant pest control problems.

RESIDENTS

Personal cleanliness is desirable for aesthetic reasons as well as for infection control. Maintaining good hygiene in the institutionalized ill aged often depends on staff performance, as many residents cannot properly bathe themselves and/or request bathing. Attendants must take responsibility for making sure that patients are clean all over—that they have clean hair, mouths, skin folds, genital and anal areas, and the like. As part of their regular observation, nursing assistants should report the discovery of cuts, bruises, rashes, swelling, and so forth, which may be sites for infection.

Clean clothes should be supplied to all residents daily or when needed, such as when they soil themselves. Because nursing home residents dress in street clothes rather than hospital gowns, it is important that each patient have a sufficient quantity of clothing to permit several changes per week (or per day if the resident is incontinent). All residents should have their own grooming and hygiene supplies: toothbrush, comb, brush, washcloth.

Educating the patient about hygiene—both routine and special precautions—is an integral part of the program, but it may be difficult if the patient is unable to understand. A common problem is that patients will store or hoard food in clothing or dressers, which inevitably will attract cockroaches and/or ants.

One of the primary and easiest steps in infection control is to separate a patient who has an acute contagious infection from those who do not. However, a confused resident may need to be restrained to accomplish this goal.

Although the nursing home cannot achieve truly sterile conditions, staff members should use antiseptic practices when they perform all treatments, change dressings, collect specimens, and so forth. Sterilized equipment will be needed for some procedures, such as insertion and irrigation of a Foley catheter or debriding a decubitus ulcer.

HOUSEKEEPING

The housekeeping staff is responsible for maintaining effective environmental sanitation to lessen the hazards of nosocomial infections. If the housekeeping staff also handles the laundry and linen, they must abide by preventive measures designed for the proper collection, transportation, processing, and storage of clothing and linens.

Routine cleaning schedules should be developed, with resident areas more frequently attended to than nonresident areas. Furthermore, areas that are more prone to contamination should be cleaned more often; for example, dust and germs fall to the floor through gravity, so floors need to be cleaned more often than walls or ceilings. Of course, shower rooms necessitate more attention than do lounge areas.

The use of both a detergent—to clean thoroughly—and a disinfectant—to kill microbes beneath the dirt layer—should be part of all cleaning procedures. These solutions may be applied separately or in combination, as many commercial solutions are marketed, thereby ensuring that both processes are completed. An Environmental Protection Agency (EPA) registration number on the bottle verifies its advertised germicidal activity and toxicity level.

For the solutions to be effective, they must be properly mixed with the correct temperature of water and applied according to directions. The two-bucket method, with one bucket containing the prepared solution and the other containing clean rinse water for the applicator, is frequently preferred when dealing with the incontinence found in long-term-care facilities. Housekeeping staff should wear gloves, although this does not eliminate the need for handwashing. Vacuum cleaners should contain a special tank or filter, which must be regularly cleaned and disinfected, to prevent germs from being expelled in the exhaust. Finally, all housekeeping equipment—sponges, brushes, mops, buckets—should be cleaned routinely.

Dirty laundry and linen are prime sources for the spread of infection and must always be kept separate from clean items. This is more true and requires greater precaution if the articles have been in an isolation room. Soiled laundry should be placed in covered receptacles for transport to the laundry room, avoiding clean utility rooms or food preparation areas, and dirty laundry should be removed before clean laundry is delivered. If any laundry is done in the facility, the process must adequately sanitize each load—that is, it must use very hot water, hot air drying, strong detergents, and often bleach. Residents' clothing laundered on the premises must be able to withstand such a harsh process; this must be thoroughly explained to families.

FIGURE 5-3
Covered Receptacle for Soiled Laundry

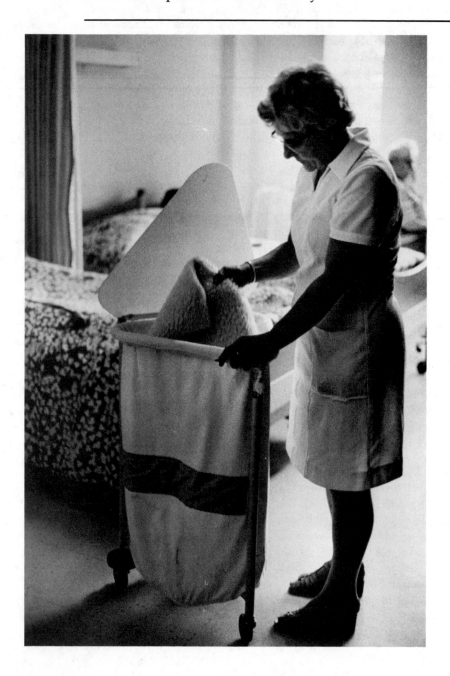

BUILDING STRUCTURE AND MAINTENANCE

Building design, layout, and materials also play a role in the infection-prevention program. Construction and building codes include specific requirements; however, a basic guide is to use materials and equipment that are durable, easily cleaned, and nonabsorbent. The building design should be such that delivery and service personnel do not have to pass through patient units or the kitchen.

The maintenance staff should systematically inspect, maintain, and repair the building and all equipment, with special consideration given to high-risk items such as foodservice equipment, for example, the temperature of the refrigerators and of the water in the dishwasher, plumbing, laundry facilities, and the autoclave. When servicing in an area where infection prevention and control is of special concern, maintenance workers should take care not to dirty any more than is necessary or to contaminate other facilities. Compounds used to make repairs should be checked for their toxicity level if they are to be used in the kitchen.

Continuous surveillance of the interior and exterior of the structure assists in insect and rodent control, implicit in a sound infection control program. In particular, it must be ascertained that all cracks and crevices in basement walls and windows and in outer walls of the nursing home are filled with caulking, concrete, or mortar. Similarly, openings around service pipes and conduits should be sealed. A qualified exterminator should service the building regularly.

Interior fissures near baseboards, window frames, or door jambs should be filled promptly. Particularly in the service or storage areas, where interior walls may be of concrete block, meticulous attention must be paid to the elimination of any openings that may harbor roaches or vermin. The grouting on tile floors and walls also requires careful maintenance department attention.

DIETARY

Enteric infections are almost always traceable to the food service. Thus care must be taken with every step of the food purchase, receiving, storage, and preparation process.

Only food of assured high quality should be purchased, with special attention given to raw food. All deliveries should be inspected to ensure that supplies are not already contaminated. Food must be stored in clean areas on shelves, and never on the floor, to allow for cleaning ease and possible flooding. Foods requiring refrigeration or freezing should immediately be stored appropriately, and cooked food should always be placed above raw food. Refrigerators and freezers must have easily readable thermometers that are accurate, with refrigerators maintained at 45°F (7°C), and freezers at 32°F (0°C). Leftovers must be properly wrapped and not kept for more than twenty-four hours.

Frozen foods should be thawed correctly, either by refrigeration or under potable water, and prepared immediately after thawing. Different food products should be prepared separately—i.e., raw meat separately from vegetables—using clean supplies and equipment in clean work areas. Sinks used for food preparation should not be used for anything else. It is essential that foods to be cooked be heated to the correct internal temperature in order to kill any bacteria present. Chilled or cold dishes must be kept between 35°F and 45°F (2°C and 7°C) to inhibit the growth of microbes, which is favored between 45°F and 140°F (7°C and 60°C).

Serving food soon after it is prepared is the best way to prevent germ growth. Food must be maintained at its correct temperature—hot foods hot and cold foods cold—and must be covered while being transported. Since food scraps must be discarded, it is important to know patient likes and dislikes to prevent waste.

All foodservice equipment facilities must be cleaned regularly with an approved solution and properly sanitized. Cleansing ice-making equipment is essential; it is sometimes forgotten that ice melts into the liquid it is cooling. For items that are small enough, the most effective method for cleaning and sanitizing is the dishwasher, which must have its wash and rinse water at specified temperatures. Cleaning should not be done while food is being prepared; in fact, the dishwasher should be placed in an alcove separate from the preparation area. After equipment, utensils, and dishes are thoroughly cleaned and sanitized, they must be handled and sorted properly so as not to make them subject to contamination.

Community dining areas must be cleaned after each meal for purposes of safety and appearance, as well as for sanitation. It is suggested not to set tables too far in advance on the unit for the brain damaged and certainly to have adequate supervision during mealtimes, as residents may pick up utensils on the recently set table or use their neighbor's fork as well as their own to feed themselves.

Trash must be disposed of correctly in plastic liners in insect-proof, nonabsorbent containers with tight-fitting covers. Daily trash disposal and garbage pickup is necessary for both aesthetic and sanitary reasons. Trash containers should be cleaned regularly.

SURVEILLANCE

In addition to specified routine preventive measures that should apply throughout the facility, the nursing home should develop a surveillance program to ensure that routine procedures are adequate and, when infection does occur, to identify what it is and where it is present so as to institute precautionary measures.

Criteria

The usefulness of routine microbiological sampling is at issue. The interpretation of the results is questionable, as there are no standards with which to compare results, for any test would yield numerous pathogenic microbes in the environment even under the best cleaning and disinfecting program. Sampling may be done to demonstrate to staff members the improvement achieved with proper disinfecting and to serve as an impetus for them to follow set procedures. Environmental sampling may be called for in order to identify and locate an infection-causing organism or to ensure that a previously infected area is now free of bacteria.

The infection control committee must develop criteria to define what symptomatology will warrant investigation for an acute infectious process. For instance, only fever over 100°F (38°C) for three days' duration will be considered for the presence of possible infection. Such a baseline is necessary to separate what is normal for the facility from what is not. Once the norm has been established, it will be easier to identify the presence of an acute infectious process.

The committee also must define criteria for determining whether a newly admitted patient's infection is nosocomial. If the patient had a temperature prior to admission but not at admission, the infection may not be considered nosocomial.

Further, the committee should develop guidelines for the external reporting of infectious disease. Communicable diseases whose presence must be made known to the authorities should be so reported by the diagnosing physician. Outbreaks of other illnesses, as documented by similar symptoms or culture returns, should be brought to the attention of the medical director for a decision as to whether it is of such magnitude as to be considered an epidemic and should be reported to the local health authorities.

With the criteria defined by the infection control committee as to what symptomatology may be indicative of an infectious process, the charge nurse can then begin documentation on the individual infection report (Exhibit 5-1). The patient's attending physician must be notified for treatment orders and recommendation of precautions. If the attending physician cannot visit the patient within twenty-four hours, the medical director should be requested to do so.

This form should be updated daily to include culture returns, treatments given, and precautions instituted to prevent the disease's spread until the symptoms have passed. A report is also given to the supervisor who is in contact with all nursing units, so he can determine whether a contagious infection is present throughout the building or just in a single nursing unit. Then, in consultation with the director of nursing and the medical director, he can take appropriate precautions. Completing the infection report does not preclude adequately documenting the nursing notes; it serves as a nursing administrative tool for supervising and evaluating the infection control program.

Precautions also must be developed for preventing the spread of infections. The infection control committee should define specific measures to impede the spread of respiratory, wound and skin, enteric, and genito-urinary infections. Precautions may range from the double-bagging of all disposables to the institution of strict isolation, depending on the seriousness of the infection. In all instances, such procedures must be communicated to the resident, neighboring residents, staff, and visitors. When the patient or patients involved are disoriented, conformance with precautionary measures is made difficult, necessitating very close management of the patients.

Isolation

Instituting the isolation technique, which requires a medical order, may be done for different reasons. An individual with a highly contagious illness may be separated from the rest of the population to prevent the spread of the pathogenic organisms to others. Conversely, "reverse" isolation may be ordered to protect a patient who is inordinately susceptible to illness—due to, say, a weakened condition, recovery from recent surgery, or a poor or nonfunctioning immune system—from disease-causing microorganisms in the environment. Skilled nursing facility patients will more often require isolation because they are contagious rather than because they are overly susceptible to illness.

To effectuate isolation, a single room with ventilation to the outside and a private lavatory and sink is necessary. To avoid displacing more patients than necessary, it is suggested that facilities in the planning stages designate one room that may be used for this purpose, although the patient's own room may be used.

As with the institution of precautions, the charge nurse's first priority should be the immediate communication of the isolation order to staff, other residents, visitors, and the patient involved. A readily available isolation room cart with all needed supplies—gowns, masks, signs, paper bags, thermometers, and so on—can then be brought to the isolation room for use. Staff members and visitors should be educated in the use of gowns and masks.

EXHIBIT 5-1
Individual Infection Report

INDIVIDUAL INFECTION REPORT

DO NOT WRITE IN THIS BOX

Met criteria as infection   Yes_____ No_____
Nosocomial   Yes_____ No_____

Patient's name _____
Type of infection _____
Physician _____   Has patient been off premises recently?   Yes_____ No_____
Date_____ Place_____

Note:
1. All information must be documented on patient's chart in detail.
2. Note date condition began.
3. Note doctor's notification, treatment program, lab tests, and results.
4. Recording nurse, please initial box.

Date							
Diarrhea							
Productive cough							
Jaundice							
Draining skin lesion Location							
Fever over 100							
Foul-smelling urine							
Foul-smelling vaginal discharge							
Purulent eye or ear drainage							

7 days

3 days

It is important to remember that everything in the isolation room, while it is used for that purpose, is considered contaminated and must be treated accordingly. All trash, linen, laundry, biological waste, and equipment must be disposed of in double bags and labeled "contaminated." Reusables must be cleaned thoroughly in the isolation room and then disinfected or sterilized; hence disposable dishes, utensils, disposable absorbent pads, needles, and the like are preferable.

Skilled nursing facilities are not equipped with a separate laundry for contaminated items, so special caution must be taken when isolation room laundry is processed. If a linen rental service is employed, procedures for contaminated linen should be clarified. The patient's clothing should be laundered separately from other linens and towels. The use of dissolving bags for the inner bag is recommended, as then the laundry staff does not handle the items directly. After washing contaminated articles, the machine should run through one complete cycle to be sanitized.

Upon medical discharge from isolation, notification must be given to all appropriate persons. The isolation room must be thoroughly cleaned, disinfected, and aired for twenty-four hours before it is returned to normal use. The housekeeping staff must wear gowns and masks during the cleaning process because the room is still considered contaminated. All equipment, including cleaning apparatus, must be treated as contaminated and must be disinfected before use elsewhere.

SUMMARY

Infection control concerns residents, staff, physicians, volunteers, visitors, purveyors—indeed, everyone in contact with the long-term-care facility.

The primary task is to identify the infection, whether the host is a resident, staff member, volunteer, or visitor. Only then can proper steps be taken to treat and to localize the infection. Sometimes treatment may be via immunization; for example, influenza injections are generally recommended for the ill aged. Alternatively, treatment may consist of drug therapy. Implicit in the facility's infection control program should be the institution of procedures designed to avoid the transmission of pathogenic microorganisms in the skilled nursing facility to the fullest possible extent.

GENERAL REFERENCES

American Health Care Association, *Infection Prevention and Control for Long Term Care Facilities: Handbook (Section I)* (Washington, D.C., 1977).

Social Service

INTRODUCTION

The primary concerns of the social service department are the successful placement of the resident in the skilled nursing facility and the psychosocial adaptation of the patient and his family to the patient's disability and to institutional living. More specifically, social service should be able to identify and minimize the patient's social and emotional problems in the separation and adjustment process by bringing effective services to residents, their families, and the staff. Because of their particular training and expertise, the social workers should be a major force in the development of the therapeutic community where individual residents, their peers, the treating staff, administration, family, and volunteers can function effectively within a protective environment. They also will be expected to develop a postinstitutional or discharge plan for the patient whenever appropriate and feasible, to accept teaching responsibilities by sharing specific social work skills with the entire staff, and to conduct research into the dynamics of family life under the stress of chronic illness and disability as they relate to the role of the ill aged in the family and the community. Finally, members of the social service department should be the catalysts to expand relationships with the health and welfare community.

STAFFING PATTERN

The recommended staffing pattern for the social service department of a 100-bed skilled nursing facility includes an experienced certified social work consultant, a full-time coordinator of social services with a baccalaureate degree, a social work assistant, and a part-time typist or the use of a typing pool. However, if the facility wishes to engage in a program of providing clinical training for social work students, the coordinator of social services must be a professional certified social worker. Although the supervision of students is costly and time-consuming, it is one method of assuring the exposure of social work students to the ill aged and their families and to the problems associated with long-term institutional care.

Social Work Consultant

The social work consultant, who serves perhaps one day per week, is administratively responsible to the administrative director and professionally responsible to the medical director. The consultant assists in the establishment, maintenance, and improvement of social work standards affecting patient care and services to patients. He advises full-time social work staff in the coordination of social work and psychological services in the nursing home. Consultation and direct participation in diagnostic and treatment services to individuals and groups of patients is one of the consultant's major functions, in addition to counseling families, individually or in groups, for problems related to patient care or adjustment to patient institutionalization. To achieve these objectives, the consultant participates in preadmission interviews, when necessary, postadmission interviews with patients and families, teaching rounds for all levels of staff, and outside educational and professional programs.

A candidate for consultant, in addition to being a certified social worker, should have broad clinical and supervisory experience. Special knowledge of family therapy, group therapy, chronic illness, and gerontology is a necessary prerequisite. Previous teaching experience is desirable, as teaching is a significant part of the consultant's role.

Coordinator of Social Services

The full-time coordinator of social services, who should have a bachelor's degree in social work with a background in gerontology and/or field experience in a health care setting, is responsible for the overall functioning of the department and works closely with the medical director. The coordinator of social services conducts preadmission interviews and evaluations, including hospital visits with the director of nursing, and assists the patient and family through the admission process. He interprets patients' rights to both patients and families and consults with the business office regarding the patients' financial status. In conjunction with other clinical staff, the coordinator develops a treatment and discharge plan for the resident and assists in the adaptation of both patient and family to the skilled nursing facility. Assisting patients and families to select, if needed, a medical specialist consultant, to make outside medical or dental appointments, and to obtain transportation to those appointments are all part of the coordinator's regular duties. At the time of discharge, he works with other clinical staff and the family to implement plans. Relationships with outside health and welfare agencies are inte-

gral to his work, and he ought to become involved in various professionally related community activities.

Social Work Assistant

The social work assistant should have some college background, preferably with field experience in a health care setting. Under the supervision
of the coordinator of social services, the full-time social work assistant
performs duties similar to the coordinator's. Rather than carrying out
separate functions—for example, one person handling all inquiries and
admissions, another person responsible for the in-house phase of patient
contact—it is recommended that each full-time department member be
encouraged to follow patients completely from admission to discharge,
thereby affording continuity in care. This is not to say that one social
worker should not be familiar with another's resident case load, but
often an intimate and trusting relationship can evolve between the initial social worker contact and the patient and his family or sponsor.
Furthermore, if both social workers are familiar with all aspects of the facility's social work program, one can relieve the other on sick days and
during vacations.

It is expedient for the coordinator of social services and the assistant
to be able to use a dictating unit to record their patient and family
reports. A typist can then transcribe the dictation, thus saving valuable
social worker time. The typist should realize that the information concerning patients and families is privileged and confidential.

SOCIAL WORK PROGRAMS WITH PATIENTS AND FAMILIES
Inquiries and Admissions

Almost without exception, plans for the placement of individuals in the
nursing home are not characterized by an orderly, planned process.
Usually a crisis of some sort precipitates plans for institutionalization.
The crisis may be physical, emotional, or psychological. An older person
who has been living a marginal existence alone in an apartment may fall
and fracture a hip; after hip surgery, he may require the continuous
nursing care and rehabilitation services of a skilled nursing facility. The
departure of a companion nurse may leave a sick elderly person totally
vulnerable. A confused, brain-damaged older person may be found wandering in the street alone at night, unable to remember where he lives.
Or the family caretaker may become ill and thus be unable to nurse his
older charge.

In the process of planning for admissions, much more is involved
than the availability of a bed. Government agencies sometimes make
futile busy work by trying to develop a mechanism whereby a daily

census is made of empty long-term beds in a particular geographic region. This may be admirable administrative methodology, but it leaves much to be desired with respect to human problems. For example, a bed may be vacant in a unit designed for mentally impaired patients, but the candidate for admission may be mentally clear and physically incapacitated and therefore inappropriate for the vacant bed. Or, even though an appropriate bed may be empty, the nursing load in that unit may be so heavy at the particular time that it would overstress the staff to admit a severely disabled patient who needs maximum nursing care.

Traditionally, initial inquiries came in via the telephone. However, this practice may be changing with the increasing use of standardized interagency referral forms mailed from the referring institution. One social worker may be assigned to respond to all inquiries for, say, a month. Thus, both staff members can remain familiar with the intake process. The intake worker must know the daily census and pertinent information about available beds — that is, whether they are male or female beds and on what units they are found.

Although most in-person initial inquiries are by appointment, about one-quarter can be expected to be unannounced. Under no circumstances should persons making inquiries be allowed to walk unaccompanied through the building "just to see it." This policy is designed for visitors who are unfamiliar with the problems of the ill aged, particularly the intellectually impaired. For these people, it is essential that an education program be provided by knowledgeable personnel at the earliest opportunity. Some arrangement must be made to assist unannounced inquirers on days when both staff members are not on duty. Responsible administrative personnel assigned to weekend or holiday duty should be trained to handle inquiries in a limited fashion. If inquirers arrive when an administrative representative is not available, the supervising nurse should be instructed to explain that no one is present to assist them and to note their names and telephone numbers so a social service staff member can later contact them.

An in-person, on-site interview with the family member or members involved is important and thus should be encouraged. Specific appointments rather than drop-in visits are preferred in order to make effective use of social workers' time and not interfere with other families or residents waiting for services and to afford sufficient time for the meeting and a tour of the building.

It is important to obtain from the family member or sponsor who makes the contact as much information about the prospective resident as possible, including a description of the crisis that has precipitated nursing home placement, the patient's medical history with emphasis on what chronic or acute problems the nursing home can anticipate, the patient's current functional level, and the patient's role within the family structure. The social worker should solicit information about family members and their expectations of the skilled nursing facility, who the family decision maker is, who will handle the patient's affairs and finances (and pay the bills), and how long the patient and/or family will be able to pay for the cost of long-term care. The family probably will not have an accurate understanding of Medicare or Medicaid, so the social worker should explain how the programs work.

Families almost always minimize the disabilities of their relatives—particularly their mental disabilities—and maximize the disabilities of other nursing home residents. It is not clear whether families do this deliberately or whether they are unaware of their unrealistic view of their parent. Often the intake social worker will hear new families commenting on how the other nursing home residents are so much sicker than their parent when in fact their parent is much more disabled than they had expressed. Families will, for example, emphasize their mother's excellent memory but will neglect to say that she remembers only the distant past and cannot name the present year. Thus the social worker must learn to be a keen interviewer, able to elicit the pertinent facts needed to plan for an appropriate placement.

Waiting lists for skilled nursing facilities can be inappropriate. Experience has demonstrated that placements in a skilled nursing facility cannot readily be delayed, in contrast to admission to a home for the aged. When skilled nursing care is required, it is required within a period of days or perhaps two or three weeks. If a potential resident and his sponsor can wait for an extended period, it is likely that the individual does not require placement or that he or his family are not ready to accept long-term-care placement.

After the initial inquiry and family interview at the facility, a visit to the prospective patient in the hospital or at his home, conducted by the social worker in the company of the director of nursing or a designee, is highly desirable. This meeting permits the social worker and nurse to meet with the patient and the hospital staff or caretaker to develop a clear picture of the patient's physical, social, and emotional needs. It can serve as the patient's first introduction to the nursing home staff and should help allay some of the older person's anxieties concerning life at the nursing home.

On the basis of the preadmission visit, the social service staff and medical director will estimate the patient's ability to function by correlating his premorbid personality structure, functional capacity, and ethnic, cultural, and religious identification with his current functional capacity and the impact of his behavior. They should consider the effect his social behavior—his possible noisiness, incontinence, unacceptable eating habits, and so on—will have on other residents.

FIGURE 6-1
Interview with Family

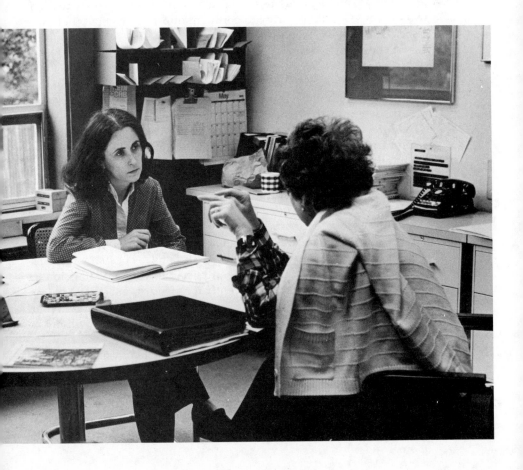

If there is any question about the patient's condition, the coordinator of social services should feel free to ask the family's permission to contact the patient's current physician for further information and then to discuss it with the medical director, particularly if the patient has an atypical medical problem. When a patient has been in a psychiatric or state hospital, the family should always be asked to write a letter to that hospital giving authorization for release of information to the nursing home and to send the nursing home a copy of this release. Prior to or upon admission, the patient and his family or sponsor should be asked to sign a medical information release form in order to collect as much written medical documentation as possible for use on the nursing home chart.

It is essential to advise the nursing staff of a scheduled admission, and it may be helpful to discuss the admission candidate at the weekly interdisciplinary meeting to acquaint key staff with the patient and his problems. Likewise, residents—particularly in the unit the new resident will occupy—should be privy to pertinent information about their new associate in order to be properly prepared.

When a married couple seek to enter the nursing home, they have a right to share a room unless it is medically contraindicated. This may pose some problems regarding placement. It is unlikely that both will be equally ill or disabled. Decisions have to be made whether placement will be determined by the more ill or by the less ill partner. Where should they be placed if one is brain damaged? Will the brain-damaged patient frighten the less disabled residents in the unit? Is it fair to place the intellectually intact person in the psychiatric unit? Thus room sharing may not always be the most desirable setup for either spouse or for the nursing home community.

If the facility has an open medical staff, the patient's own physician may continue to care for him. If the physician will not follow the patient into the nursing home, the nomination of a new attending physician is the responsibility of the patient and/or his family. They should be informed that it is mandatory for the physician to visit on admission, at least once a month, and more frequently if necessary, and that physician fees usually are separate from the nursing home's per diem rate. When the skilled nursing facility has full-time staff physicians, this will not be the case.

The social worker may assist the patient or family in selecting a doctor by making specific suggestions according to his perception of the resident, the family, and physicians available in the area. After providing the names of local physicians, the social worker should request that the family contact its choice before admission to make certain that that particular doctor will serve as the attending physician. Alternatively, the social worker may attempt to contact the physician by telephone with the family in the office if the family cannot reach him.

In the literature, there is a good deal of discussion about the stress of relocation into nursing homes, which is sometimes called transplantation shock. Understandably, the act of changing one's residence and way of life, and of acknowledging that one is ill and therefore dependent, is stressful. However, it is important to remember that this process of dislocation is superimposed on an individual who is physically and, probably, emotionally and socially disturbed. Naturally, if he is ill enough to need the care provided in a skilled nursing facility, he will be subject to additional strokes or exacerbation of medical problems. These incidents cannot be attributed specifically to the process of relocation, but rather to his medical status.

Families can help ameliorate the stress by being truthful with their relative. Social service staff members should be firm in advising families to be explicit about where their relative is going and why. Families sometimes tell their relative that he is going to a hotel for a few weeks. Such deception makes the adaptation more difficult and causes strain between patient and family members. The result may be that the angry, deceived resident will make a scapegoat of the nursing home.

In-residence Phase

When a patient is admitted or readmitted from a hospital, the nursing home should receive a copy of the hospital interagency referral form from the ambulance driver or the relative accompanying the patient. Upon arrival, the patient should be greeted by the social worker and the charge nurse of the unit, and escorted to his room. The family or a staff member should bring in his luggage. While the patient is helped to settle in his room, the social worker should complete the necessary forms with the help of the family and receive funds for the first month of care if the resident is not covered by Medicare or Medicaid.

Shortly after admission, a social service staff member should meet with the new resident to help acquaint him with the facility and the daily routine, to familiarize him with patients' rights, if appropriate, and to answer any questions. During the course of the interview, the social worker should assess the patient's functional and intellectual abilities to develop the initial social service summary.

The social service summary (Exhibit 6-1) should be a descriptive guide of the patient, maintained on the chart. It should note who supplied the information, who the patient is, what his current problems are, and who his family is and their apparent relationship with him. It should include the patient's past and present medical history and psychosocial status, his current functional status, and any other pertinent information.

Specific social problems should be identified and methods of management suggested for implementation by treating staff. Private material that in any way impinges on the confidential relationship the social worker has with the patient and/or his family should not be placed on the chart but maintained in a private file in the social service office. As the condition of the patient or his family changes, new social service summaries should be written and placed on the health record. Such updating should be done quarterly at minimum even though no change is noted.

Within two weeks of admission, the social worker should complete the social service section of the patient care plan. This plan of action identifies the anticipated limitations of the patient, the goals for treatment, and the kinds of social work services needed to achieve those goals. The care plan should emphasize developing the patient's strengths and assets rather than reiterating his losses and deficits. The resident's potential for discharge into the community or other health care setting should be indicated and—if this is an imminent possibility—plans for discharge should be elaborated. The patient care plan should be reviewed monthly at the interdisciplinary meeting, with changes made when indicated.

The social worker should become involved in helping residents to adjust and to resolve social problems such as conflicts with roommates or unsatisfactory dining room seating arrangements. Sometimes the social worker will have to seek out the "good" patient—the quiet one who does not assert himself and makes no demands—for he in fact may need the most help. The social worker can become the patient's advocate by helping him sustain relationships with family members by attending family events and going out with the family regularly. He may need to help the new resident with laundry problems, or with relations with a particular staff member or other residents.

Often the original room plan made for the resident needs modification. For some people, the single room is the only possible alternative. For others, an appropriate roommate is helpful to both: frequently two people living together in a symbiotic relationship function at a higher level than each would alone.

The nursing home has the right to move a patient within the facility in the best interest of the patient and the rest of the nursing home community. When a patient becomes displeased with living accommodations or a room companion, the social worker, charge nurse, director of nursing, medical director if necessary, and other professionals should discuss the basis for such discontent and explore a remedy. When a room change is considered, the family and attending physician should be informed of the contemplated change prior to finalizing a move, since both must be kept informed about the management of the patient and also since a room change often means a change in rate. A change in the patient's financial status may necessitate a room change because Medicare and Medicaid usually do not cover the cost of a private room. As the patient is a focal point of the move, it is essential that he be included in the planning.

Family Relationships

It is important to identify as soon as possible after admission whether the resident and his family agree about the nature of the resident's disability. Sometimes the resident will see himself one way and family members will see him another; or the patient may look very sick to one son but not to the other. It is crucial that there be agreement among patient, family, and nursing home staff about the patient's level of disability and about realistic physical, social, and emotional goals. If family members are not in accord with the nursing home, the placement will be unstable and will be reflected in the patient's behavior.

Family members often will state that all they want is "for mother to be happy." They forget that mother recently lost her spouse of fifty years, that she has lost her home, that she is ill and, of course, that she is depressed. For mother to be happy, it would be necessary to turn back the clock, and even the best qualified professional staff cannot perform miracles. What they can offer is professional and personalized care commensurate with the patient's present needs. The social service staff should encourage residents to bring their own furniture and personal belongings to ease the transition from home to institution.

Often the nursing home staff will witness role reversal: children will act as decision makers for their ill parent. This is particularly difficult and sensitive, especially when the older person was once the "oak" and the stalwart member of the family, accustomed to making his own decisions or even decisions for his children. The patient–family relationship has been conditioned years before nursing home admission and thus the role reversal comes only with great pain. Families really suffer through such experiences, and social workers can help family members accept this responsible role without treating their relative like an infant. It is especially important to have the older person participate as much as possible in planning for his future.

Nursing home social workers cannot help but become involved in a host of family reactions following the institutionalization of their relative. For some families who have not functioned as a family and who have real schisms in their relationships, the placement of their parent is particularly traumatic. Sometimes nursing home placement is the vehicle that once again draws the family together, as its members face a common problem.

EXHIBIT 6-1
Social Service Summary

SAMPLE INITIAL SOCIAL SERVICE SUMMARY

Mrs. Mary Jones
February 15, 1979
Social Service Summary

Mrs. Jones is an eighty-eight-year-old white, Protestant female who will be admitted to the skilled nursing facility on Thursday, February 16, 1979, at 10:00 A.M., by ambulance from the Community Hospital, Morgan City, New York.

Medical History

This eighty-eight-year-old female was reported as well, without any significant medical history, until the age of eighty-five, at which time she is reported to have become forgetful and intermittently confused. In the opinion of her family physician, she became unable to continue to live alone in her own apartment in New York City. She subsequently moved into the home of her daughter, Mrs. Eva Smith, of 37 Deep End Lane, Morgan City, in 1975. The patient reportedly "did well" until six weeks ago, at which time it is reported she fell while getting out of bed and sustained a fracture of the left hip. She was subsequently hospitalized on January 3, 1979, at the Community Hospital and sustained surgery for hip-pinning. Following the surgery, the patient became markedly forgetful, confused, and disoriented, and she required special duty nurses around the clock for management in the hospital. Her physician, Dr. John Barnes, has suggested that the patient may have sustained a cerebral vascular accident following surgery. No paralysis is reported. Hearing and vision are reported intact. No other significant medical information is reported.

EXHIBIT 6-1 (cont.)

Functional

The patient was seen in an interview at the Community Hospital on Tuesday, February 13, 1979, at 10:00 A.M. Present at the interview were the patient; her special duty nurse, Miss O'Gosh; her physician, Dr. John Barnes; her daughter, Mrs. Eva Smith of the Morgan City address; our director of nursing, Mrs. Martin; and this interviewer.

The patient presented as an attractive, white-haired lady who looked somewhat younger than her stated age. She was seated in a chair and was dressed in a hospital gown and bathrobe. Although her social affect remained intact, the patient was unable to state accurately where she was or why she was there. There was complete denial of or forgetfulness about the recent surgical experience. The patient was confused about time and place and was able to identify her daughter only after many errors. She seemed pleasant, good-natured, and cooperative. She appeared to have a memory content of somewhat less than five seconds. Miss O'Gosh reported that the patient can feed herself, is intermittently incontinent of urine and not incontinent of feces, and is quiet and cooperative with nurses in nursing management. The patient must be watched or she will attempt to ambulate independently, which is not recommended at this time.

Dr. Barnes presented the patient as six weeks postsurgical repair of a fractured left hip; possible cerebral vascular accident. Dr. Barnes recommended placement in a skilled nursing facility for patient management. He wishes a program in physical rehabilitation with independent ambulation as a goal, if the confusion and disorientation permit.

EXHIBIT 6-1 (cont.)

Social Service Summary (continued)   -3-

Social History

    The patient is a college graduate, was married at age twenty-two, and lived in New York City with her husband. The couple had one child, Mrs. Eva Smith. The patient's husband was employed by a toothbrush company as a vice-president and died in 1973 following a brief illness. Following his death, the patient remained in the New York apartment alone until 1975, at which time she moved in with her daughter.

    The daughter appears to be genuinely interested in providing a great deal of care and nursing attention for her mother. The daughter also seems extremely anxious about her mother's medical status and especially worried about the possibility of the recent cardiovascular accident. Although the daughter is aware her mother has been forgetful and confused for at least three years, she is very much upset by the recent events and will probably need a great deal of reassurance from her physician (whom she trusts) that "I am doing the right thing." The daughter is having difficulty in permitting herself to understand that the patient is, and has been, ill for some time and is no longer the strong and vigorous maternal figure of previous years.

Plan

    Mrs. Smith has acquired power of attorney for her mother's affairs. The patient will be transferred from the Community Hospital to the nursing home on February 16, 1979. Mrs. Smith has been invited to participate in the next series of family group therapy programs, beginning in one week.

    The patient care plan for Mrs. Jones should include physical therapy for reambulation. The patient should be encouraged to participate in the appropriate activities program. This department will offer support to the patient to ease the adjustment process.

EXHIBIT 6-1 (cont.)

Social Service Summary (continued)   -4-

    There is no discharge plan at this time. It is anticipated that
this will be a long-term placement. However, should the patient's physical
and mental status improve significantly, the discharge plan will be
reevaluated for possible discharge to a lesser level of care. At that
time, the social service department will become involved in effecting the
plan.

                                                  _____

                                                  Ann Weeks, A.C.S.W.
                                                  Coordinator of Social Services

For some families, patient deterioration after nursing home placement will rouse all kinds of guilt, as the family blames the nursing home
for their parent's continuing progressive illness. For other families, continued illness and deterioration are beneficial in that the family feels
justified in having placed their parent in a long-term-care facility. Some
families place their relative in a nursing home only when they have
completely given up. In effect, they see the nursing home as a place to die
and they begin a premature mourning process upon placement. If their
relative improves, the family may respond in anger or confusion. Thus
the professional social worker must be completely apprised of the condition of both patient and family at all times and must be dedicated to help
both accept changes in the patient's physical, psychological, and mental
functioning.

Group Process

Group work with residents may occur in several departments, particularly social service and activities. However, leaders in different services
should be exposed to the value of the group process. For example, in a
discussion about placement, a resident may feel more comfortable speaking with hostility toward his daughter, who did not wish him to move
into her own home, when he hears another resident voice similar feelings. Often residents who would hesitate to share their feelings on a one-
to-one basis will, with proper guidance from the group, learn to express
themselves and thus be helped to sort out their feelings and problems.

Problem-centered groups could include groups of new residents
who meet for a specified period to learn about living in a nursing home
and to discuss and work through problems inherent in group living,
such as mass-prepared meals. Since males are generally in the minority, a
special mens' club could be useful to men who wish to exchange ideas
about sexuality without embarrassment. For long-term residents,
therapeutic group discussions can center around the increasing illness of
a peer and the advisability of his transfer to another unit, or the impend-
ing death of a highly revered colleague. Learning to live with newly
admitted patients who present with overt anger, total withdrawal, or
continuous complaining as well as irritating personality characteristics
can also be a subject for group exploration.

Social action groups can provide a meaningful outlet to residents
and a way for them to continue to participate in the outside community.

Groups can also be therapeutic for families struggling with their
guilt in a social structure that is changing but that still values the principle of honoring parents. New family members should be invited to a
series of family integration sessions that orient them to the nursing

home and give them an opportunity to be helped in the process of accommodating to separation from their relative and to his new status as a resident of an institution. On a continuing basis, groups may be organized for spouses of residents, who have their own special set of problems and often overwhelming guilt. Families can be organized to provide a social support system for their relatives.

Extreme caution must be exercised in such therapeutic group endeavors, however. Only the qualified group leader should be permitted to work in this complicated area. In most instances, groups should be within the purview of the social work consultant or other social worker who has had specific training.

Certainly, other people can lead groups for other purposes. For example, the administrator may meet with groups of families to apprise them of matters related to administration, such as rate changes, but the social workers should attend even those meetings because matters unrelated to the topic of the meeting will inevitably arise and need to be handled. The administration must be sure to respond to the problem, not the manifestation of the problem. For instance, since it is acceptable to complain about institutional meals, families may criticize the food when indeed that is not the problem at all.

Financial Arrangements

The social service staff should be aware of the financial status of all patients and of any anticipated changes in that status. This includes conversion from Medicare to private, private to Medicaid, and Medicare to Medicaid.

As part of the intake process, the social worker should review the Medicare and Medicaid programs, emphasizing that Medicare is an insurance plan with limited coverage while Medicaid is financial support for those who are medically indigent, and clarifying the eligibility requirements for both programs. Families (sponsors) must understand that Medicare coverage in a skilled nursing facility is minimal and that, when benefits cease, the patient immediately reverts to private sponsorship, or to Medicaid if approval had previously been granted. Furthermore, families (sponsors) should be made aware that the processing of a Medicaid application can be very time-consuming; therefore they should not wait until their funds are totally depleted, but should approach Medicaid several months prior to that time.

When a patient who has been receiving Medicare benefits is notified that he is no longer covered by Medicare, the social worker must make sure that the business office, pharmacy, and nursing department are provided with the full name and address of the patient's sponsor.

FIGURE 6-2
Therapeutic Group

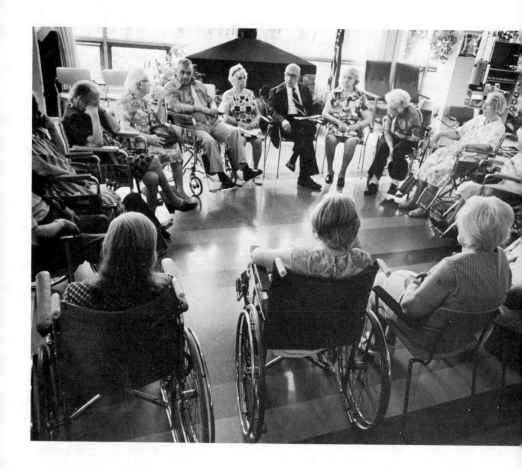

When families (sponsors) of patients on private status inform the staff that patient funds are running low and that Medicaid coverage may be needed, the social worker must be notified so he can determine the status of the patient's current account with the business office and his medical and nursing status. Arrangements should be made for an interview with the family (sponsor) to discuss the conversion to Medicaid, and the administration should be notified. The social worker should assist the family (sponsor) in contacting the Medicaid office, located in the patient's prior county of residence, and in completing the necessary forms regarding the patient's need for skilled nursing care. During the interim period when the patient and family (sponsor) are awaiting the approval of Medicaid benefits, the social worker should remain familiar with the progress of the application for Medicaid and the condition of the patient's account. Only upon receipt of an approved budget by Medicaid, with the effective date of coverage, should the patient be considered covered by Medicaid.

Discharge

Discharge planning is the joint responsibility of social service, the attending physician, and the interdisciplinary staff. Along with the development of and monthly review of the patient care plan, the discharge plan is amended as needed. Final planning requires the approval of the family and/or sponsor and/or attending physician.

If the patient and/or his family inform the institution—or if the institution informs the family—of the need to have the patient discharged, the social service staff should be notified of those plans at least two weeks prior to the date of discharge. A conference should be held with the family to determine the basis for the planned discharge and to provide counseling on procedure and future plans. Assistance may be given to the family in locating the appropriate facility and in arranging transportation. If the discharge is counter to the professional recommendations of the nursing home staff, the responsible family member should be asked to sign a statement to that effect. Any refusal to do so should be noted in writing and witnessed by two staff members.

At discharge, the social worker completes the appropriate section of the interagency referral form and writes a final social service note for the health record. When a Medicaid patient is discharged or expires, the social service staff must notify the appropriate Medicaid office. In the case of a private patient or a patient covered by Medicare, the family (sponsor) must decide whether to reserve the patient's bed during any hospitalization, necessitating the continuation of payment during the absence. The decision for holding the bed for a discharged Medicaid patient lies with the local Medicaid office, which may reserve the bed in conformity to local guidelines.

The social service staff should make certain that the family is informed of an emergency discharge and the reason for it. The disposition of the patient's personal effects and petty cash should be noted on the chart. For example, readmission plans should be documented, along with a statement that the patient's belongings are remaining in his room. Special attention should be offered to residents without family nearby or with uninvolved family, perhaps by requesting a hospital social worker to greet the patient upon arrival and to assist him through the admission process. Irrespective of the availability of family members, the social worker should remain in contact with the resident and should make every effort to visit him during his hospitalization.

In the event of a patient death, the social worker should confirm with the nursing staff that the attending physician has reached the family with news of the death. In the course of the condolence phone call, the social worker should verify that the family has contacted a funeral director and should make arrangements with the family for the removal of the deceased's effects from the premises.

RELATIONSHIP WITH COMMUNITY AND GOVERNMENT AGENCIES

The social service department should assist in developing and maintaining integration of the skilled nursing facility within the health and welfare community by personal and telephone contacts with other social workers and with health and welfare agencies both within and outside the community. This integration can be augmented by visits to the hospital and other health care facilities for preadmission interviews with patients. Attendance and participation at meetings, conferences, seminars, and courses pertaining to social work that are sponsored by private organizers, educational institutions, other health care facilities, professional associations, state and federal agencies, and professionally related community activities should be encouraged. Resource files for patient and family referrals should be updated when needed in order that the social work staff will always be knowledgeable regarding services available elsewhere in the community.

RECORDS

Each patient should have his own file in the social service office containing information that constitutes the basis for ongoing work with the patient and family. These records must be current as to the responsible family member, the patient's financial status, and summaries of interviews held with the patient and family members. As this file may include confidential information, only the social service staff should have access to it.

In addition to individual files, the social service department is responsible for maintaining separate admission and discharge registers with the appropriate demographic material about each patient in chronological order.

Specific information on all inquiries should be noted on a record-of-inquiry card, which elicits demographic material about the patient; information about his current situation, diagnosis, functional capacity, anticipated date of admission, and accommodations requested; and the name, address, and telephone number of the inquirer. These cards should be maintained for three to four months and then filed for future reference. Sometimes months elapse between contacts, and it is useful to be able to refer to the initial contact.

All persons inquiring about possible placement—whether via mail, by telephone, or in person—should be given a copy of the nursing home handbook. In addition to providing a description of the facility's programs, the handbook should offer pertinent information for residents, families, and visitors, including a suggested clothing list.

The admission record card should be a multiple-copy form, which can be distributed to various departments that require the information it contains.

Monthly department reports should be submitted to the administrative director on a standardized form to aid in evaluating the allocation of social service staff time, for instance, how much time is spent in the intake process versus counseling versus staff conferences. Also, a record is then available of the number of intake interviews, revealing whether they were initiated in person or over the phone, by whom they were referred, and how many actually resulted in admission; all this information can be helpful in assessing the nursing home's role and impact in the community.

The initial social service summary should be a very complete medical, functional, and behavioral description of the patient, his family history and current position within the family structure, and discharge plans, if any.

The quarterly social service progress report should assess changes in the patient's status since the last report, highlighting his present situation and listing revised goals for treatment. The patient's discharge plan should also be reviewed for any changes.

The continuing care contract, sometimes known as the admission or basic services contract, is the agreement that the patient's representative and/or sponsor (depending on the patient's financial status) signs upon admission. It should clearly describe the services the skilled nursing facility provides under the per diem rate, any services that incur an additional charge, and the process for charging for both. It may be expedient to describe the Medicare and Medicaid programs, and the facility's and family's roles in securing payment from these third-party payers. Conditions for admission and the procedure for both admission and discharge should be delineated. Most important, the continuing care contract should highlight the responsibilities of the patient and his representative and/or sponsor during his stay and the obligations that the skilled nursing facility has to the patient. It is helpful to include the designation-of-dentist form and the authorization for release of medical information, as these forms require the signature of the patient or his representative and should be completed at admission. Separate signature pages for representatives of Medicaid patients and the representative/ sponsor of a private patient is recommended, thereby defining the representative's financial and ethical responsibility for the patient. The patient's representative may also confirm the receipt of the Recognition of Patient Rights on this form if the patient is unable to do so.

FACILITIES AND EQUIPMENT

The nursing home administration is responsible for providing the proper physical environment for the social service department. Although discussions with residents and families should be private, the social workers' offices should not be too removed from the traffic pattern of residents. They should be situated in an area that is easy for patients to reach on their own, and families should be able to drop in informally. While families and patients should make appointments and be seen regularly, residents and families should feel at ease about seeking help before a crisis erupts.

A comfortably sized office should be available to the social service staff, with the necessary number of desks and telephones per worker, ample file cabinets, typewriter and table, dictating equipment, and bookshelves. Three or four comfortable chairs around a table may be preferable to opposite sides of a desk for conferences, and such a setup may promote a more relaxed environment for such meetings and interviews. A large bulletin board in the office simplifies the posting of facility information that should be known to families and patients, as well as messages and important telephone numbers.

SUMMARY

Social work is the link between the patient, the family, and the community. Nursing home social workers have the unique opportunity to work with their clients prior to institutionalization, during the in-residence phase, and in the discharge process. Such a broad exposure mandates that social workers develop clinical expertise about patients and their families. Only by spending more time studying the physical, social, and emotional needs of their patients and families will they graduate from being pencil pushers to being professional social workers and enhancers of the therapeutic community.

Rehabilitation Services

INTRODUCTION

Patient rehabilitation is a major goal of the skilled nursing program. Staff members should be trained to conduct daily activities with particular emphasis on helping patients to maintain and improve their functioning on all levels—physical, psychological, and social. This is especially true for personnel who have direct contact with patients, such as members of the nursing, social service, and activities departments.

Staff members are the key to a successful rehabilitation program. They need to set goals that are achievable while continuously assessing the changing functional status of residents. They must be encouraged by being aware of positive, but often intangible, results of their efforts, for improvements in the ill aged can be slow and barely perceptible.

Rehabilitation is more than helping patients achieve their maximum levels of functioning via the professional services of physical and occupational therapy, speech pathology, and audiology. It is more than attempting to meet social and psychological needs through programs such as reality orientation (a rehabilitation technique for people with memory loss and confusion related to time and place, in which concrete information is reinforced with regularity, by staff members and by the use of clocks, calendars, and announcements over the public address system) and remotivation (a methodology to stimulate institutionalized persons to think about the real world and to help them relate to each other by discussing such matters).

Indeed, rehabilitation does not occur at specific times with specific therapists. For rehabilitation to be of permanent value, the philosophy of encouraging patients to perform at their highest level must permeate the entire program of the facility. It is not sufficient for the physical therapist to train a person to ambulate on the parallel bars. The nursing staff must follow through by encouraging and almost insisting that the patient walk to meals, to the lavatory, and to activities, even though it may be easier and faster to use a wheelchair. Likewise, it may take less time and be less messy for a nurse to feed a stroke patient than to encourage him to feed himself, but he certainly will not do so unless he is given ample opportunity to relearn such basic functions. The same is true of brushing teeth, dressing, speaking, and so on.

All clinical areas of the skilled nursing facility should be planned with the rehabilitation process in mind. Items such as handrails and grab bars in lavatories and bathing areas encourage disabled patients to help themselves.

It is useful to recall that a patient whose stroke has injured the right side of the brain may present with paralysis to the left side of the body. He may also have residual problems related to spatial perception, such as an inability to judge position, distance, or speed.

A patient who has sustained a stroke to the left side of the brain may be paralyzed on the right side. He may also demonstrate difficulty with speech and language. Most aphasic patients experience difficulty in speaking and comprehending words, although some can understand more than they can speak. Often an aphasic person is regarded as more disabled than he really is. If he cannot speak, it may be incorrectly assumed that he does not understand. Conversely, it may be incorrectly assumed that an aphasic person can comprehend because he shakes his head and smiles when addressed, even though the nodding and smiling bear no relationship to his ability to understand. Staff members generally will be able to perceive language problems. However, they may incorrectly classify a person with speech perception difficulties as uncooperative when in fact they have failed to identify the perceptual problem.

PHYSICAL THERAPY

The physical therapy program in the skilled nursing facility should be oriented toward both prevention and treatment. Whenever possible, patient function should be maintained, developed, and restored with major emphasis on avoiding or correcting deformity and alleviating pain at joints, muscles, or nerve centers. Implicit in the administration of a successful physical therapy program is an understanding of the psychosocial needs of the physically handicapped patient. The patient's positive motivation is a necessary prerequisite if the treatment team is to develop an optimistic attitude toward effecting a successful rehabilitation program for the chronically ill aged.

Physical therapy is essentially the skilled treatment of disabilities, disorders, and injuries, and the prevention or arresting of deterioration through the selective use of physical agents, procedures, and techniques prescribed by a physician. This includes the application of physical

FIGURE 7-1
Joint Exercises

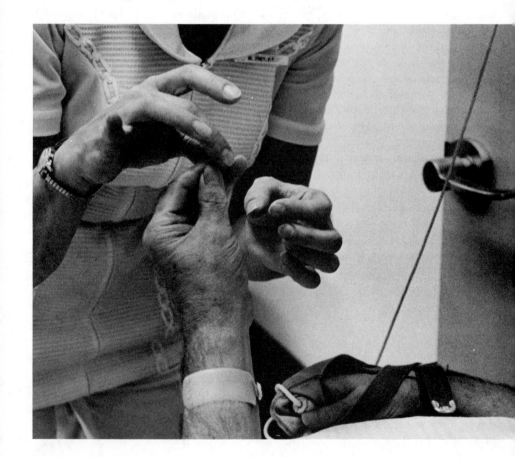

agents such as heat, light, water, and electricity by means of specialized equipment, therapeutic exercise and massage, training in ambulation and stair climbing with appropriate aids as necessary, and training in activities of daily living, transfer, and wheelchair use with appropriate assistive devices as necessary.

Supplemental Nursing Rehabilitation

A coordinated program between physical therapy and nursing should be developed, particularly for the benefit of patients who do not have a medical prescription for physical therapy. In this way, the nursing staff may consult with the physical therapy staff regarding techniques for lifting, ambulating, and transferring and request physical therapists to observe patients' functional abilities. This working relationship can augment a progressive restorative nursing program: both staffs can work together to design and carry out a rehabilitation program with the goal of maintaining patients at their current functional levels.

The supplemental nursing rehabilitation program, as it may be called, can serve as a safeguard against decline in patient performance after discharge from a formal physical therapy program due to the sudden absence of the one-to-one contact during treatment sessions. If the physical therapist observes regression, he may intercede with appropriate action before the patient totally relapses. If the physical therapist observes a recently admitted patient in the supplemental nursing rehabilitation program who might benefit from physical therapy, he could speak to the attending physician to request physical therapy for that patient.

Location of Treatments

The supplemental nursing rehabilitation program is only one example of how physical rehabilitation should be integrated into all aspects of the therapeutic community. Physical rehabilitation should not end once the patient leaves the treatment session with the physical therapist; rather, it must be considered every time the patient moves or is moved.

Therefore conducting physical therapy treatments throughout the building in various community or activity areas rather than in one designated room may be beneficial to staff members and residents. Staff members would then be able to observe the physical therapist's techniques in terms of treatments rendered and the psychosocial aspects of such care, and they could also learn about the patients' capabilities. Such interaction between disciplines can be very helpful and enlightening when assessing patient performance and response to treatments. Furthermore, allowing staff members the opportunity to observe physical therapy techniques helps them incorporate physical therapy into the entire nursing home program instead of leaving it solely to the physical therapy room.

Patients, too, benefit from receiving their physical therapy treatments in community areas throughout the facility, for observing the progress of peers may encourage a patient to do better. Inspiration from nearby staff members can be beneficial, as can the patient's desire to demonstrate improvement to favorite staff or family members.

Staffing Pattern

The physical therapy department of a 100-bed skilled nursing facility should be staffed by two full-time employees: a licensed physical therapist and an assistant or aide. Consideration should be given to having one position held by a male and the other by a female, for experience has shown that some patients respond better to a woman's touch while others feel more secure with a man. In a very large long-term-care institution, the physical therapy department may be directed by a physiatrist, a physician who specializes in physical medicine.

Under the supervision of the medical director, the licensed physical therapist is responsible for the overall physical therapy program in the facility. When ordered by a physician, the physical therapist develops a restorative program of physical therapy based on an initial evaluation of the patient. He supervises the conduct of each treatment session, instructs the assistant or aide in proper technique, when necessary, and maintains documentation on the health record, care plan, and department records.

The physical therapist coordinates the physical therapy program with the other disciplines, especially nursing, and the attending physician. Consultation with the nursing staff on both physical therapy and supplemental nursing rehabilitation provides continuity of care and is augmented by frequent instruction to nursing personnel, who carry out the supplemental nursing rehabilitation procedures. With medical approval, the physical therapist orders appropriate orthopedic aids and appliances for patients.

The physical therapist should be a college graduate of an approved American Medical Association and American Physical Therapy Association school. In addition, he should have had clinical training in a recognized rehabilitation center and should be licensed by the state, if required. The therapist must be familiar with state and federal health codes regulating restorative services in the skilled nursing facility, and he should regularly review and amend facility policies and procedures to conform to them.

The physical therapist should translate the physical therapy program to professional and nonprofessional personnel so that there is continuity in the total rehabilitative effort. In a geriatric setting particularly, motivating patients to perform at their maximal level is the biggest challenge to physical therapy personnel.

The physical therapy assistant or aide must have a genuine interest in working with the ill aged. The physical therapy assistant is a graduate of an associate degree program for physical therapy assistants approved by the American Physical Therapy Association. Although the physical therapy aide does not have a specialized degree, post–high school education may be desired, especially education in body mechanics. A candidate for this position must be able to clearly express himself verbally and in writing.

Under the supervision of the licensed therapist, the assistant or aide conducts physical therapy treatments after the therapist performs the initial evaluation and develops the treatment plan. When requested, the assistant or aide consults with nursing staff to demonstrate and/or conduct supplemental nursing rehabilitation procedures.

Program

Often patients arrive at the skilled nursing facility from a rehabilitation center with documentation indicating that they have reached a plateau in the rehabilitation process. This can be misleading, even untrue. Improvement frequently continues, although at a much slower pace than is generally anticipated with younger patients. Hence a rehabilitation center may discharge a patient who is seen as having achieved his potential, whereas at the skilled nursing facility the patient continues to progress under physical therapy treatments. The progress may not be evident for six months or even a year, but it is all the more rewarding to patient and staff when it does occur.

For patients who do indeed achieve their maximum level of functioning, the physical therapy program in a skilled nursing facility is concerned with encouraging mobility, teaching safety, and observing for change.

Upon the admission of a new patient who appears to be a candidate for physical therapy, it is helpful if the physical therapist is present during the initial physical examination given by the attending physician. This will give him an opportunity to learn first-hand of the patient's general condition and of any precautions to be observed in the physical therapy program. Also, the physical therapist and the doctor can discuss the patient's goals and review together the prescription for physical therapy.

In some instances, if the attending physician has requested consultation by a specialist—for example, an orthopedic consultant for a hip fracture—the physical therapy prescription would be completed by the specialist. Whenever a patient has had a recent fracture, an x ray must be taken before any physical therapy is begun to ensure that the fracture is healing properly, or that the pin is set correctly. If the patient has a fracture of a lower extremity, the physician must specify on the prescription form the degree of weight bearing permitted.

After completing the prescription, the physical therapist evaluates the patient—his strength, range of motion, transfer ability, ambulatory status, long- and short-term objectives—and recommends a treatment plan. This information should be communicated to the attending physician within two weeks of the order date. However, if the evaluation reveals a treatment course that differs from the doctor's order, the physical therapist should verbally discuss his findings and recommendations with the physician and obtain approval for the new prescription and plan.

As with all other physician orders, telephone orders must be countersigned within forty-eight hours, and all orders must be renewed every thirty days. If the attending physician does not appear on the premises to sign orders, the physical therapist should request the medical director to review and sign the prescription forms.

Appropriate information contained in the physical therapist's evaluation—the patient's needs, long- and short-term goals, and the plan of approach—also should be noted on the patient care plan. In addition to a log of treatments for each patient, notes should be written on the chart at least weekly indicating the patient's progress to date and conferences held with staff and the attending physician. As the licensed physical therapist cannot personally care for each patient and part of the treatment load is assigned to the physical therapy assistant or aide, consideration must be given to allowing the assistant or aide to document information on the chart with the licensed physical therapist countersigning. It is reasonable to assume that the physical therapy assistant or aide would know more about individual cases on a daily basis than the therapist, and thus his observations would be more valid. This practice alleviates part of the record-keeping duties of the licensed therapist, who would need input from the assistant or aide anyway in order to write notes on the aide's cases.

Once a month, however, the licensed therapist should reevaluate the patient, noting any significant changes in his condition, his progress in treatment, and revisions in objectives based on the patient's current status. In conjunction with the monthly reevaluation, the patient care plan should be amended as needed.

The preparation for discharging a patient from therapy should be described and especially elaborated on if the patient will be discharged from the facility. At this point, the physical therapist may discuss the patient's transition into the supplemental nursing rehabilitation program with recommendations about what treatment modalities the patient should receive and how frequently. The supplemental nursing rehabilitation program should be clearly defined and should include such treatments as a maintenance exercise program, maximum assistance in ambulation, transfer training, and wheelchair manipulation, with emphasis on the patient receiving individualized attention from the supplemental nursing rehabilitation aide.

The nursing home should stock a reasonable amount of personal use equipment, such as wheelchairs, walkers, and canes. However, when a patient requires an assistive device (prosthesis, brace, splint, wheelchair, cane, walker) for his exclusive and continuous use, the physical therapist should contact the patient's attending physician to request an order for it. Following the physician's prescription, the physical therapist and/or social worker should notify the patient's family and/or sponsor of its need and cost and the option of rental or purchase. The family should be discouraged from purchasing the item directly without professional advice, for special measurements must be taken by the physical therapist or equipment vendor to ensure that the device is adequate and therapeutic for the patient.

Treatment is generally offered on an individual basis, but group ambulation and exercises may be instituted for appropriate cases. The location of treatment often depends on the location of the equipment utilized; it can take place in various areas throughout the facility even if a particular treatment room exists.

Like nurses, the physical therapy staff members must be sensitized to the often subtle changes in patient function that are symptomatic of a changing medical status, and they should report these observations to the charge nurse. This is especially true with brain-damaged patients, whose ability to communicate pain or illness is hampered, or who may not even experience pain when injured. Geriatric patients may need to be more closely supervised when receiving treatments that involve heat and cold, for their sensitivity to either extreme may be diminished.

With the physician's assistance, the physical therapist must learn to differentiate between inability to ambulate and unwillingness to do so. In addition, the physical therapist must be able to identify when a patient is purposely creating false barriers to inhibit his improvement. For instance, a sitting patient who is instructed to get up may place his feet too far forward to balance himself and therefore be unable to rise unaided.

One difficult issue is when and how far to push a patient who is capable of doing more but refuses. The physical therapist must seek the counsel of other professional treatment staff and the physician to determine the appropriate level at which the patient may stabilize.

After a fracture, an elderly person is almost always afraid to begin walking; the therapist must deal with this fear calmly but firmly. It may take several weeks for the patient to develop confidence and trust in the physical therapist, but it may evolve as the patient realizes he is improving and that the physical therapist is trying to help him get better.

Conversely, some patients may be reluctant to end physical therapy because they enjoy the personalized attention or because they fear that their functional ability will decline without the therapy. If a patient is to be discharged from the program, the therapist should gradually reduce the number of his weekly treatments rather than immediately cut them off. During this time, the therapist may instruct the patient or the nursing staff in the exercise or routine ambulation program that the patient should follow to maintain his current functional status. Continued interest in the patient by the physical therapist is beneficial for the patient's morale and for maintaining his present level of functioning.

A physical therapy department in a skilled nursing facility should be prepared to conduct the following modalities of treatment: active and passive exercises, ambulation, massage, and the use of whirlpool baths, infrared lamps, diathermy, hot and cold packs, tilt tables, stall bars, shoulder wheels, parallel bars, door pulleys, sandbags, trapeze frames, and traction apparatuses.

Payment for Services

The nursing home should bill the patient's sponsor for non-Medicare-covered physical therapy. For patients who are receiving Medicare Part A benefits, covered physical therapy is included on the Medicare claim form. The facility should pursue Medicare Part B benefits for eligible patients. Medicare eligibility for physical therapy–covered benefits depends on the patient's potential for rehabilitation and his demonstration of functional improvement during the course of treatment.

Frequently, a family will protest a prescription for physical therapy or request the physician not to order it due to the increased charges. As this clearly is not in the patient's best interest, the nursing home may consider not charging extra for physical therapy. In this manner, all patients who should be receiving physical therapy will receive it regardless of their financial status. Physical therapy is an important part of the treatment program for the chronically ill aged and should not be denied because of cost.

Records

The individual physical therapy prescription (Exhibit 7–1) should list the different modalities available at the skilled nursing facility. On this form, the physical therapist should describe goals for the patient and identify any precautions to be taken.

FIGURE 7-2
Parallel Bars Assist Ambulation

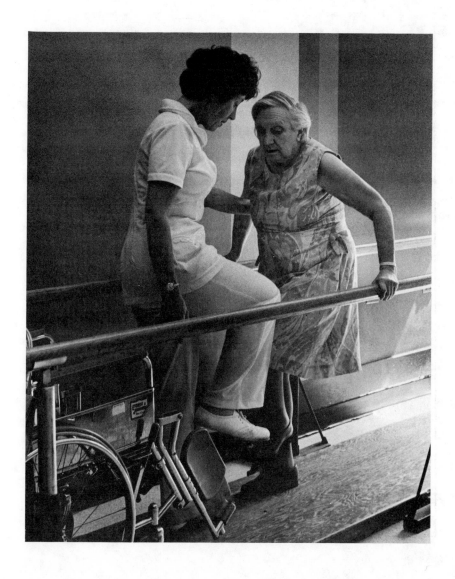

EXHIBIT 7-1
Physical Therapy Prescription

PHYSICAL THERAPY PRESCRIPTION

Patient's name _____ Attending physician _____ Month/Year _____

Check Treatment Requested:

1. Evaluation   ____   8. Diathermy   ____

2. Exercises: 9. Microtherm   ____
    Strength
    Range   ____   10. Ultrasound   ____
    Balance
    Coordination   ____   11. Electrical stimulation   ____
    Active-assistive
    PRE (progressive resistive) ____   12. Cold packs   ____

3. Ambulation   13. Pulleys   ____
    In parallel bars
    With walker   ____   14. Shoulder wheel   ____
    With quad cane
    With regular cane   ____   15. Whirlpool bath   ____

    Independent   ____   16. Tilt table   ____
    With supervision
    With assistance   ____   17. Massage   ____

    Stairs   18. Positioning   ____

    Full-weight-bearing   ____   19. Traction apparatus   ____
    Partial-weight-bearing
    Non-weight-bearing   ____   20. TNS (transcutaneous
                                              nerve stimulation)   ____
4. ADL (activities of daily
    living) training   ____   21. Biofeedback   ____

5. Hot packs   ____   22. Breathing exercises
                                              and postural drainage   ____
6. Infrared lamp   ____
                                         23. Splinting   ____
7. Ultraviolet lamp   ____
                                         24. Other _____   ____

Goals:

Prognosis:

Precautions:

Physician's signature _____ Date _____

The physical therapy record form should provide a check-off area to see at a glance the number of treatments the patient received during a month and also a space for written notes.

The physical therapy monthly report form, which should be submitted to the administrative director, identifies the month's physical therapy census, briefly describes treatments rendered to each patient, lists recommendations, and indicates which personnel were involved, how many patients were admitted and discharged from therapy, and how much physical therapy time was spent in meetings, consultation, and educational programs.

The master log of treatments should document the frequency of treatments for every patient on the physical therapy census. It should be completed daily and kept in the physical therapy office for reference.

Facilities and Equipment

In a 100-bed skilled nursing facility, one area should be designated for physical therapy, where some of the large equipment may be permanently maintained and where smaller items may be stored when not in use. Parallel bars (and possibly a shoulder wheel and stall bars) should be located in a general activity area to encourage patients to practice frequently, with nursing assistance, between physical therapy sessions.

The following equipment should be maintained for physical therapy use in a skilled nursing facility:

> whirlpool bath (either a separate item or a portable unit that
> can be placed in a tub)
> infrared lamp
> diathermy machine
> hot packs and hydrocollator
> tilt table
> stall bars
> shoulder wheel
> parallel bars
> door pulley
> wheelchairs
> walkerettes
> canes
> crutches
> traction apparatus
> trapeze frames

The licensed physical therapist should regularly examine the condition of physical therapy equipment and report needed repairs or replacement.

OCCUPATIONAL THERAPY

Occupational therapy is involved with the medically prescribed treatment of patients through the use of selected activities in order to improve physical and mental functioning in the activities of daily living.

The goals of the occupational therapy program in the nursing care facility should be closely related to those of the physical therapy and total rehabilitation programs, with emphasis on encouraging patients to help themselves: to perform the functions of daily living as independently as possible with specific focus on feeding, dressing, and bathing. Occupational therapy should be preventive and remedial and should promote and sustain the patients' social and psychological well-being by discouraging social withdrawal and by assisting the patients in becoming adjusted to the environment, to the staff, and to patient peers.

Staffing Pattern

A licensed occupational therapist should be retained in a 100-bed skilled nursing facility for at least three days per week, six hours per day. The occupational therapist is professionally responsible to the medical director for the patients under his care and for the occupational therapy services provided in the facility.

Upon physician's orders, the therapist evaluates the patient and develops an occupational therapy treatment plan. He performs specific treatments and directs nursing and activities personnel in carrying out supplementary treatments. He interprets occupational therapy's role in the treatment of patients who are physically and psychosocially disabled and integrates occupational therapy into the entire therapeutic program of the skilled nursing facility.

The therapist's administrative responsibilities include maintaining the proper individual patient care records and departmental records. He must be familiar with government regulations in order to review and modify facility policy and procedures pertaining to occupational therapy. Attendance at outside professional conferences, meetings, and classes is expected, as is involvement in community health organizations.

Considerable initiative and judgment is required of the occupational therapist in adapting programs to meet the needs of individual patients. One of the therapist's major assignments is to secure the cooperation of patients, many of whom are psychosocially disturbed, to participate in programs he designs or to use an adaptive device.

The occupational therapist should have a degree in occupational therapy from a four-year program and should be licensed by the state. A geriatric and psychiatric background is preferred, particularly one with exposure to the multidisciplinary approach to rehabilitation.

Program

Occupational therapists serving as consultants to the activities department offer the value of developing therapeutically oriented activities based on training in and knowledge of the physical disabilities and psychosocial needs of geriatric patients. Activities are an important part of the therapeutic program and are designed to improve the general welfare of the residents. Considering that most of a resident's day is spent in leisure time, the nature of an activities program can be critical to the value of the overall nursing home program.

It is unfortunate when occupational therapists refrain from this role and primarily emphasize the functional aspect of occupational therapy. Enrichment of the activity program by ensuring a rehabilitative approach should be an important objective of an occupational therapist in a skilled nursing facility.

Functional therapy entails a treatment program to increase the patient's ability to participate satisfactorily in various daily tasks. A functional treatment program that includes activities of daily living and/or kinetic therapy as well as psychosocial input should be considered for any patient whose evaluation indicates a potentially higher level of functional ability. Treatment may be conducted individually or in groups, as in an activity program.

A program of activities of daily living (ADL) should be designed to help patients achieve a maximum degree of independence in such routine functions as dressing, feeding, bathing, grooming, and transfer. After evaluating a patient's performance of such activities, the occupational therapist plans a self-help retraining program. The occupational therapist should instruct both the patient and the nursing staff in the techniques to be used so the program can be carried out daily, with the occupational therapist observing and revising the plan when necessary. Self-help devices for dressing, eating, and bathing may be used to increase the patient's independence in these areas.

The ongoing reality orientation program is one part of the activities of daily living program that the occupational therapist could be assigned to implement, although some believe it is properly the responsibility of the activities coordinator or other qualified staff member. Experts in rehabilitation have long recognized that psychosocial and emotional rehabilitation must be achieved concurrently with physical rehabilitation in order to sustain long-lasting improvement in the disabled patient. The confusion and disorientation frequently seen in the geriatric patient may be of physiological or emotional origin; in either case, it can be alleviated by an intense effort focusing on the basic realities of the world around the patient. By increasing the patient's awareness of his

FIGURE 7-3
Therapeutically Oriented Activity

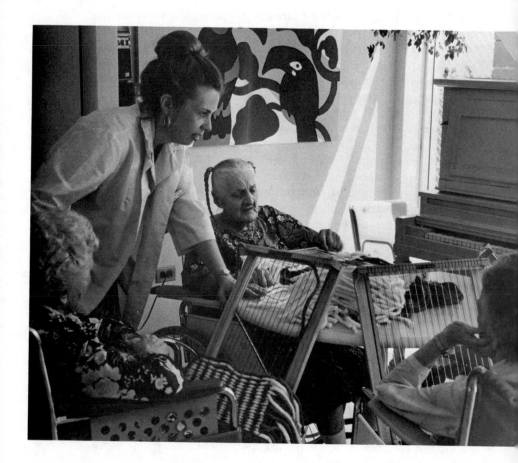

surroundings and of himself and by reaffirming the meaning of those surroundings, the therapist helps the patient become more actively involved with events, people, and objects affecting him.

The key to a successful reality orientation program is consistency; therefore the occupational therapist must train all personnel who come into contact with patients, even those in the ancillary services. Families, too, must be familiarized with the program's purpose and techniques. Emphasis must be on the repeated and regular affirmation of person, place, and time. Staff members should be encouraged to communicate with the patient whenever they are in the patient's presence, always emphasizing the objective facts of the situation—time of day, year, season, the patient's name, their own names—and should never participate in the patient's confusion.

In addition to ongoing reality orientation during the course of the day, classroom experiences for residents should augment the program. Specially trained staff members—perhaps the occupational therapist or other professional personnel—should be assigned this duty on a routine basis. Again, consistency is the key—same people, same time, same place—and the group should be limited in size, generally from six to ten participants. The actual number of participants will depend on the level of confusion and degree of input required for each group member. These organized situations can be centered around sensory identification, remembering basic life experiences (occupation, hometown), and reaffirming time, place, and person by answering questions, reading, and writing. The patient should always be rewarded for a correct response. The attention span of this patient population is limited, so the correct response must be given in a minimal amount of time to constitute a learning experience. Patients who are progressing with the basic program should be advanced to more sophisticated concepts.

A successful reality orientation program will do more than decrease patient disorientation and withdrawal. It will boost staff morale as they see patients improving as a result of their combined efforts and assisting more in their own daily activities. Initially, reality orientation requires a substantial time commitment in terms of training, but in the long run, the time involved is little because the staff will need to spend less time attending patients in their daily activities.

Kinetic therapy is aimed at restoring maximum joint and muscle function to the upper extremities to prevent deformity and disuse and to increase work tolerance. The occupational therapist specifies activities to produce the desired result as part of the treatment plan. The activities department can carry out these activities after training and under the supervision of the occupational therapist.

The occupational therapist may be requested, on doctor's orders, to design and apply a splint for preventing or correcting a deformity of an upper extremity.

Both restorative and maintenance occupational therapy are components of a skilled nursing facility program. The patient must first be elevated to his highest functioning level by a restorative program and then be assisted to continue at that level through a maintenance plan of care.

To implement an order for treatment and to develop a care plan consistent with the physician's prescription and established goals, the occupational therapist should receive a thorough briefing on the patient's medical, social, and psychological history from the director of nursing and the coordinator of social services before doing an evaluation. The results of the evaluation and the occupational therapist's treatment plan should be communicated to the attending physician within two weeks. In addition, the occupational therapist should complete the appropriate section of the patient care plan, noting the patient's problems and needs, the long- and short-term objectives of treatment within specific time frames, and the plan of care designed to achieve those objectives. It should be clarified, when appropriate, whether the treatments are to be conducted by the occupational therapist or carried out by nursing or activity staff after thorough training by the occupational therapist.

Every thirty days, the physician must reorder occupational therapy and should review the patient's course of treatment via the occupational therapy material on the health record. Proper documentation of the patient's progress, including a monthly reevaluation of the patient's status in relation to original goals, is the therapist's responsibility. At the same time, the patient care plan should be updated. When discharge from treatment is anticipated, the therapist must define the steps to be taken to prepare the patient for discharge and must ensure that nursing home personnel are familiar with the patient's present functional level and routine.

In addition to treating patients directly, the occupational therapist spends valuable and needed time observing all nursing units frequently and making recommendations to staff and patients. On-the-spot in-service for all involved personnel is the most effective method of training and incorporating the concepts and skills of occupational therapy into the nursing home program.

Payment for Services

As with physical therapy, the family or sponsor may protest an extra charge for occupational therapy and thus the patient will be denied the therapy. Including occupational therapy as one of the services covered in the daily or monthly rate of the nursing home ensures that all patients will receive treatment without concern for the ability to pay.

Records

The completed occupational therapy prescription form (Exhibit 7–2) should include precautionary information, the patient's rehabilitation potential and prognosis, and the physician's objective for occupational therapy. The order must be renewed in writing every thirty days. A well-designed form can be particularly helpful to the attending physician who has limited exposure to the specifics of occupational therapy.

The occupational therapy evaluation is noted on a form that allows the attending physician to signify his approval or to make comments or changes in the stated plan of care. Because the physician may not visit before the thirty-day limit, the occupational therapist should send the report to the physician for review within the two-week period and also maintain a copy of the report on the patient's chart.

Occupational therapy must have its own progress note form, which always should be kept on the patient's health record.

Patient participation and progress in the reality orientation program should be documented. This may be done on the nursing progress note form, particularly if a nurse is conducting the classroom experiences. Or a separate reality orientation form may be developed for use by the occupational therapist or team leader.

Facilities and Equipment

Self-help devices for the activities of daily living should be available in the facility for testing and training. If a patient requires a device for personal use, however, the family or sponsor should purchase it. Assistive devices for dressing include elastic shoelaces, long-handled shoe-horns, and buttonhooks; eating aids include flatware for the handicapped (swivel spoons, built-up-handle utensils, long-handled spoons and forks), compartmentalized dishes, utensil holders, plate guards, and glass holders; personal hygiene is promoted by elongated toothbrushes or handles modified by placing an elastic band around the toothbrush to slip on the hand of patients with arthritis and limited arm movement, flexible shower arm attachments, hand brushes with rubber suction cups, and soap mitts. Other useful devices are book butlers, scissor-type pickup sticks, wheelchair trays, wheelchair brake extensions, and card holders.

Because occupational therapy is concerned with the patient's ability to function in all aspects of usual daily tasks, treatments can take place throughout the facility—in community and activity areas, dining areas,

EXHIBIT 7–2
Occupational Therapy Prescription

OCCUPATIONAL THERAPY PRESCRIPTION

Patient's name _____ Room _____ Age _____ Sex _____

Diagnosis _____

_____

_____ Date of onset _____

Precautionary information _____

_____

_____

Rehabilitation potential and prognosis _____

_____

_____

Objective of occupational therapy:

_____ Evaluation

_____ Activities of daily living

_____ Upper extremity functional activity

_____ Splinting

_____ Blind technique training

_____ Upper extremity prosthetic training

_____ Reality orientation

Attending physician _____ Phone no. _____

Date _____

FIGURE 7-4
Adaptive Card Holder

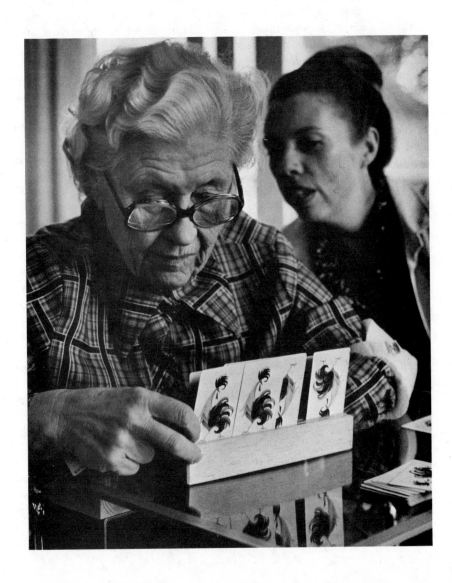

patient bedrooms, and lavatories. An equipped kitchen should be available to retrain those who will be returning home. In facilities where vocational rehabilitation is a major thrust of the occupational therapy department and special mechanical equipment is necessary, occupational therapy should be designated a room or area to carry out treatment.

SPEECH PATHOLOGY AND AUDIOLOGY

The goals of speech pathology and audiology are closely related to the total program of patient rehabilitation. Since communication relates to all activities, emphasis should be placed on improving speech intelligibility. Formal speech pathology treatments must be integrated into the comprehensive care plan to help the patient function as a social being to the best of his ability.

Speech pathology is principally the diagnosis and treatment of speech, language, voice, and hearing disorders in order to improve the communication abilities of the communicatively handicapped. Audiology is the evaluation of a patient's hearing thresholds for pure tones and speech. Audiology also is concerned with the conservation of hearing and rehabilitation for auditorily impaired patients in the form of hearing training and lipreading.

In a setting of chronically ill aged patients, two types of language disorders resulting from organic brain damage present major challenges. Dysarthria is a disorder of articulation due to the impairment of the part of the central nervous system that directly controls the muscles of articulation. Since such patients cannot form words with a reasonable degree of clarity, the goal of therapy is to improve intelligibility. Dysphasia is partial or complete loss of the ability to speak and/or understand spoken and/or written language due to lesion(s) in certain areas of the brain. Improving written and spoken language comprehension and expression is the objective with the dysphasic patient.

To be able to communicate effectively, it has been suggested that a nursing home resident needs to know about sixty words, including nouns for relatives, kinds of clothing, names of foods, cutlery, transportation, communication items (such as *book, car, newspaper, telephone, radio, television*), and certain adjectives (like *hot, cold, hungry,* and *thirsty*).[1] The nursing home staff should be instructed to keep the patients' conversations simple and direct but not childlike.

Victims of recent strokes may revert to their native language temporarily; in some cases this condition may persist. Speech pathologists assert that less-educated patients are more likely to show greater improvement than the more highly educated as a result of the treatment process. Those with less education who performed manual work before their illness had less need for highly descriptive vocabularies. Professionals, such as teachers and physicians, did need extensive vocabularies in their daily lives, so they become more disheartened with limited means of communication. Thus the better educated may be less motivated in language retraining and thus make slower progress than the less well educated.

Staffing Pattern

One consultant in audiology and speech pathology should be available when needed to treat individuals or groups of patients and to participate in the nursing home educational program. It is preferable to have one person perform both speech pathology and audiology functions due to the part-time nature of the service. Two persons would have even less opportunity to become integrated into the total program of care. Under the supervision of the medical director and upon physician's orders, the speech pathologist/audiologist evaluates a patient's speech or hearing deficit and prepares a remedial program. He keeps the staff informed of patients' progress in order to maintain a continuity of total rehabilitation efforts and advises them on methods to assist patients to express themselves and to understand more effectively.

In conjunction with treatment sessions, the speech pathologist/audiologist maintains documentation on the health record. He guides the facility in current government regulations and professional standards in this area of rehabilitation and submits monthly reports to the administrative director.

The speech pathologist/audiologist must be a college graduate who is currently licensed and registered by the state. As for all therapists dealing with the disabled, a unique ability is required to encourage patients to improve especially when, by societal standards, they believe their improvement may be in vain. The speech pathologist/audiologist must have an understanding of and training in the multidisciplinary approach to a comprehensive rehabilitation program.

Program

In a 100-bed skilled nursing facility, it can be anticipated that less than 10 percent of the patients will present stroke-related communication problems; perhaps several other communications problems will have different causes. Many more residents are hard of hearing. While residents who are hard of hearing should be identified by attending physicians at the initial physical examinations, the audiologist may have to review them after admission.

Hearing is an important aspect of the entire rehabilitation program. Loss of hearing in the elderly results from deterioration of the eighth cranial nerve, which causes an increasingly limited perception of high-frequency sounds.[2] Hearing loss develops slowly, offering the older person the opportunity to make a gradual adjustment to his handicap. If such persons have normal vision, it is helpful for them to learn to lip-read. If their vision is impaired, a hearing aid is essential. Often they need to learn lipreading as well as use a hearing aid. Nursing home patients should be fitted with the simplest hearing aids with the fewest controls; intellectually impaired residents may not be able to use such devices at all.

Instruction in lipreading should be held several times a week with a volunteer instructor trained by the audiologist. Pictures in magazines, which are ideal for this purpose, can be used as the basis of classes.

As with other rehabilitation services, therapeutic sessions in speech pathology and audiology may be more effective for some residents on an individual basis; others will find greater stimulation through group activities. Certainly the speech pathologist/audiologist makes better use of his time in group treatments, but he should consider the patients' abilities to perform in front of their peers as well as the privacy that individual sessions offer.

Because the speech pathologist/audiologist is not on staff at the nursing home, the professional treating staff must be attuned to recognize patients who have potential for speech or audiological therapy. This necessitates an understanding of the objectives and rehabilitation prognosis for patients who undergo treatment, which is the consultant's responsibility to impart to the staff. The consultant should hold sessions to describe the physiology of speech/hearing disorders and the methodology used in treating such disorders at least two times a year to varying levels of treating personnel. It is particularly useful if these sessions can be focused around patients who are currently undergoing therapy.

The interdisciplinary committee meetings provide an excellent setting for the consideration of patients for care by the speech pathologist/audiologist. The medical director should participate in this decision-making process. Of course, the order must originate from the attending physician.

Particularly in the case of private paying patients, it will be necessary to inform the family or sponsor of the order for treatment and/or hearing aids. The speech pathologist/audiologist might agree to conduct an initial evaluation with treatment and equipment recommendations and prognosis at a modest fee in order to present the family with a recommendation for treatment based on facts rather than conjecture. Once again, it is mandatory for the family's expectations and recommendations to be a part of the overall treatment process. If progress is not what they were led to believe it would be, the family may discourage the continuation of treatment or the use of assistive equipment.

As in physical and occupational therapy, the sooner that the patient with communication problems begins a therapeutic program, the better the potential for recovery. It is incumbent on the director of nursing to inform the speech pathologist/audiologist of a physician's prescription for treatment. With the assistance of the coordinator of social services, the director of nursing should then meet with the therapist to review the patient's medical, psychosocial, and emotional problems and needs, along with the comprehensive plan of care for the patient.

Prior to the onset of therapy, the speech pathologist/audiologist should undertake a complete evaluation of the patient's reading, writing, hearing, and vision. He should note the patient's problems, the plan of care, and objectives of treatment on the patient care plan Kardex as well as on the evaluation form maintained on the health record. Ongoing progress notes, including a monthly reevaluation, are part of the patient's record. When discharge from therapy is planned, the therapist should note steps being taken to prepare the patient, the progress noted, and the prognosis. Pertinent and succinct information should be exchanged between the therapist and other nursing home staff, keeping in mind that the therapist is a consultant and that he cannot observe the patient during the course of the day.

One of the problems encountered with individual practitioners whose main relationship to the nursing home is to provide a service when ordered by a physician is to maintain their interest during periods when their treatment census is low or nonexistent. Involvement in the in-service education program is one method to enhance their interest. A second opportunity is to invite their participation at weekly rounds, which offer professional interaction and stimuli not available to the lone practitioner who operates primarily in an office setting. The speech pathologist/audiologist should be invited to attend interdisciplinary committee meetings when patients under his care or prospective treatment candidates will be discussed.

Payment for Services

The services of the speech pathologist/audiologist should be on a fee-for-service basis, with the therapist directly billing the patient's sponsor. Sponsors of patients eligible for Medicare Part B benefits would then seek reimbursement from Medicare.

For patients whose stay at the nursing home is currently being covered by Medicare Part A benefits, speech pathology and audiology is added to the billing form transmitted to the fiscal intermediary. Therefore the speech pathologist/audiologist must verify the Medicare status of all patients under treatment for the purposes of billing. After the nursing home is reimbursed by Medicare for the services, the speech pathologist/audiologist is paid by the nursing home.

In addition to payment for direct treatment, the nursing home should develop an arrangement for reimbursing the speech pathologist/audiologist for his time in conducting in-service programs.

Records

A simple lined form for notation of evaluation findings, recommendations for treatment, and patient progress is adequate for the speech pathology/audiology chart record form. Alternatively, the individual practitioner may want to use forms developed to record results from specialized testing equipment.

Facilities and Equipment

Ideally, an audiometer to test hearing should be available for use in a soundproof room. If the nursing home does not provide it, however, the patient may need to travel to the audiologist's office for testing.

A quiet office or room that will accommodate half a dozen people is needed for both individual and group therapy sessions.

A tape recorder and sets of cards and tapes should be available. A small electric typewriter, which can be used as a communication tool, should be provided for use by some residents. Sets of illustrated word cards and toys used to simulate objects such as clocks and cars are also necessary tools for the speech pathologist/audiologist.

SUMMARY

Rehabilitation therapists in a nursing home must possess the technical skills of their professions, but even more important, they must have the personal qualities needed to work with the chronic ill aged. These include the ability to motivate a depressed patient, and the perseverance to continue a program despite little immediate success. Each therapy program must be designed with realistic goals for the patient that agree with the goals of the family and the nursing home. Therapists in a 100-bed facility need to be self-starters, since they are not continuously supervised as they would be in a larger organization. Finally, therapists must have a true understanding of the workings of the interdisciplinary team for their treatment plans are carried through and/or are supplemented by other staff members on a daily basis.

NOTES

1. Ralph W. Jones, "Communication Problems of the Client in a Nursing Home or Rehabilitation Center," in S. Schneiweiss and S. Davis, eds., *Nursing Home Administration* (Baltimore: University Park Press, 1974), p. 134.
2. Langdon Hooper, M.D., and Paul McWilliams, eds., "Speech Therapy," *Care of the Nursing-Home Patient* (Boston: Little, Brown and Company, 1967), pp. 169-170.

Activities and Volunteers

INTRODUCTION

Activities represent a key segment of the total rehabilitation program in a skilled nursing facility by encouraging patients to function socially in pursuit of a meaningful way of life. A planned and diversified schedule of recreational and social activities should be designed to help patients use their physical and mental capacities to the fullest. Successful diversional therapy should engender self-confidence and should prevent the withdrawn attitude often typical of the aged ill by promoting participation in group activities commensurate with the individual patient's ability to perform.

Developing an effective activities program is not a science but a skill. The identification of patient needs and the selection of specific therapeutic systems are essentially empirical exercises, not supported by objective, quantifiable criteria. The fact that the program works is more important than the rationale for its working. What works is dictated by the physical, social, and emotional well-being of the patient in response to the therapeutic modality offered.

STAFFING PATTERN

For the hypothetical 100-bed facility, a minimum of two full-time activity personnel is suggested, with the assumption that there will be a backup of five or six volunteers—three or four mature volunteers in the mornings and two or three junior volunteers in the afternoons.

Activities Coordinator

The coordinator of activities and volunteers reports directly to the administrative director. His responsibility is to plan, develop, and implement an activities program that assists in maintaining each resident's highest functioning level. The activities program must be incorporated into the general nursing home program, with the staff understanding the role of activities and its relationship to the other patient care services.

In consultation with the treatment team, the activities coordinator develops a plan of care for each resident's participation in the activities program, unless it is medically contraindicated. In addition to the planning function, the activities coordinator is responsible for keeping up with new trends, for attending occasional professional meetings, for maintaining liaisons in the community designed to recruit groups and individuals to augment the activities program, and for establishing relationships with the various clergy who conduct religious services.

In a skilled nursing facility where volunteers primarily are involved with the activities program, the coordinator of activities and volunteers is assigned the additional task of recruiting, orienting, supervising, and evaluating volunteers in the nursing home, and for using the volunteers in the most effective manner for the patients and the nursing home program. Regular contact with volunteers—individuals or groups—and recognition of services rendered is necessary to reinforce their relationship with the nursing home.

The coordinator of activities and volunteers should comply with any state qualifications for the position. A very important requirement is broad exposure to the abilities and disabilities of the ill aged. A special aptitude for drawing residents out, for working with them on an individual and group basis, is more crucial than the ability to engage in specific craft and recreational pursuits. The coordinator can always recruit volunteers with specific technical skills, but he must have the human skills. Formal educational training in therapeutic recreation or group social work, with additional courses in the techniques of activities planning for the ill aged, would be desirable.

The activities coordinator must establish good interpersonal relationships with residents, families, volunteers, community representatives, and especially with other staff members. For example, he should communicate with the nursing aides and conscientiously try to follow their suggestions regarding patient participation and scheduling to avoid complaints about a lack of cooperation between the nursing and activities staffs. Also, the frequent tension between activities and dietary personnel can be alleviated if the activities coordinator gives advance notice of special needs to the dietary department rather than waiting until the last minute. If he seeks suggestions from the staff rather than gives orders, he will engender a spirit of cooperation.

Activities Assistant

The activities assistant is under the supervision of the coordinator of activities and volunteers and in the latter's absence serves as acting activities coordinator. The assistant performs duties as assigned by the activities coordinator; these might include developing individual resident care plans, documenting records, ordering supplies, supervising volunteers, and planning, coordinating, and implementing activities programs.

The activities assistant should have a high school education, preferably augmented by additional courses in activities programming for the handicapped. A desire to work with the institutionalized ill elderly should override all other qualifications, but it must be complemented by an understanding of and training in their physical, psychosocial, and emotional problems. It is helpful if the activities assistant also meets state requirements as an activities coordinator, to facilitate the operation of the department in the coordinator's absence.

Activities Consultant

If there is a consultant to the activities program, he should be considered the agent of change or the facilitator. The consultant should act as interventionist to evaluate the program, to change the focus of the program, to identify problems in the program, and to help resolve the problems. He should provide continuing education for all staff regarding the importance of activities, and he should lend a rehabilitative approach to the activities program. A consultant may be either an occupational therapist or a therapeutic recreation specialist, and may be mandated to provide consultation in order to meet state requirements if the activities coordinator's qualifications do not comply with federal and state standards.

Activities Volunteer

During the summer months, when activities staff members schedule vacations and when the regular corps of volunteers is diminished due to vacation plans, one full-time volunteer should be recruited for an eight-week period. Or it may be necessary to employ a student, preferably in recreation or occupational therapy, to assist in carrying out a full array of programs. In this manner, the skilled nursing facility is participating in educating future health care paraprofessionals to the special needs of the chronically ill aged.

PROGRAM

If only three hours per day per patient are utilized for nursing care and rehabilitative services, it is obvious that meaningful activities are needed for a considerable part of each patient's day. To plan intelligent programs suitable for long-term-care residents, the activities staff must have a clear picture of the nature of the patient population in the particular facility. Six different groupings of residents have to be considered:

1. the substantially physically and intellectually intact
2. the physically disabled and intellectually intact
3. the ambulatory resident with advanced organic brain syndrome

4. the severely physically handicapped with organic brain
syndrome
5. the intellectually intact, ambulatory terminal patient
6. the terminal patient who is intellectually intact but
severely debilitated

Terminal patients who are physically debilitated and not intellectually
intact are not candidates for participation in activities programs.

Of particular concern to activities personnel is the diminution in
perceptual and sensory perceptions of older people. Declines in their
visual acuity, particularly their ability to discriminate among details,
should be compensated for by the use of large, clear visual aids. In
addition, activities personnel should ascertain whether residents can
really see projected images such as films or slides.

In addition to visual losses, losses related to auditory acuity and
sensitivity often occur with nursing home residents. Thus it is helpful
for activities personnel to discipline themselves to speak slowly and with
sufficient loudness and to position themselves so that residents can look
directly at them to observe their lip movements and facial expressions.[1]
Staff members must be careful not to underestimate the residents' intel-
ligence and abilities due to their hearing and vision losses.

Such factors as motivation, life experience, educational and cultural
background, and ability to communicate are superimposed on sensory
and perceptual changes and affect the older person's desire or ability to
participate in the activity program.[2]

The activities staff should also be alerted to the profound effects of
immobilization on nursing home patients. Depression, social withdrawal, apathy, and even stupor are among the more severe behavioral
characteristics resulting from immobilization; the physical effects include contractures, decubitus ulcers, incontinence, and weight loss resulting in malnutrition.[3] The physical and behavioral symptomatology
should underscore for all activities personnel the urgency that nursing
home patients continue to be physically mobile and participate in various activities.

After analyzing the composition of the resident population, activities personnel are faced with the dilemma of making certain value judg-
ments. They must decide which grouping of residents merit the most
attention. The natural tendency of activities personnel is to pay the most
attention to residents who are most responsive, who can speak for themselves, who participate in residents' councils, and who in general are the
most able to relate to their peers, to the staff, and to volunteers. While
such residents may be the most appealing, they do not necessarily represent the most deprived segment of the typical nursing home population.

The intellectually intact resident, mobile or wheelchair-bound, as a

FIGURE 8-1
Participation in Physical Exercise

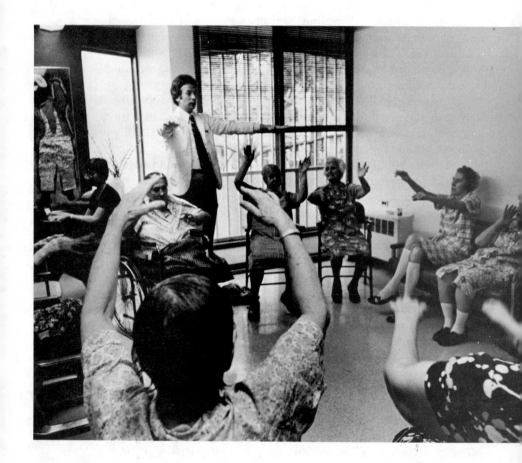

general rule leaves the nursing home premises more frequently for a greater number of events with friends, volunteers, and family members than does the intellectually impaired patient, who leaves the premises rarely, and then only with family members. Similarly, visiting patterns to residents demonstrate that behaviorally handicapped patients receive briefer and more infrequent visits than do the intact residents. Thus the main thrust of the activities program should be directed toward the most disadvantaged group: the intellectually impaired residents who have fewer resources within themselves and within and outside the nursing home community.

The quality of life in long-term-care institutions is largely reflective of the activities program, the role that activities can play in helping overcome the ill effects of institutionalization and/or immobilization. For example, when the patient does not follow medical orders for movement, the activities program may prove to be a more positive influence than medical or rehabilitative services. It is necessary to find the appropriate type of activity to challenge and stimulate each patient.

Activities can be helpful only to a patient who participates. If a patient will not participate, obviously he cannot be helped. Activities personnel need to decide whether to coerce or force residents to participate in activities when it is quite certain that such pursuits will prove therapeutic. The interdisciplinary team must resolve the dilemma of whether staff members have an obligation to insist on participation or whether the patient has the right not to participate even though such participation would be helpful to him.

The activities program needs to emphasize the participant's strengths while not neglecting his social, physical, and emotional needs. The staff should be supportive, even demanding of a resident's performance. Staff satisfaction with poor performance will guarantee continued poor performance. Making demands on patients may, in fact, encourage achievement.

The participation of residents in the planning process is an essential component of program development and the therapeutic community. Indeed, experimentation in activities is useful and should be carried out with the guidance of the activities program committee. The coordinator of activities and volunteers should meet with the committee members monthly to review the upcoming month's schedule and to discuss new programs or the elimination of current programs that are poorly received.

Therapeutic Activities

The range of activities in a skilled nursing facility is limited only by the staff's creativity. By adapting everyday tasks or well-known games to give them a rehabilitative orientation, the staff can produce a wide variety of programs.

Programming for the confused and/or withdrawn patient population should emphasize reality orientation, sensory stimulation, and remotivation, with basic and more advanced programs conducted depending on the degree of patient disability. Singing familiar old songs, playing "name that tune," and dancing are activities that even the most intellectually impaired residents can enjoy and will willingly join. Adapting religious services to make them shorter due to the residents' limited attention spans and concentrating on hymns and chants that are easily remembered also elicit an active response from this patient group. Many patients enjoy Bingo, which can be modified to become "Singo," a game in which song titles are written on the cards and players mark appropriate boxes when they recognize the songs played. Card Bingo, which uses the figures on playing cards, may be substituted.

A spelling bee can be organized and conducted for residents with diverse intellectual levels; it can become a truly competitive event for intact residents. Anagrams, a variation of spelling, also can be a stimulating mind-teaser for alert residents. Playing Password and finding multiple words within a single word also encourage participants to use thought processes that frequently lie dormant in nursing home residents. Not announcing the week's word game until all the participants have assembled adds even further stimulation.

"Horse Racing," a game in which figures are moved according to the roll of dice, coordinates both mental functioning and gross motor activities. A rhythm band provides the residents with sensory stimulation (hearing, touch), general body movement and exercise, and a lot of fun.

Activities staff members can read aloud to individual patients or to a group of residents; patients with impaired sight especially appreciate it. Newspapers, magazines (including current events magazines), or books (particularly biographies) should all be considered for this activity, which may be conducted by a volunteer.

Gardening offers many therapeutic benefits and can be modified to the intellectual level of the residents involved. It allows many residents to continue an activity that was a hobby for them before their admission, to have responsibility for a project that necessitates continued involvement, and to have pride in the results of their efforts.

As often as is necessary, perhaps weekly, a "Getting to Know You" hour, where new residents are introduced to their peers and describe their backgrounds and interests, should be held. A sunshine committee, comprising only residents, can be organized. Committee members would welcome new residents or those recently returned from the hospital, visit those who are roombound or hospitalized, and send get-well

FIGURE 8-2
Indoor Gardening

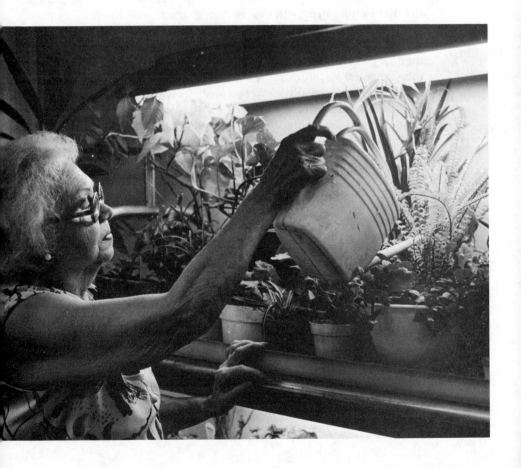

cards to hospitalized residents or condolence notes to the families of recently deceased residents.

Food and dining can be the focus for many lively and creative activities. A gourmeteer club can be organized for residents who have a special interest in cuisine. The members might plan a special monthly meal, perhaps participate in some of the cooking, and, of course, eat the specialties prepared. The general patient population can also enjoy a monthly luncheon or cookout for which they determine the menu. Coffee socials, planned for Saturday or Sunday afternoons when many families visit, can provide a warm ambience for both residents and visitors. A festive occasion that draws together staff, volunteers, and families is an international buffet for which everyone is requested to prepare a dish— from appetizers to desserts—of an international origin. The cooks will take pride in their delicious results and everyone will benefit from the communal effort.

At least once a month, the activities coordinator should arrange for the dietician to meet with the resident group to plan menus for upcoming special events. This will also afford the residents an apportunity to comment on the current menu and to make suggestions for future menus. Direct contact with the dietitian to discuss these matters is another manner of affording residents a voice in determining their lifestyle, and it is especially important since food and mealtime are primary focuses for institutionalized persons. If issues relating to dietary are raised in the monthly residents' council meeting, they should be promptly referred to the dietitian. Alternatively, the dietitian may be asked to join the meeting to resolve them immediately.

Large functions—like a luncheon, a holiday open house, and a grandchildrens' pizza or ice cream party—should be planned regularly throughout the year to afford an opportunity for all staff, and especially families, to join in the activities program and to work together for the enjoyment of the entire nursing home "family." Residents take a great deal of pride in showing off their relatives at such occasions, especially when family members are recruited to provide entertainment at these parties. A photographer should be present at such events to record the happenings: pictures can then be given to family members as mementos. These are particularly meaningful because they are often the only recent photos of aged relatives.

Maintaining a boutique cart that contains a few cosmetics, stationery, stamps, candy, and so on gives the residents a small-scale shopping experience at a time in their lives when almost everything is done for them. Junior volunteers can provide manicures, which may help reinforce a positive self-image and build morale for the women.

Community Involvement

Many residents enjoy the sense of community involvement and volunteering that community service projects offer. The Red Cross, Salvation Army, Boy Scouts, and various service organizations may all be contacted for such projects. During summer months, the residents could conduct a weekly reading hour for area children, giving the mothers some free time for themselves. This type of activity may have been an integral part of the lifestyles of many residents, and men may be more willing to join as they may not consider this "women's work."

During election season, the League of Women Voters should be contacted to provide campaign information, and candidates should be asked to speak at the nursing home. As responsible citizens, residents who are able to should exercise their right to vote. It becomes the activities staff's responsibility to make certain that residents are properly registered and that absentee ballots are received, distributed, and returned in due time.

Outings

Outings should be planned as often as possible, for it is important that residents know they are still viable members of the community and are able to venture out into the community. The microcosm of the nursing home will eventually become stale and unstimulating for some residents (others will fear to leave its protective environment). A refreshing look at a new surrounding, not to speak of the thrill of getting dressed up "to go out," can be a morale boost.

The benefits for institutionalized persons in visiting homes, with their evidences of family life, are inestimable. Families of residents often welcome the opportunity to entertain groups of residents in their homes because of the pleasure experienced by their relatives with their peers. Volunteers and, indeed, some staff also may be encouraged to invite residents to their homes.

Individual and Specialized Group Activities

It is not necessary to delineate activities that patients may pursue on a solitary basis. It is appropriate, however, to emphasize the value of the life-review process. It can help the elderly to accept their age, disability, and eventual death and to realize that their life has been worthwhile, that they have made achievements, and that they have overcome adversities and losses. Life review can be an individual or group activity. A foreign-born resident might recall life in the "old country" to a staff member or a volunteer or to a small group of residents, staff, and/or volunteers. Likewise, the celebration of particular religious or ethnic

FIGURE 8-3
Bandage-rolling Project

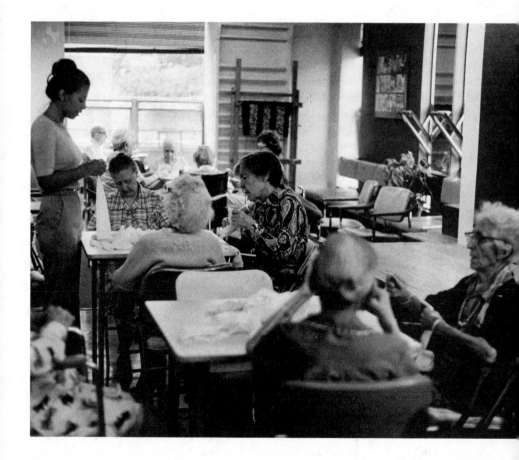

holidays can be part of life review; audiovisual and musical material can be used to encourage residents to recall these past experiences.

While individual programs can be organized to meet the needs of the individual resident, group programs also can be developed to meet the different needs of the group. Life task groups can be devoted to residents' special interests, such as sewing and cooking. Other groups can direct their attention to adaptation to institutional life. Men's clubs can be fruitful for the generally outnumbered males in a nursing home, who may wish to discuss problems, or to share traditionally male-oriented interests such as sports, woodworking, or card playing. A couples' group and a widows' group are other possibilities. Patient volunteer groups who perform in community service activities for organizations outside the nursing home or who serve as friendly visitors to other more handicapped residents should not be overlooked.

Resident self-government units can be beneficial to those who are intellectually able to handle such responsibilities. Social action groups are beginning to grow in popularity in long-term-care institutions as the number of aging persons in America grows and as the voice of the elderly commands more attention from government agencies and political leaders. Older people are concerned about problems such as Medicare and Medicaid, and together they can hold discussions and write letters to their legislators concerning specific issues.

ACTIVITIES PLAN

Upon the admission of a new patient, the activities coordinator ascertains from the attending physician whether the patient is medically permitted to participate in the activities program. After that, he should regularly check with other appropriate professional staff members on the patient's ability to participate. Shortly following admission, he should meet with the patient to learn the patient's interests and previous hobbies, his current needs, and his capabilities in order to develop an appropriate plan for individual (solitary), group, and independent (without staff assistance) activities. The coordinator may have to solicit the history from the family if the patient is unable to relate it.

The resident should be requested to give written consent to the jointly prepared activities plan, thus signifying his commitment to participate and his involvement in the decision-making process regarding his daily activities. The activities coordinator should review this plan with the resident quarterly. Should the resident refuse, or not be able to sign his name, or be unable to participate, his family or sponsor may be contacted to sign the plan, offering proof that the resident cannot participate in the program.

When the attending physician approves, the activities plan, which outlines the short- and long-term goals for the resident, is then incorporated into the total patient care plan, which will be reviewed monthly or whenever the condition of the patient warrants.

LIBRARY

There are two points of view vis-à-vis the patient library in a long-term-care facility. Some people believe that a permanent patient library does not serve the needs of long-term residents who eventually will tire of the same books. Those opposed to a permanent patient library suggest developing an arrangement by which the local public library will loan a certain number of different books each month, thus affording residents the availability of a continuously changing supply of reading material. For this arrangement, a special room is not needed; a mobile book cart is sufficient.

Others believe that this arrangement is useful but that a permanent library in its own room affords residents and families the opportunity for another activity removed from the group. A permanent library tends to receive donations of books and magazines. These should be examined ruthlessly and disposed of after a reasonable length of time if library volunteers find that they are just taking up space.

Certainly, arrangements should be made with the public library to loan out large-print books and magazines such as *Reader's Digest*. Individual residents may enjoy reading the large-print edition of newspapers such as the *New York Times*. All residents who are able should be encouraged to read newspapers, and appropriate arrangements should be made with local distributors for their delivery.

Most books that are circulated from the local public library to outside facilities are mysteries, humorous books, short stories, poetry, light romantic novels, autobiographies and biographies, histories, and psychology books. Subjects of least interest, judged by circulation lists, include books about nature, religion, animals, sports, westerns, and science fiction. These choices may be attributable to the traditional reading tastes of the predominantly female population in the skilled nursing home.

A book's popularity may also depend on its condition. If a book is new, not too big or heavy, or not too small for balancing and turning pages, generally it will be more appealing to the reader.

EVALUATION

Change is an essential component of a viable activities program—changes to meet the changing physical, social, and emotional needs of new and old residents and changes to combat the inevitable sameness of long-term care. Activities can compensate for the rigidity of institutional life and can provide a special opportunity for creativity, flexibility, and stimulation. The success of programs should not be measured by the numbers of participants but rather by their involvement.

Activities staff members should ask themselves and their resident program committee the following questions:

Are the intellectual needs of the residents being met? Or are the programs failing to stimulate their minds? Are the religious needs of the intellectually impaired being met by brief, specially designed services, or are such residents being excluded from the overall religious programs because they are noisy and disturbing to others?

Are music and dance—which are so useful for communication, the release of tension, socialization, and reality orientation—being used in the activities?

Are there opportunities for passive activities where the patient pursues his own interests, and active programs where the participant reaches beyond himself?

Are new programs added monthly or at least bimonthly?

Are the intellectually alert residents encouraged to perform community service for outside organizations and to visit and communicate with other patients inside the nursing home?

Do residents who are able join in outings once or twice a month?

RELIGIOUS ACTIVITIES

The religious program in a skilled nursing facility can become an important part of the fabric of the institution. If the patients in the facility represent the three major faiths, the nursing home should make contacts with community-based clergy. It is far preferable to have clergy in area churches and synagogues include the nursing home in their activities than to recruit out-of-area clerical students or unaffiliated clergy.

The local rabbi, minister, or priest will undoubtedly call on different groups and members of his congregation to supplement the nursing home's religious services. For example, he may ask volunteers to accompany the nursing home service on the piano or distribute prayer books, or he may call on the church's youth groups to participate in certain special holiday services. The unaffiliated clergyman does not have an available volunteer personnel pool. Ladies' auxiliaries and mens' clubs may become involved with the patients either by visiting the nursing home or by inviting residents to specific events—such as special religious celebrations, auxiliary luncheons, and breakfasts—at their houses of worship.

FIGURE 8-4
Religious Services

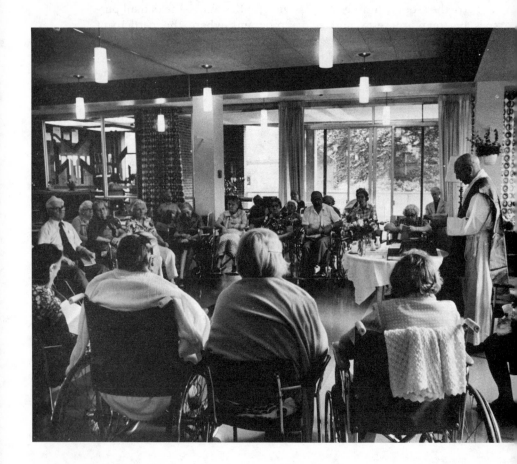

In some communities, the practice of performing services in long-term-care facilities is shared by each religious denomination. For example, Protestant ministers may take turns so that each performs services once a month or three times per year. It probably is easier to recruit volunteers for this kind of an undemanding schedule but the religious program would then be reduced to religious services. Unless the clergy have the opportunity to become acquainted with the residents by establishing a continuing relationship, it is unlikely that residents or family members would feel comfortable in seeking pastoral counseling. Even staff members would be less likely to draw the clergy into the therapeutic program if they were faced with a succession of different ministers, priests, and rabbis each week. When clergy have year-round assignments at the nursing home, they will arrange for substitute clergy during vacations or other times when they are unable to fulfill their duties.

The clergy are busy, overcommitted, and often underpaid. It would be helpful to them if the nursing home were to offer them honoraria for their services, at least enough to cover certain small expenses. With such an arrangement, the nursing home staff will feel more comfortable about seeking help for particular patients and special situations. Otherwise, they will always worry about taking advantage of volunteer clergy and overstepping their time limitations.

The clergy should be alerted to newly admitted residents, patients transferred to the hospital, discharges, and deaths of residents via written memoranda, except in an emergency. They should be encouraged to check with the social workers each week to determine whether help is needed with certain residents and/or their families.

Two or three times per year (and more frequently, if possible) the clergy should be invited to attend interdisciplinary meetings. Both staff members and clergy can discuss suggestions for improving the quality of life at the nursing home via spiritual intervention. Full-time staff members may have suggestions for improving the religious program with respect to such mechanical matters as length and time of services. In addition, problems and concerns can be identified and resolved via a mutual exchange of information.

At such meetings, the participants might want to consider holding two services for each religious group. The intellectually intact residents are often disturbed by the antisocial behavior of the mentally impaired residents during religious services. The staff will tend to select only quiet residents to attend religious services, and thus the spiritual needs of the more confused and noisy residents will not be met. Brief ritualistic services with the emphasis on singing familiar hymns can be of great value to intellectually impaired residents, and they can serve as meaningful exercises in reality orientation.

Of course, conducting two services and allowing time for postservice visiting and some individual pastoral counseling and conferring with staff enlarge the time commitment for the clergy. If congregational volunteers attend the services, sometimes they can take over the responsibility for less complicated tasks without intruding in the special relationship between patient and clerical representative.

The clergy may be able to guide the staff in how to handle the death of a resident with fellow residents. Pro forma they will conduct appropriate services at the regular worship service in memory of a recently expired patient. They can be helpful by encouraging staff and residents to acknowledge deaths of residents in other meaningful ways, such as mentioning the death in the facility newsletter and discussing feelings about death at group meetings.

Besides weekly worship services of the three major faiths, traditional foods and decorations should be added to the special holiday services to replicate the patients' preinstitutional experiences. Worship services can be enhanced by group Bible study and religious and ethical discussions. Choir and choral groups composed of residents and/or staff and volunteers can add still another dimension to the religious program. On occasion, some residents may be assisted to attend outside religious services.

While some facilities are fortunate in having a chapel on the premises, many nonsectarian institutions need to use general activity areas for worship services. Although portable altars are available, an alternative is to place ritualistic items on tables covered with white cloths. If general open areas are used for services, some special planning is required to preserve the dignity of the service. For example, the public address system should not be used during religious services except in an emergency. Similarly, staff members and visitors should be urged to modulate their voices. Elevator and corridor doors should be closed as infrequently and as quietly as possible.

Some clerical representatives will wish to use certain prayer books or request that the nursing home staff reproduce portions of services. When possible, this material should be typed in large print or in capital letters to help the visually handicapped read it. Religious articles should be stored in a conveniently located area so they can be used at any time.

Both residents and clergy have mixed feelings about the wearing of religious vestments. Some prefer this kind of ritualism; others do not find it necessary or even appropriate. Presumably, the individual clergyman should wear whatever is comfortable. Some residents (Jewish males and females of various faiths) prefer to wear hats to religious services, and they should, of course, be encouraged to wear whatever they feel is proper.

VOLUNTEERS

Volunteers are not needed in skilled nursing facilities to replace full-time staff, but rather to develop interpersonal relationships with residents on a different level than exists with professional staff and to enhance and broaden the therapeutic program. Indeed, facilities that develop a volunteer program in the hope of cutting costs will be sadly disappointed to learn that the program requires a full-time director or responsible person who will be charged with recruiting, interviewing, screening, orienting, training, assigning, and evaluating volunteers.

In the hospital, with its shorter patient stay, volunteers are task oriented: they deliver mail, care for flowers, direct visitors. In the nursing home, with its longer patient stay, volunteers can be more patient oriented. Continuing interaction between long-stay residents and volunteers offers volunteers more specialized and interesting possibilities for service. If 50 to 70 percent of the skilled nursing facility patients are characterized by behavioral disabilities, the need for a broad range of activities is obvious; however, in the 100-bed facility, it is not financially feasible to employ more than two or three activity staff members. Therefore volunteers are needed to offer specialized activities and to visit with residents for whom professional staff members do not have time.

Volunteers perform their assigned duties under the supervision of the coordinator of activities and volunteers. Interdepartmental associations concerning the volunteers' role should be handled by the activities coordinator except in emergency situations. If staff members are apprehensive about the abilities or performance of an individual volunteer, they should direct their concerns to the coordinator, who has the personal relationship with the volunteer needed to discuss the problems and to reach an acceptable understanding. The coordinator should always make sure that a staff member is assigned to activities programs carried on by a volunteer in order to attend patients who need assistance.

There are moral and legal considerations as to appropriate assignments for volunteers. For instance, professional tasks should be performed only by professionals. Vital and continuous patient-related assignments must not be relegated to volunteers. Volunteers can be exposed to patient records only after careful orientation and should understand that their awareness of a patient's condition is offered in confidence.

Benefits of a Volunteer Program

Volunteer service in a skilled nursing facility can also reap rewards for the volunteer who derives satisfaction from service to others. Volunteers often utilize service as a means of working through personal problems with siblings, job situations, and parental figures. Middle-aged mothers use volunteering to get over loneliness they feel after all their children have left home, and retired people may turn to volunteering to regain a feeling of purpose. Serving in a nursing home may help an older volunteer accept disability and view long-term care in a more positive light. For the younger volunteer, it can provide the impetus to enter a helping profession.

Nursing home volunteers have the opportunity to relate to residents on a continuing basis, and they can observe firsthand the meaning of chronic disability and long-term care. Volunteers will view and participate in patient improvement or in the attempt to maintain the status quo and will observe patient deterioration and even death. Furthermore, they will witness the unfolding of family history as they observe residents, their children, and grandchildren. They will see all these things in conjunction with an educational program, so that they will come to view aging, illness, and death with less fear and more maturity.

Many benefits accrue to the skilled nursing facility in the development of a volunteer program. On an organized basis, it can constitute an effective technique for relating the long-term-care facility to the community, which is particularly important since the ill aged are rejected in our youth-oriented society. Volunteers can engender positive feelings among the staff so that the nursing home is considered an environment for living rather than dying, a place for engagement rather than disengagement.

Thus long-term-care volunteers can help both residents and the entire nursing home program. They can improve the knowledge of the nursing home within the community and, in fact, can help themselves as they contribute to the care of the ill aged.

Who Does Volunteer Work

Some skilled nursing facilities have developed successful volunteer programs sponsored by a particular social or religious agency. For example, the auxiliary of a church may adopt a nursing home and provide volunteers for religious services, for craft activities, for friendly visiting, for shopping, for monthly parties, and so on. In effect, the auxiliary or coalition of several clubs serves as the volunteer agency. Alternatively, the nursing home may develop its own volunteer program under the aegis of a staff member.

The volunteer corps presenting itself today has some marked socioeconomic differences from years past. The middle-class homemaker who fifteen years ago would have put her free time to good use in a socially acceptable activity is today earning a living; if she does continue volunteer work, it is scheduled into a crowded time frame. Retirees now compose a growing segment of the volunteers in nursing homes. Among others, large corporations have begun to impress upon their employees that they have an obligation to become involved in the community and to assist the less fortunate. In addition, many schools and colleges are encouraging students to devote some of their time to volunteering in community agencies by offering academic credit for their experiences.

The nursing home staff must be mindful of the changing nature of the volunteer corps and adapt its volunteer policies and program to meet the current needs and character of its volunteers. Due to the changing socioeconomic status of volunteers, the facility should provide smocks for volunteers rather than ask them to purchase and launder their own. The coordinator of activities and volunteers may be required to spend time completing reports to students' supervisors and teachers. Program scheduling may have to reflect the availability of the volunteer leader rather than the most convenient time for the activities staff.

The most desirable personal attributes for volunteers in the long-term-care setting are warmth, enthusiasm, flexibility, sensitivity, and a sincere affection for older people. Potential volunteers must demonstrate self-discipline and self-awareness, a strong sense of responsibility, and an ability to accept training and supervision. In addition, they should have specific skills for nursing home work, such as painting, singing, piano playing, or chair caning.

The most effective nursing home volunteers tend to be middle-aged men and women who do not appear to be threatened by the residents' disabilities and illnesses. Relatively few people in their twenties and thirties serve as individual volunteers, although they may well constitute a part of one of the volunteer groups of entertainers who perform at the facility. The exception may be psychiatrically handicapped or retarded persons, who, with a great deal of support, training, and continuing supervision (as well as acceptance by the residents and nursing home staff) can be effective and loyal volunteers.

Young people in their mid-teens can also prove to be assets in the nursing home environment. Their youth and enthusiasm are generally well received by the patients, who view the teen-agers as surrogate grandchildren. In this era of dissolving family relationships and population mobility, many young people have limited contact with their grandparents or other elderly persons. The nursing home experience affords youngsters a chance to relate to older people on a meaningful level.

Volunteer Selection and Orientation

The coordinator of activities and volunteers should carefully interview the prospective volunteer to ensure that he is familiar with all pertinent aspects of the skilled nursing facility, including the philosophy of the institution, the nature of the patient population, the purpose and scope

FIGURE 8-5
Junior Volunteer

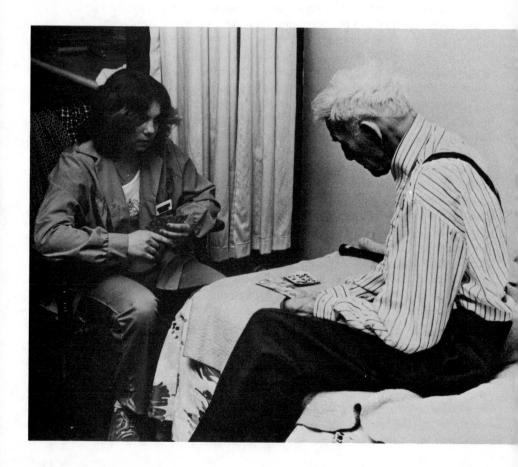

of the activities program, and the expectations of volunteer service. The potential volunteer should receive a copy of the volunteer handbook and should be given a tour of the facility. If arrangements are made with a group to visit the nursing home, it is helpful if the handbook can be distributed to them for their perusal and brief orientation prior to their visit.

Sufficient time should be allowed for the individual to determine if long-term care is the appropriate field in which to channel his desire for volunteerism. Once that is affirmed, the volunteer should have a careful orientation to familiarize him with the facility, staff, and patients (particularly those with whom he will have the most contact). Volunteers must learn about the patients' clinical problems, the process of separation from families, the adaptation to disability and institutional living, and the separation problems of guilt-ridden families. They need to be trained in the correct method of transporting patients in wheelchairs, of walking with patients who are unsteady on their feet and need assistance, and of relating to confused and disoriented residents.

Volunteers can be a negative voice in the community if they are uninformed, misinformed, or ill informed. If they are uninformed about the patients' physical and mental disabilities, they may think that, say, using an authoritarian voice to encourage disabled patients to bear weight in order to walk is disrespectful, when it is actually completely necessary to motivate the resident to do for himself. Similarly, volunteers may not comprehend the omnipresent depression of chronically ill aged nursing home patients, which is often apparent in their refusal of food and medications. Personnel may have to be forceful to make certain that patients do eat and do accept needed medications; volunteers should realize that this does not represent cruel treatment but rather interest and concern. Volunteers may consider nurses heartless if they insist that patients do not remain in bed even though they profess that they are tired, whereas experienced rehabilitation-oriented staff members know that immobilization and prolonged bedrest can be deleterious and even lethal for ill elderly persons. And although volunteers may view nasogastric tube feeding as inhumane, the alternative is allowing the patient to starve to death.

However, the informed, educated, and trained volunteer can be an ambassador of constructive information to the community. At least annually, the nursing home should hold an extensive interdisciplinary seminar that reviews the physical, psychosocial, and emotional problems in the nursing home population, how patients are treated, and the volunteer's role in that treatment. Such a program can be held in conjunction with a community education program with the hope of recruiting additional volunteers.

Volunteer Recognition

Just as years of service of personnel are acknowledged and honored on an annual basis, so should the service of volunteers—both individuals and groups—be recognized by the nursing home community. This experience is useful for everyone—it is a warm way to show appreciation to volunteers—and it permits each volunteer to observe the scope of the entire volunteer program, which he may not see if he comes only once a week. It also heartens residents, families, and staff to see how many people are helping others altruistically for only inner rewards.

Traditionally, volunteer award days are held in late spring or early summer before the vacation period. For the skilled nursing facility, the event is best scheduled in the autumn. At that time of year, the event can serve as a reminder to volunteers to renew their service, whereas the summer is more likely to represent a period of volunteer inactivity. Similarly, the fall volunteer ceremony offers an opportunity for recruiting volunteers.

Patients should attend and, ideally, present some awards and/or give speeches. Volunteers, too, may wish to speak briefly about their personal rewards from volunteer service.

Since all patients will attend, only one event should be held to honor both junior and adult volunteers. Not only the volunteers, but also their spouses, children, and parents should be invited.

The formal part of the event should be brief, avoiding the individual calling of scores of names out of courtesy to the residents and the older volunteers. A printed program can include names and numbers of volunteer-hours given.

Some facilities prefer to have such events in the evening; older volunteers generally favor daytime events. A Saturday luncheon would be a good choice for most of these people, and it would also be desirable for residents and families. Since the cadre of volunteers undoubtedly will include young people, old people, and an increasing number of males, the traditional tea-party-and-speech ceremony is inappropriate.

RECORDS

All records maintained by activities personnel will help the physician in prescribing or in contraindicating the need for activities, in reviewing the individual's current situation, and in evaluating the progress that he has made so that future care can be planned. The records also aid nursing and other professional staff in determining what is to be done for the patient when he is in their charge. They assist the nursing home administrator in evaluating the procedures used for the program in the facility

FIGURE 8-6
Volunteer Recognition

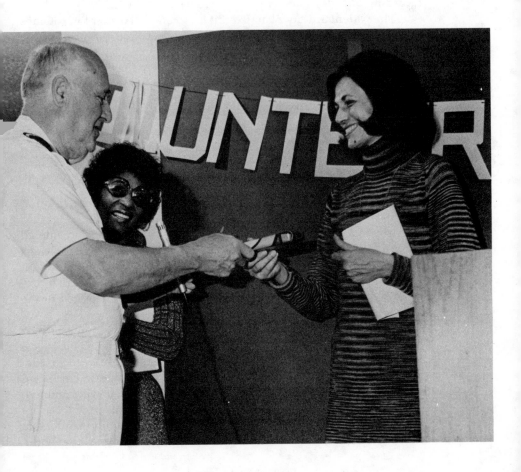

and in planning for the future, and serve as proof of what has been done with and for the individual. Often families or friends who visit at odd hours doubt that their relative or friend has participated in a particular program, but the written record will serve as verification. Activities records may aid organizations such as occupational therapy groups, therapeutic recreationalists, those involved in long-term-care administration, and social and health agencies in planning for the future course of programming in long-term-care institutions.

Two types of records should be maintained: patient records and departmental records.

Patient Records

Resident records include the record card received by the activities director from the admitting office, which includes demographic information about the patient. This card should be filed in a cabinet and used for recording birthdays, family phone numbers, and the like.

The patient activity plan (Exhibit 8-1), completed after the patient's admission, documents the patient's life interests and the plan for his participation in the nursing home program. The resident's signature is required to affirm his awareness and agreement to the proposed plan.

The patient report is completed quarterly or whenever changes occur in the patient's condition. It contains general information regarding his social behavior, disability, personal habits, and response to the program. It is maintained in the patient's chart so that other professional personnel, particularly physicians, can learn the course of the patient's activities. (See Exhibit 8-2.)

The patient's activities program participation record is also a daily activity attendance record for each resident.

Departmental Records

Departmental records include a large monthly calendar, centered around individual and group needs, showing activities planned at least a month in advance and listing each activity by hour, date, and type with the names of the volunteers or outside person(s) involved in that program. Because this is a working document, it should be posted in the activities coordinator's office.

A weekly program should be written up at the beginning of each week, starting with Saturday, and be prepared for distribution on Friday. It should list all the week's activities by time, date, and place to be held, and the name of the responsible volunteer (if applicable), all extracted from the master calendar. This program should be posted in a prominent spot so that residents, staff, visitors, families, and volunteers will be sure to notice it. Copies should be distributed to all nursing units in order that nursing staff will be able to encourage residents to join specific events.

EXHIBIT 8-1
Patient Activity Plan

PATIENT ACTIVITY PLAN

Patient's name _____ Room no. _____

Life Interests:

Clubs and organizations: _____

_____

_____

Political interests: _____

Hobbies and other activities: _____

_____

Activities Plan:

Religious services	Movie/slide presentations ____
Jewish	
Protestant ____	Sunshine committee ____
Catholic ____	
Friday evening vespers ____	Getting to Know You ____
Arts and crafts (specify type)	Gardening club ____
	Reading group ____
_____	Players' group ____
Music appreciation ____	Body movement sessions ____
Chorus ____	Current events discussion group ____
Rhythm band ____	
Sing-along ____	Residents' council ____
Entertainment ____	Games
Social/cocktail hour ____	Bingo ____
Gourmeteer club ____	Lotto ____
Mens' club ____	Scrabble ____
	Checkers ____
Individual volunteer visits ____	Cards (specify) ____
	Spelling bee ____
Group interaction ____	Anagrams ____
Off-premises trips ____	Password ____
Activities program planning committee ____	Resident volunteer committee ____
	Community projects ____
	Other (specify) ____

_____   _____ _____
Resident's signature   Activities worker's signature Date

EXHIBIT 8-2
Patient Report

ACTIVITIES PROGRAM

PATIENT REPORT

Resident's name _____ Room no. _____

Contraindications for program participation as indicated by the attending

physician: _____

Participates in planned programs: regularly _____   occasionally _____
                                    rarely   _____   never   _____

Pursues activities independently: yes _____   no _____

Indicate those activities in which the resident participates: _____

_____

_____

Disability: _____

_____

Response to program (including attitude): _____

_____

Interpersonal relationships: _____

_____

Social behavior: _____

_____

Intellectual behavior: _____

_____

Emotional behavior: _____

_____

Verbalization: _____

_____

Appearance: _____

_____

Personal habits: _____

_____

Activities worker _____   Date _____

The administrative director will want to receive monthly and annual statistical data from the activities program. The monthly activities program record is kept daily and lists all activities for the day; the duration of each activity; the number of staff members, volunteers, residents, and families participating; and the name of the particular volunteer group, if applicable.

Another departmental record is a monthly activities summary, which synthesizes the month's activities by listing the number of times an activity is held, the number of residents participating, and a brief evaluation of the activity, if appropriate. This summary is then used to develop the annual report for the department, which lists the number of entertainers by month, the number of entertainment hours by month, the number of professional meetings and seminars attended by the activities staff, the special events of the year, new programs, the changes in departmental procedures/policies, a listing of the major programming areas, and the number of times specific activities have been held within the year. This report is forwarded to the administrator and a copy is kept in the activities coordinator's file.

Finally, the consultant to the activities program should prepare a monthly report telling how and with whom he spent time, including in-depth interviews with all new residents, a list of meetings attended, an outline of changes within the department, and recommendations for improving the service.

Other Records

In addition to attending physician's permission for a patient to leave the premises, the patient must also have the permission of the responsible relative. Whenever the range of activities, the modes of transportation to the activities, and their distance from the facility increase, so do the risks of accidents for nursing home patients. For the protection of the facility, staff, and volunteers, a release-of-responsibility clause should be included in a permission form even though public and professional liability insurance can provide coverage for all those factors in all settings. Rather than have the relative or sponsor give blanket permission at the time of the patient's admission, it is recommended permission be requested for each outing, thereby taking into account the changing nature of the patient's condition.

The resident, or his responsible relative or sponsor if the resident is unable to do so, must grant permission to use his name and/or photograph in news releases concerning nursing home activities. Such release forms should be updated with each news or feature story in which the patient is mentioned or pictured.

Volunteers should be asked to complete an application form and present a health record. Junior volunteers should be required to have working papers as well as written permission from their parents to serve as volunteers. Each volunteer should have his own sheet in the volunteer hours book to record each visit.

FACILITIES, EQUIPMENT, AND SUPPLIES

At least two large areas for group programs will be needed: one for programs for the intellectually intact and one for programs held simultaneously for the intellectually impaired. Activities can also be held in community rooms or dining areas that are located throughout the units. Individual resident rooms can be used for independent activities or volunteer visiting if residents are unwilling or too ill to leave their rooms. An outdoor terrace or patio that is at least partially shaded should also be available for activities in good weather. The main activity areas and/or visitor lounge areas should have a display cabinet and bulletin board for showing residents' works.

Large locked cabinets for the storage of supplies—especially bulky items such as folding tables and stacking or folding chairs with arms—a piano on wheels, and a built-in film screen should be located within or nearby the main activity rooms to facilitate setting up for programs. Care must be taken, however, to store valuable equipment such as projectors and cameras in a secure area. In addition to locked storage cabinets and bookshelves, a rack for volunteer uniforms and coats must be provided in the activities/volunteer office. If full-length lockers are not available for volunteers' belongings, the facility should provide small lockers for valuables. If the facility is fortunate enough to have a kiln, it may need to be located in the maintenance room with sufficient shelf space to place projects that are not yet complete. Seasonal decorations should be carefully labeled when they are stored for easy accessibility the following year.

The activities coordinator must keep a careful watch on the use of supplies. When the upcoming month's schedule of events is planned, the coordinator should make sure that supplies are adequate and, if not, order what is needed. Advance planning and ordering will be needed for special programs where the supplies are not usually stocked and may be hard to find.

Some facilities find that the display and sale of residents' arts and crafts helps finance the activities program. Of course, unsolicited donations of items such as books, wallpaper and fabric samples, craft materials, and yarn are useful in cutting expenses.

FIGURE 8-7
Activity Brought to Patient's Room

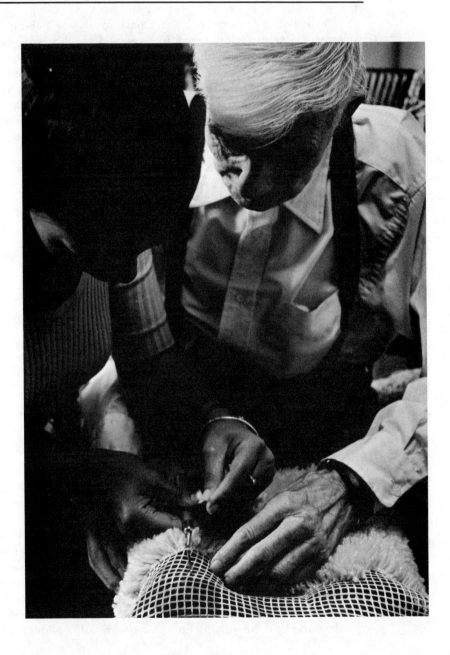

The purchasing director in the business office should purchase supplies for the activities department. If the activities coordinator pays cash for last-minute purchases, he should be reimbursed from petty cash upon presentation of a receipt for the purchase.

The activities department should have for its use a 16-mm sound projector, a slide projector, a record player, and possibly two cameras—an instant camera for individual patient photographs to be placed on the health record, and a 35-mm camera for recording special events so that reprints can be made—and a portable microphone, which is particularly useful for outdoor programs. Religious supplies—which may include candles, tablecloths, prayer books, wine cups, a holy water container, or other items requested by clergy—should be stored in a safe but accessible area for use when activities personnel are not on duty.

According to the scope of the activity program, activities supplies would include, but not be limited to, the following:

> arts and crafts materials and tools
> games (Scrabble, Lotto, Bingo, backgammon, checkers, etc.)
> game tables
> shuffleboard court (painted on the activity room floor or on
>   an outside patio)
> outdoor cooker
> lectern
> record albums
> party tablecloths
> flower containers
> plant cart and supplies
> sewing, knitting, and crocheting supplies
> bookmobile with magazines
> small portable film screen
> large bulletin board and lettering for posting the week's
>   activities
> paper supplies

SUMMARY

An analysis of how patients spend their day will underscore the number of hours spent in activities, one of the services that deals with residents primarily as people, not as patients. It is advantageous however for activities to be therapeutic, and the occupational therapist can advise the activities coordinator to this end. Also, since residents infrequently have the opportunity to leave the premises, it is important to introduce the outside world into the nursing home via community volunteers.

NOTES

1. J. C. Hallburg, "The Teaching of Aged Adults," *The Journal of Gerontological Nursing* 2, no. 3 (May–June 1976): 15.
2. Ibid., p. 17.
3. M. B. Miller, M.D., "Iatrogenic and Nurisgenic Effects of Prolonged Immobilization of the Ill Aged," *The Interdisciplinary Role of the Nursing Home Medical Director* (Wakefield, Mass.: Contemporary Publishing, 1976).

CHAPTER 9

Consumerism

INTRODUCTION

Nursing home consumers are sometimes classified as insiders and outsiders. Residents and their families are the "insiders," while sponsors and community organizations are the "outsiders." Volunteers in skilled nursing facilities are the liaison between these two groups.

Individual consumers may be their own advocates or they may serve as advocates for their relatives, friends, clients, or charges. But groups of consumers (composed of insiders—such as residents' councils, committees of friends and relatives of residents, auxiliaries, and volunteer committees—or of outsiders—such as advisory councils, community boards, citizen groups, public interest and research groups, ombudsmen, patient advocates, and monitoring teams) form potentially more powerful constituencies than do individual consumers.

The patients' rights movement is an example of social progress where providers acknowledge, promote, and protect the residents' concerns. Emphasis on the rights of individuals or groups of residents represents a struggle against the negative aspects of institutionalization, depersonalization, sterility, indifference, and insensitivity.

THE RESIDENT AS CONSUMER

The federal government has promulgated a Bill of Rights for patients in Medicare and Medicaid skilled nursing facilities. The Bill of Rights includes prerogatives concerning residents' personal, environmental, health, and legal rights, such as the right to be treated as intelligent and sensitive human beings, the maintenance of religious and civil liberties, and the freedom of choice and decision making consistent with the facility's philosophy.

Personal Rights

Personal rights include rights to courteous and impartial treatment, dignified care, and special consideration for the communicatively handicapped (including non–English-speaking residents), as well as the right to keep a reasonable number of personal mementos. Physical and emotional privacy, confidential telephone and mail communication, private visits with friends and families, opportunities for personal growth, and community service to contribute volunteer efforts when deemed therapeutic are stressed, as is the availability of physical, psychological, and spiritual counsel. Perhaps the most important right in this area concerns the opportunity to have one's suggestions considered by staff, administration, and others who have a genuine interest in improving the quality of life of nursing home residents.

The right to confidential mail and telephone communication is important for intellectually intact residents. If patients are intellectually impaired, paranoid, or otherwise acting-out individuals, it may be advisable or even necessary to monitor their correspondence or telephone calls at the request of their families or attending physicians. Such patients may, for example, wish to make telephone calls during the night, or contact their physician ten times a day, or their children every hour, since they may have no concept of time or memory recall. However, such monitoring must be periodically reviewed to determine its appropriateness to changes in patients' conditions.

While having personal mementos and even furniture is deemed highly desirable for residents, it is surprising how few personal things patients bring into skilled nursing facilities. It may be that a considerable number of residents have not lived in their own homes prior to entering the institution and therefore have few remaining possessions aside from clothing. Or it may be attributed to a patient's or family's reluctance to give up a residence and with it the possibility of the patient's returning to it.

The most effective mechanism for considering suggestions of residents is via a residents' committee or council, where openness and frankness will encourage a free interchange of ideas. Often residents' suggestions are helpful and can be easily implemented. Other times, residents do not realize the implications of their suggestions, and open discourse between them and the facility staff is a healthy process.

Environmental Rights

Environmental rights refer to safe, healthful, and aesthetically pleasing indoor and outdoor physical accommodations with areas for entertaining and visiting privately with family and friends. Environmental rights extend to physical security in case of natural disasters and protection against the theft of personal belongings. The facility should provide a safety box for the storage of residents' personal valuables and spending money, although residents and families should be discouraged from leaving large sums of money or irreplaceable items at the nursing home.

The resident should acknowledge, in writing, the receipt of money or valuables from the safety box.

It certainly is desirable to have areas to entertain family and friends, but problems would ensue in most nursing homes if half or even ten residents needed such areas simultaneously. A certain amount of mutual consideration between roommates can help. For example, when one roommate has visitors, the other may leave the room. Privacy during conjugal visits, however, is easier to describe than to implement. If a resident lives in a private room, there is no problem. In a semiprivate room, the roommate's rights will be abrogated if he is displaced. Furthermore, is closing the door really an issue of privacy or actually an announcement of what is happening?

Various courses of action are possible regarding the sexual practices of inpatients, which perforce will include homosexual and heterosexual activity between intellectually intact and/or brain-damaged residents. The nursing home may prefer a hands-off attitude because sex is a private matter, or a laissez-faire policy that encourages residents to "do their own thing." The nursing home may act *in loco infantis*—in place of the residents' children—and act according to the children's wishes (though the children may not always agree or may feel differently about the activities of their mother versus those of their father). The skilled nursing facility may encourage sexual fulfillment as an important means of communication, or it may impose restraints on sexual practices, believing that sex is unnatural for the elderly, and therefore undesirable. Obviously, the opinions of residents, families, personnel, volunteers, board members, professionals, and citizens in the community influence long-term-care policies concerning sexual activity in the nursing home.

An important aspect of resident rights regarding sexual activity concerns the confused ill aged, who may have lost impulse control in social situations. Morally, should not nursing home management ascertain that intellectually impaired residents behave in the way they would have behaved when they were well? This, it would seem, is part of the unwritten contract between the sponsor of the patient and the nursing home. Husbands of female residents may have particularly strong feelings about these matters.

The safety of personal belongings presents certain difficulties with respect to confused residents who have been known to dispose of dentures or rings in the toilet, or who may rummage and pilfer belongings in the closets and drawers of others. In addition, if families take things home without informing other members of the family or nursing home staff, patients may become convinced that such items have been stolen. However, these factors in no way should preclude emphasizing in staff orientation and continuing education the importance and sanctity of all personal belongings.

FIGURE 9-1
Resident Signing for Receipt of Cash

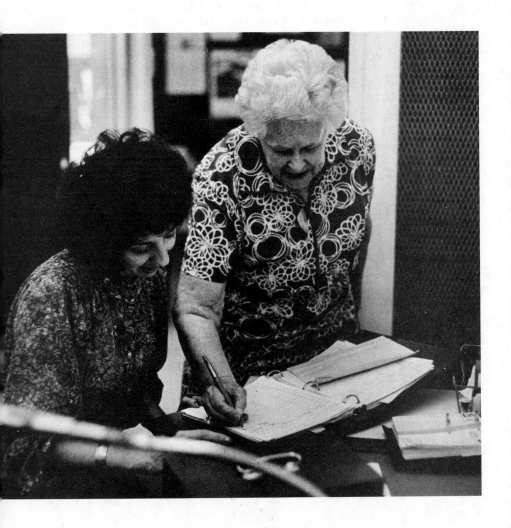

Health Rights

Health rights include being properly informed about one's medical condition and receiving prompt treatment from qualified personnel, with the assurance of privacy and confidentiality of records. In addition, patients should not be physically and/or chemically restrained except when medically authorized, and they should be allowed to exercise self-determination regarding their medical treatment and participation in experimentation. Except in an emergency, due notification must be given to the resident and/or his family if his health status mandates a transfer from the facility.

These health rights point up some interesting issues. For example, the uninformed liken the use of physical restraints to cruelty and indifference to patient welfare, when it can be more cruel to permit a severely debilitated patient to sit in a wheelchair without the proper support to prevent him from toppling out of the chair and injuring himself. Thus, while the use of restraints may have an unappealing connotation to the public, their judicious use is clearly required in some instances. Staff members and nurses who are in continuous contact with patients often better understand such needs than do attending physicians who visit patients briefly and intermittently.

The right to self-determination opens a Pandora's box, especially when the right to prompt medical treatment is considered. Is the nursing home staff obligated to follow medical orders that do not include the use of antibiotics when it is obvious that the patient is suffering from a reversible situation such as a urinary tract infection? Nurses and nursing attendants in skilled nursing facilities also are reluctant to permit patients to starve when nasogastric tube feedings would provide the needed nutrients. Such issues become even more complex when the patient is brain impaired and his family is making the decisions. Family members themselves often do not agree, or they change their minds often. For example, they may request no tube feeding on Monday and change their minds on Wednesday when they realize that their relative is starving. It is intriguing to consider who should be the final decision maker—the family, the physician, or the nursing home staff, who in some instances have become an extension of the resident's family.

Legal Rights

In the legal category, nursing home residents or their sponsors should have complete information in writing regarding fees, services, and regulations, while the facility reserves the right to request discharge for nonpayment of bills. A periodic accounting of funds held by the nursing home on behalf of the resident should be provided to the resident and his sponsor.

Legal prerogatives also include the right to leave the premises if medically appropriate, the right to present grievances to nursing home personnel without fear of reprisal, and, in some states, the right to pursue class action suits or individual legal assistance for acts and injuries for which the skilled nursing facility is responsible or liable under statute or case law. Finally, the skilled nursing facility should accept and acknowledge accordingly the admission of patients without regard to race, color, creed, marital status, sex, sponsor, national origin, or handicap.

The nursing home administration is responsible for investigating and assessing the validity of grievances. A structure for resolving grievances should be established, perhaps via the residents' council or a special committee designated solely for this purpose that is composed of residents, staff, and perhaps family members and disinterested parties such as clergy and/or consumers.

The pursuit of legal and class action suits may accomplish little more than harassment of the already highly regulated and supervised nursing care facility. Indeed, such litigation may serve to increase tension and ill will rather than to develop effective means of resolving problems and grievances. In the final analysis, legal suits really underscore a breakdown of communication between resident, family and/or sponsor, and nursing home management.

RESIDENTS' COUNCIL

A residents' council, a committee for the rights and welfare of residents, or a residents' advisory forum is composed of a group of patients living in a long-term-care facility who organize to protect their rights of self-determination by active participation in all affairs that affect their daily lives. The presence of such an organization can be beneficial because it enables residents to be active participants in decisions that affect them and because it offers expert guidance to administration on certain management decisions.

A residents' council should not be confused with therapeutic resident group meetings, which provide participants an opportunity to work out problems of adjustment to congregate living, to disability, to loss of spouse, to separation from family, to loss of role, and so forth. A trained social worker or other therapist skilled in group dynamics is essential to lead this type of therapeutic program.

A well-functioning residents' council increases the individual resident's morale, as he expresses opinions to assist in policy determinations, provides administration with feedback, and helps staff by lessening the anger and complaints of residents. Dealing with operational problems once again exposes patients to the realities of community living.

FIGURE 9-2
Residents' Council Meeting

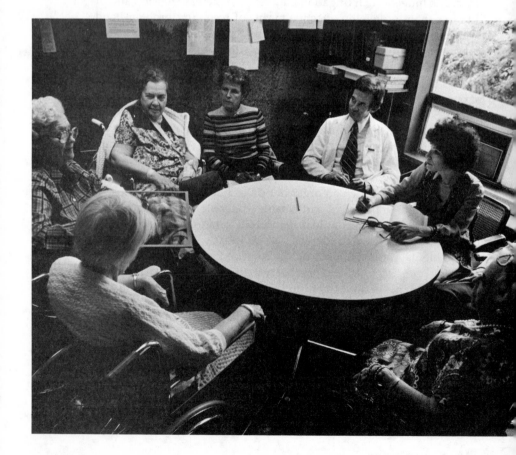

The composition of a residents' council can take various forms. Obviously, only residents who are intact intellectually can participate in this kind of activity, leaving a great number of residents with no representation. Most council members are elected or chosen according to the geography of the facility: each unit, floor, or wing may be allowed a certain number of delegates. Members at large who have contact with patients residing in units for the intellectually impaired may be asked to speak for their less intact peers at council meetings. Some councils have regular members and invite one or two guests to attend each meeting to familiarize them with the purpose of the group. It is suggested that one member represent no more than twenty-five residents in large skilled nursing facilities, but a council should have at least six members to allow for absences, illnesses, and deaths.

Some councils are composed of residents exclusively, although others also have administrative members to permit the immediate resolution of problems and/or to help provide some needed structure when residents are more disabled. The membership of residents' advisory committees occasionally includes family members, clergy, and interested but impartial consumers. Although skilled nursing facility residents indicate a strong preference for excluding relatives or outside consumers, such outside representation may be appropriate for facilities whose residents are preponderantly brain-damaged and thus unable to speak for themselves.

Councils frequently have working committees such as a foodservice committee, a welcoming committee for new residents, an activities committee to advise on recreational programs, and a resident-staff relations committee to resolve grievances from both groups. Other possible committees are housekeeping and laundry committees (missing laundry is often a matter for discussion in institutions) and a sunshine committee.

Minutes must be recorded and distributed to all interested parties and perhaps summarized in the facility newsletter. After problems are discussed, the administrative liaison should make absolutely certain that decisions are implemented with dispatch. For purposes of credibility, it is essential that there be no breakdown in effectuating administrative promises.

Such matters as bylaws, rules for group discussions, officers, elections, and special meetings should be dealt with according to individual facility needs. An exception relates to the resident-staff relations committee, which should develop a procedure whereby special meetings can be called promptly to resolve reports or incidents of patient and staff abuse. Such matters should not await a regular monthly meeting.

Meetings should be held regularly and should last a maximum of an hour, or else they become wearisome and ultimately less effective. If a critical matter needs further airing, another meeting can be scheduled.

The administration should be alert to certain problem areas that may become apparent. Sometimes one group of residents, such as the longest-stay residents, will remain on the council too long and will behave autocratically instead of encouraging democratic processes. Some residents may inappropriately use meetings to discuss personal problems that are not relevant to the group and more correctly should be brought to the social workers. In some instances, the residents may not be interested in forming a council. In that case, at group therapy meetings the social worker or social work consultant should urge residents to assert themselves in a positive way to enhance the welfare of the group.

The rewards for the successful functioning of a residents' committee redound upon patients, whose energies are redirected to constructive activities; to staff members, who will find allies when residents understand problems, and to administration and governing bodies, who will benefit from direct, open two-way communication.

However, the governing bodies and administration of nursing homes must remember that once invited into the inner circle, residents will rightfully insist on remaining there. Resident participation in decision making cannot be episodic. Consistency and continuity are necessary for an effective democratic process.

RESIDENT ADVOCATES

Involvement in nursing home councils is the most obvious way for residents to pursue issues of self-determination. Other mechanisms, too, exist for resident participation on behalf of peers. For example, serving as contributing editor for the facility newsletter provides the opportunity to use the press for reform, change, and exchange of information. Writing letters to board members, legislators, and other power brokers is always a possible course of action open to residents. Other means for resident involvement are lobbying for more helpless residents who have no functioning family structure and contacting families or sponsors of fellow residents to influence the nursing home management to effect desired changes.

Skilled nursing facility residents often have sponsors other than family, such as old friends, former neighbors, or attorneys who act as conservators or guardians. Too often conservators and court-appointed committees have only a financial involvement, in effect leaving the resident with no advocate.

A resident advocate is an intercessor—one who pleads the cause for a resident. A family member or a sponsor may be classified as a resident advocate, but in general this title is given to a disinterested party who may be a volunteer in the facility who has developed a close attachment with one or two patients. A friendly volunteer may evolve into a resident advocate after learning of the frustration that some institutionalized elderly people experience. An advocate may also be a non–nursing home volunteer such as a member of a church auxiliary that has "adopted" the nursing home population or a so-called foster grandchild who has an ongoing relationship with an individual resident.

A professional facilitator, pathfinder, or case manager whose specific job is to locate existing resources for the ill elderly and to assure integration of needed services may serve as a resident advocate. Such a case manager would be the advocate of the person he helped place in the skilled nursing facility by providing the single continuous contact for advice and assistance, thereby cushioning the patient against unresponsive staff in the facility or disinterested social welfare bureaucrats.

FAMILIES AS CONSUMERS

It would appear that families or sponsors of patients in skilled nursing facilities would be ideally qualified to act as monitors of the quality of their relatives' care. Family members would have a genuine interest and, in all likelihood, would have experience with the problems of caring for the chronically ill aged. Relatives would engage in the monitoring process while visiting with the patient.

This type of family involvement has disadvantages, however. Families may be smitten with guilt about placing their relative in the nursing home and may criticize the facility to mask their own feelings. Families may be so emotionally involved with their relatives that it is virtually impossible for them to act objectively. In fact, relatives may become so overbearing in their advocacy role that an impossible rift may develop between them and the staff.

Just as resident councils have been developed to encourage participatory management and an open communication system, similar objectives may be realized with a family council or advisory committee. Instead of waiting to call general family/sponsor meetings when specific problems arise or when a rate increase is anticipated, it is preferable to have a functioning family advisory committee that meets regularly and tries to anticipate and prevent problems from occurring. As is the case with resident councils, such groups offer the administration the opportunity to educate families about the intricacies of long-term-care institutions—about government intervention, about Medicare and Medicaid, about third-party reimbursement, and so on. Educated families can be the best nursing home advocates because they understand the nature of the problems encountered better than most other concerned citizens.

Meetings with families can be administratively oriented meetings, such as with the family advisory committee, or therapeutic meetings. Therapeutic meetings might be orientation meetings for families of newly admitted residents to help them adjust to institutional life and associated concerns. They could be organized to deal only with families whose relatives are brain-damaged or to help the spouses of the institutionalized ill aged deal with their feelings.

Sometimes families wish to become involved with the nursing home community but need help in beginning. They can be encouraged to develop a pattern of group visiting; for example, they can entertain residents who have no families and visitors and can help families who find it troublesome to visit confused, disoriented relatives on a continuing basis. Indeed, it may be equally trying to pay regular visits to nonbrain-damaged residents because their lives are so circumscribed that they have little to discuss during visits. Of course, some residents do manage to continue interests outside themselves and thus remain stimulating conversationalists.

Some spouses or relatives enjoy the opportunity to serve as volunteers, although occasionally patients will not wish to share their family members and will become resentful of such activity. Volunteering gives the relative something more to do during regular visits and has the salutory effect of giving the resident a sense of importance because his relative is helping others. Families can help residents and even themselves by feeding patients, by accompanying residents on trips outside the facility, by driving residents to outside medical appointments, by helping in the recreation program, and so on.

Staff members will need some education along these lines, as they may be reluctant to give up patient care responsibilities. They may feel it is easier for them to feed patients than to have critical families around at all hours to observe, to ask questions, and generally to interfere with staff routines. If personnel learn how useful such volunteering is for families and how it affords them a sense of worth, they will be more patient with and understanding of such "interference."

Informed families can be the best liaison to state and national elected officials. Their collective clout represents votes to legislators, and it is therefore essential to keep them informed about developments in long-term care so that they act in the best interests of nursing home patients.

The facility should seriously consider including educated, interested, and willing family members or volunteers in the governing body. Due to their firsthand knowledge of the daily activities and problems of the nursing home, they will provide insight for the rest of the board and bring to its attention concerns of the nursing home community that might not otherwise be presented.

FIGURE 9-3
Family Advisory Committee

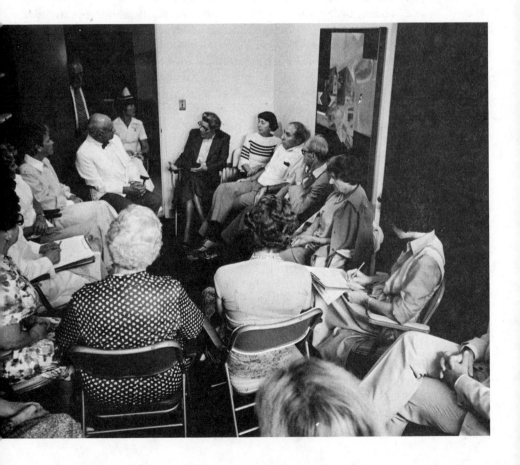

COMMUNITY INTERVENTION

In spite of the presence of various mechanisms to assess and upgrade the quality of care in skilled nursing facilities—such as state licensure, certification to participate in Medicare and Medicaid, and accreditation by the Joint Commission on Accreditation of Hospitals—the news media tend to feature horror stories about nursing homes, which has prompted concerned community members to want to become involved in improving the quality of nursing homes. Groups of citizens as varied as the Gray Panthers (elderly activists), the National Council of Senior Citizens, the AFL–CIO, and the American Jewish Congress are encouraging their membership to remain consistently involved with the problems of the ill aged rather than engaging in only intermittent crisis intervention.

Some community groups declare that skilled nursing facilities receiving government funding should be mandated to have lay governing bodies to analyze expenditures and evaluate care. They emphasize the use of community volunteers to conduct and publicize surveys in order to enhance public knowledge concerning the problems of skilled nursing facility patients. Advisory committees, youth groups, and other volunteer consortia can enhance public understanding of the long-term-care system by being well informed and spreading word-of-mouth support. It is critical, however, for such advocate groups to be more than well meaning; they must be educated about nursing home patients, their families, problems, needs, and prejudices before they assume activist roles.

The most obvious place for outside citizen groups to begin their programs of assuring quality in long-term care is at the referral source. If hospitals, social welfare and family agencies, and other nursing home referral organizations were to provide the continuity of care they publicly espouse, these agencies would follow their patients to the skilled nursing facility to determine the correctness of the original placement and the course of the patient's recovery or deterioration, and incidentally they would be exposed to the quality of care provided. Such a quality-assurance program would build on existing relationships and patterns of patient movement and could be a learning experience for all those involved.

Older citizens in the community are probably the next most logical group to have a vested interest in nursing homes and nursing home patients. Various so-called senior citizen groups have developed nursing home ombudsman programs. Ombudsman is a Scandinavian word to denote a government official who investigates complaints of citizens against the government or its bureaucrats. In such a program, volunteers supplement government surveys of a nursing home by investigating complaints and seeking recommendations from nursing home patients during weekly visits to the facility. The rationale for weekly visits by ombudsmen is to develop a cadre of informed volunteers who may be able to resolve problems directly and quickly by working with nursing home administrators.

In addition to involvement with patients, ombudsman committees at the local community level provide a vehicle for members of civic organizations, business groups, unions, religious leaders, families, and patients to work together to monitor and elevate the standards of care offered in skilled nursing facilities. It is suggested that unions affiliated with nursing homes and nursing home administrators be excluded from councils due to their vested interests or biased views.

Volunteer ombudsman programs have different approaches in urban and rural areas. In urban areas with many facilities, where the ombudsmen are probably strangers to the facilities and their patients, formal written complaints are the usual modus operandi. In rural areas, which generally have few facilities and few volunteer ombudsmen, the approach is less formal, less structured, and based on long-standing relationships between the ombudsmen and the providers and residents.

Alleged complaints can be categorized as follows:

1. The nature of institutional life: residents disturbing to other patients, drunken relatives disrupting facility while visiting, patients being left on bedpans too long, missing clothing and personal possessions, tipping, bathing of two sexes together, opening of personal mail, male residents "spying" on females, men and women sharing lavatories

2. Gaps in formalized programs: lack of in-service education for staff, lack of activities for residents, lack of reading materials, hardships of transferring patients as their conditions change

3. Gaps in professional technical services: insufficient physical therapy, untreated decubiti, slow or nonexistent dental services, shortage of staff, administration of medications by unqualified aides

4. The quality of services provided by unprofessional staff: patients verbally abused by aides, rough handling of patients by aides, difficult patients neglected, lunch brought into the room with dirty linen

5. Financial matters: unreasonable laundry charges, patients billed for Medicaid-covered services, refunds not given family after death of patient, accounting not given on request

6. Legal problems: eviction of patient without notice, no facilities for safekeeping of personal valuables

7. Nursing home rules and policies: failure to notify family
of patient stroke or accident, no grievance mechanism,
patients not permitted to leave premises, facility not
providing needed transportation for patient, nursing home
refusing to give physician telephone number, intact resident
wishing intact roommate
8. Dietary: food served cold, patient not receiving special
diet, residents given TV dinners on cook's day off
9. Poor physical facilities: urine odor, roaches, call bells out
of patients' reach, inadequate space for wheelchairs in
patient's bedrooms

Many of these issues warrant further explanation. For example, the policy of not permitting the patient to leave the premises may well be correct. Confused or debilitated patients cannot safely leave the premises unattended. Not having informed the family of a patient's stroke or accident may well relate to the dictum that the attending physician relay medical problems to the family. Urine odors among a severely handicapped patient population are understandable—even the most attentive staff cannot anticipate every incontinent act.

The nonexistence of dental services is an ever-present problem that relates to such factors as poor reimbursement for the dentist and the disinterest of families and sponsors in providing their relatives with dentures.

The criticism about transportation services underscores a problem area. For the facility to provide transportation, two people are needed: the driver and someone to assist the patient out of the car and up the stairs to the office. One person cannot handle this. If two persons are taken off the floors, who cares for other residents while they are gone?

These few instances underscore the need for an ombudsman educational program. Some of the criticisms are clearly valid and would be easily resolved; others are valid but difficult to resolve. And a portion are valid only in the eyes of uninformed, well-meaning amateurs.

Other structured citizen-based organizations devoted to handling complaints on behalf of aged patients and improving care are being tested. Families and friends of institutionalized aged have participated in the formation of membership organizations devoted to monitoring nursing home care and learning how to deal successfully with personnel and administrators in the prompt resolution of problems.

At the same time, such organizations perform an educational function by exposing friends and relatives to what constitutes quality nursing home care—and to federal and state requirements. This is accomplished by training friends and relatives to investigate and attempt to resolve complaints of other families in facilities where they do not have relatives. The investigators then have a certain detachment, although they still are consumers. It is essential that such groups have the professional expertise of physicians, psychiatrists, nurses, and social workers readily available to them to act as consultants and teachers.

Other approaches are the use of telephone hotlines that residents, staff, families, and visitors use to make direct complaint calls to a centralized government agency. This system, however, has proved less than satisfactory. It elicits many anonymous unsubstantiated calls, all of which must be followed up in the local areas, with great expenditures of time and money. While some reports may prove accurate, this methodology facilitates making complaints without personal accountability or investment on the part of the complainant.

Written complaints by consumers to government agencies and representatives require little more effort than hotline telephone calls. These practices encourage an adversarial relationship between the government representative investigating the complaint and the provider of service, as the nursing home is often assumed guilty until proved innocent.

Perhaps a more constructive approach is possible through existing relationships. Nursing home–hospital transfer agreements offer the hospitals who refer patients to a nursing home the opportunity, and indeed the responsibility, to become familiar with the services, practices, and staff of the nursing home. The hospital discharge coordinator and the hospital patient representative also could perform this service. In some instances, specially trained hospital volunteers are assigned this follow-up duty.

An extension of this function is the development of directories of area long-term-care services. Such a directory is usually formulated from data gleaned from planned visits to all facilities and the facilities' responses to a uniform questionnaire. Whether done by professional persons or by volunteers, due to time and experience limitations, this directory generally provides a rather superficial body of information.

Hospital staff physicians can also provide a quality mechanism by serving on the medical staffs and utilization review committees of the nursing homes with which the hospital has a transfer arrangement.

Possibly the most desirable and effective approach to community intervention in nursing home affairs is the appointment of community representatives to nursing home governing bodies so that each and every facility will have its own concerned consumers.

The importance of integrating the nursing home into the community, particularly with the help of volunteers, has been stated. However, for the community to be informed of the purpose, programs, and problems of the skilled nursing facility and of the ill elderly people in its care, the nursing home must assume responsibility for the educational process. It is unrealistic to expect the public to come to the nursing home to seek this knowledge; therefore the nursing home must reach out to the public.

The creation of a committee composed of professional staff, family members, volunteers, and other interested persons whose purpose it is to share this information with the community is one method to achieve the goal of public education. Representatives of the committee would arrange to speak to various organizations to discuss the process of aging, the problems it poses, identifying when an older person needs help, what financial assistance is available, nursing home placement and the alternatives, family expectations of their relative and the institution, and a host of other related topics. A committee with consumer members would provide a very personal approach; individuals could share their own experiences to help guide others who are or may in the future face similar problems. Naturally, professional supporting expertise should also be available.

SUMMARY

Nursing homes must move away from the closed view of the institution—dedicated to the convenience of staff—to a more open system allowing ease of communication and surveillance by interested members of the lay and professional communities.

Dietary

INTRODUCTION

In the eyes of residents, families, and community members, nursing home food service is often the primary factor in rating the skilled nursing facility. Visitors cannot readily evaluate the quality of professional services such as nursing or medical care, but everyone feels competent about judging food. Residents may focus their attention on the meal service and may be inordinately critical when what they are really experiencing is pain and desolation at having been placed in an institutional setting.

While it is acceptable to criticize the food, it is not generally acceptable to criticize, say, one's daughter for not caring for her parent at home. Likewise, families who are suffering from feelings of guilt because they have allowed strangers to provide care for their relatives, often overcriticize the nursing home dietary service to hide their own emotional struggles.

Food service also significantly influences staff morale. The serving of attractive and nutritious meals will reinforce to staff that the nursing home is not cutting corners in this crucial aspect of patient care. Likewise, the food service provided to employees can be a major factor in successful employee–management relations.

Large nursing homes may contract their entire foodservice operation to an outside company, along with full responsibility for its operation within a prescribed budget. This, of course, means that the nursing home may dispense with its own personnel; however, the dietary staff will then have its allegiance to the foodservice company rather than to the nursing home. Also, the nursing home will have to consider whether the personalized approach is being compromised by the use of a commercial service. The skilled nursing facility is still responsible for ensuring conformance with all prescribed government codes and regulations regarding dietary service, no matter who the provider is.

UNIQUE ASPECTS OF NURSING HOME DIETARY SERVICE

Although both are health care institutions, the nursing home foodservice is faced with different concerns than is the hospital foodservice. The hospital dietitian may never see patients on regular diets unless a problem arises. In the nursing home, however, the dietitian is involved with every patient and must develop a nutritional plan of care for each. The range of therapeutic diets available in the hospital is greater than in the skilled nursing facility, but the hospital patient follows the diet for a far shorter time so that there is little need to adapt the diet to the patient's preferences. Conversely, residents in nursing homes on special diets may remain on those diets permanently; therefore the diet must be made compatible with the resident's likes and dislikes.

In essence, the differences in providing a hospital or nursing home foodservice chiefly relate to the patients' length of stay. Since the skilled nursing facility is the patient's home, meals *must* be consistently good, and with sufficient variety so as to minimize the effect of institutional meals. The dietary staff must deal with personal food preferences and eating habits effectively to the satisfaction of the physician, the patient, and the staff, remembering that food patterns established over a lifetime are not easily abandoned. The staff will also have to consider religious and cultural customs when developing a nutritional plan for a long-term-care patient.

It may be necessary to consult with residents' families to explain to them the reasons for different diets and to request their cooperation, for family members may try to assuage their relative's complaints by bringing in a favorite food that is not permitted on the patient's diet.

Adequate nutrition is extremely important in the ill elderly population. A constant surveillance of weights must be carried on to alert the treating staff when a patient is losing weight, for a ten-pound weight loss can be critical. Indeed, feeding may become a life-saving treatment for some patients.

PATIENT DISABILITIES

Physical illness and psychosocial stresses influence nutritional stability. Diminished sensory perceptions, especially smell and taste, can radically affect the elderly's interest and enjoyment of food. Chronically ill older persons present further dietary constraints because their disabilities often affect their eating processes.

Perhaps foremost of these physical changes is the incidence of dentures found in the institutionalized aged population. Commonly, nursing home residents reject wearing their dentures. For some, poorly fitting dentures due to weight loss cause discomfort that may be remediable only via the purchase of new dentures.

For patients who do have their own teeth, keeping them in good repair can be important to their eating ability. A toothache of several days' duration may make chewing too painful. And if the patient does not chew enough, he may have trouble with swallowing and digestion.

For a patient who is unable to masticate properly due to loose dentures or lack of teeth, food may have to be mechanically altered to a chopped or pureed state. This in itself may be unappealing to the resident and cause him to reject food. Therefore it is important both for the patient to have proper dentition and for meals to be served in the proper consistency to each patient.

Foods should not be pureed for the convenience of the staff. A periodic reassessment of patients on pureed diets should be conducted to ascertain whether the patient is capable of progressing to chopped food, which may be more time-consuming for the feeding staff although more appetizing for the patient.

Attendants who feed patients pureed foods must be trained to do so properly. Individual pureed foods—meat, vegetable, potato—should not be mashed together with ice cream and then fed to the patient as one indescribable concoction. Each item should be fed separately, to allow the patient to experience the taste differences.

Poor vision may also be an impediment to the eating processes of nursing home residents. A visually impaired resident may be trained to feed himself independently via the clock method of locating food on his dish and items on the table. He may become discouraged and embarrassed to eat with his peers if he is always spilling and making a mess of himself and his plate; or, as so often happens with blind patients, he may revert to eating with his fingers.

A hearing loss can affect a patient's interest in eating, just as it may discourage his participation in other activities. Hard-of-hearing people may become social isolates, characterized by withdrawal and its associated behavior, including a diminished desire to eat.

Certainly, limited range of motion in arms and hands (as is found in arthritic patients or in those with recent fractures) or lack of muscle strength (common in stroke patients) poses severe restrictions on the ability to feed oneself. Retraining is necessary, perhaps with the help of adaptive devices. While it is important that these patients be encouraged to feed themselves, they will need close supervision and possibly assistance to make sure they are eating adequate quantities.

Perceptual deficiencies that are commonly encountered with brain-damaged patients may be incorrectly identified as noncooperation.

Apraxia, the inability to conceptualize an act and/or execute it upon command, may severely limit a patient's ability to feed himself. A careful, thorough treatment plan must be carried out to retrain such a person, although its success will depend on the degree of brain damage.

Intellectually impaired patients must be thoroughly supervised during meals. They may nibble a little at their food but not eat sufficiently, or they may eat their neighbor's meal rather than their own. A certain percentage of these patients will need total assistance in feeding.

Residents may express emotional difficulties through their eating habits. For example, a resident with a dependent personality may insist on having staff assistance to eat when he is perfectly capable of self-feeding. Behavior modification may be needed to train such residents to feed themselves.

It should not be overlooked that changes in medication can decrease appetite and thus influence food intake.

Finally, residents may manifest depression by not eating. This may occur in varying degrees—some may just pick at their food and some might totally refuse to eat in an expression of a death wish. These patients must be properly supervised, perhaps by receiving substantial between-meal nourishments in addition to encouragement during regular mealtimes. Involving these people in a whole range of activities as part of the treatment plan should be stressed so that they will take an interest in themselves that includes feeding themselves. The insertion of a nasogastric tube is, of course, a more extreme alternative for feeding a patient who cannot or will not take any substance orally.

The results of a cross-national study of skilled nursing facilities revealed that about 75 percent of all residents required some assistance with their meals and that 24 percent needed self-help feeding devices.[1]

STAFFING PATTERN
Consulting Dietitian

A 100-bed skilled nursing facility will require a consulting dietitian for twenty-hours per week to provide the professional guidance necessary in the operation of the institution's dietary facilities. As a health professional involved in patient care, the dietitian is responsible to the medical director; however, his guidance in the operation of the foodservice department necessitates reporting to the administrative director on those matters.

The consultant dietitian's primary role is to assess, evaluate, and plan each resident's nutrition program. The dietitian has ongoing contact with residents from the initial development of each resident's nutritional history to the preparation of the patient for discharge from the facility. The dietitian reviews all physician diet orders, confers with the physician when needed, and, in conjunction with the nutritional history information, develops each resident's dietary plan of care. Regular consultation with the nursing staff is necessary to monitor patient tolerance of the diet and to determine patient improvement. The dietitian may recommend changes in the consistency of the diet or suggest a change in physician's orders.

The dietitian must also develop therapeutic diets and instruct staff in how to prepare and integrate them with the regular house diet. In addition, he should prepare a four-week-cycle menu for each season of the year, which he should continually review and change according to the availability and cost of food and patient tolerances.

The dietitian and the foodservice supervisor should confer routinely to review the daily operation of the dietary service, including the preparation and serving of all diets, the standardization of recipes, procedural changes to enhance personnel or food efficiency, and the maintenance of proper sanitation and infection control techniques in all aspects of the foodservice. The dietitian should take an active role in determining the quality and quantity of food to be purchased and must always know current food costs. Finally, the dietitian should participate in recommending and selecting new supplies and equipment.

The dietitian coordinates the dietary service with other patient care services. In-service education directed to both dietary and nursing personnel is a vital part of the dietitian's role, particularly as he is not a full-time staff member.

Qualifications for a consultant dietitian would include a bachelor's or graduate degree, with a major in food, nutrition, or institutional management, from an accredited institution. In addition, the dietitian should be a member or a qualified candidate for membership in the American Dietetic Association. Specific knowledge of geriatric dietary needs and supervisory experience in a health care setting are both highly desirable. Considerable initiative and judgment are required in developing and adapting diets to meet individual needs and preferences.

Foodservice Supervisor

Several staffing alternatives are available for the full-time foodservice supervisor. A dietetic technician may be recruited for this position. This person should have an associate degree, should meet definitive qualifications of the American Dietetic Association, and should be skilled in foodservice administration or nutrition care. With consultation from the registered dietitian and the administrative director, a dietetic technician can plan menus for regular and therapeutic diets and be responsible for all other operational aspects of the foodservice—purchasing, personnel, sanitation, record maintenance, and so on. Since a dietetic technician is trained to participate in the professional area of patient nutritional care, this position would be of great help to the consultant dietitian by providing continuity on the days when the dietitian is not on duty.

If not a dietetic technician, the foodservice supervisor must be a graduate of a foodservice management program that provides special training in foodservice administration, nutrition, therapeutic diets, personnel management, and sanitary regulations. Furthermore, the foodservice supervisor must remain current on dietary techniques and health code regulations.

If the foodservice supervisor assumes cooking duties, his title should then be changed to "cook manager" to indicate the two functions. This position is directly responsible to the administrator but receives required supervision and consultation from the dietitian.

The daily operation of the dietary department is the foodservice supervisor's responsibility. This includes selecting and supervising all dietary personnel, purchasing all food and supplies, receiving orders, properly storing all items, and maintaining cleanliness in the foodservice area. The foodservice supervisor plans and performs or directs the preparation and serving of all meals to residents and staff. Keeping required records of invoices, meals served, inventory of all goods, and the Kardex of patient dietary needs is assigned to the foodservice supervisor.

The position of foodservice supervisor is critical in terms of conforming to dietary standards within a prescribed budget and providing tasteful meals. Special requirements of a foodservice supervisor include alertness and attention to detail in observing dietary and sanitary standards and good judgment and initiative in all aspects of ordering, preparing food, supervising personnel, and adapting menus and procedures when necessary. Because the foodservice supervisor serves a vital function in relation to residents and staff, he must be able to work effectively and maintain a spirit of cooperation with all facility constituencies.

Assistant Foodservice Supervisor

The appointment of a competent and responsible assistant foodservice supervisor is necessary to ensure the smooth operation of the foodservice when the supervisor is not on duty. The assistant should also be a graduate of a food supervisor's course and thus be able to assume full responsibility for managing the kitchen when so scheduled.

Other Personnel

The foodservice supervisor should follow certain guidelines when scheduling department personnel. He should determine that the most capable and best trained chef or chefs are assigned to the noon and evening meals. The breakfast cook need not be so skilled but must be completely reliable, as it is his job to come in early and begin the breakfast preparations. The foodservice supervisor needs to be sure that the staff is capable of preparing the menu items, utilizing mechanical aids when necessary and prepared foods when feasible.

The number of other dietary positions required, either full- or part-time, depends on providing a sufficient number of staff members for each meal of the day. On a regular basis, at least three people are needed for breakfast, five for the noon meal (if it is the dinner meal), and three for supper. More staff members are needed at mid-day because dinner is a more involved meal and feeds more people when considering guests and staff. Also, preparations are going on simultaneously for meals other than dinner: making supplements and nourishments for the afternoon and evening, making initial preparations for the following day's menu, ordering supplies, receiving deliveries, baking, and preparing the supper according to the day's menu selections.

Additional staff may be scheduled on days of special activities, parties, or luncheons, when heavy cleaning is planned, when large deliveries are due, or if new staff members are being trained to allow sufficient time for them to be adequately familiarized with the routine.

The kitchen is like a well-oiled machine when it is functioning well. Because it is labor dependent, however, it is very vulnerable to breakdown. Proper leadership from the foodservice supervisor and guidance from the consultant dietitian, naturally, play a big role in its efficient operation, but the ability of each individual to do his job and of the entire kitchen staff to work together cooperatively is basic.

Dietary staff members can be difficult to recruit because the nature of the work attracts unskilled, often unsettled, people who also may hold a second job to augment their income. The candidate's attendance and longevity record at previous jobs, his initiative to perform job duties without constant follow-up, his cleanliness, and the degree of his cooperation with fellow employees should be checked. Most of all, it is imperative to impress on potential employees that reporting to work when scheduled is essential, for otherwise their work becomes a burden to others.

The following sanitation practices need continuing emphasis for dietary personnel:

    the absolute necessity for personal cleanliness and frequent
        handwashing
    the prohibition of handling of food by personnel with
        abrasions, pimples, or infections
    acceptable cleaning of all utensils and equipment

proper inspection of food on delivery
correct storage of raw, packaged, or cooked food
approved method of washing of fresh foods
correct use of utensils rather than fingers in food preparation
picking up utensils by handles and bases, not by food-contact
    or drinking surfaces

DIETS

After considering the medical problems predominating in the skilled nursing facility population, the dietitian should develop or review the range of diets provided regularly in the facility. Consultation and, indeed, final approval of the standardized diets of the nursing home must be obtained from the medical director or medical staff (if it is organized).

Diet Manual

The house and therapeutic diets should be fully described in writing in the diet manual, which should be available at each nursing station, in the kitchen, and in appropriate offices. The manual should describe each diet in full, its purpose, its nutritional breakdown, a suggested meal plan, permitted foods, and general rules in following the diet. By reading the manual, physicians, nurses, the dietitian, and the dietary staff should have a mutual understanding of the diets available.

Should a physician order a diet that is not listed in the diet manual, the dietitian must be informed so that he can develop it and direct the staff in its preparation. In some instances, the dietitian may be able to suggest simply modifying a diet that is already listed in the manual.

Nutrition

Nutrients needed for life and health include proteins, vitamins, minerals, carbohydrates, and fats. All are available in foods and, although invisible to the naked eye, can be calculated chemically and weighed in grams, ounces, and pounds. Calories are a unit of measurement that express the energy value of a food. Although the Food and Nutrition Board of the National Academy of Sciences–National Research Council has established recommended daily allowances of calories for healthy people, there are no special allowances for the ill aged. We know only that they need fewer calories because they are less physically active.

Proteins are the basic material in every cell of body tissue and are needed for growth, repair, and renewal of tissue. Convalescent patients may require extra protein for producing new tissue and repairing damaged tissue.

House Diet

The regular, or house, diet should be designed to meet the nutritional needs of older persons who have no dietary restrictions while maintaining the caloric content at 2000 calories (approximately 75 percent of the calories needed by the average person) and providing variety in food color, texture, temperature, and flavor. Consideration should be given to restricting the sodium content of the regular diet to 2.5 grams daily due to the high incidence of circulatory problems and heart disease among chronically ill aged people. No additional salt should be used in cooking, and physician approval should be sought before allowing patients to add salt or a salt substitute to their food at meals. If necessary, the dietitian can develop a special diet that restricts salt even further.

All these restrictions do not mean that meals must be tasteless and unflavorful. The efficacious use of herbs, spices, and lemon juice can serve as salt substitutes to provide palatable meals.

For patients who like to add salt to their food, but for whom it is restricted, supervision should be provided so as to prevent its excessive use. The reasons for monitoring salt intake may be a topic for discussion at the residents' council meeting.

Mechanically Altered Diets

Diets may be modified to meet varying nutritional needs. A mechanically altered soft diet should be offered to those who have difficulty in chewing due to dental problems or as a result of a stroke; it may also be necessary for certain gastrointestinal disturbances. A soft diet is typically a regular diet with chopped or pureed meat and chopped or mashed vegetables.

Both clear and full liquid diets may be ordered. A clear liquid (broth or jello) diet has little nutritional value and must be ordered only for a very short period. It should be used in a nursing home only if a patient is unable to hold down any other food. Full liquid (milk) diets in the skilled nursing facility are ordered for patients who are unable to chew or swallow solid food. It, too, is low in nutritional value and should be used for a brief period only. The patient should progress to puree as soon as possible.

Nasogastric Tube Feeding

Nasogastric tube feeding is considered a method of treatment when a patient is unable to eat or is not eating adequately. The feedings, obviously, must be liquid enough to pass through the tube. While prepared tube feedings are available, they sometimes cause diarrhea in the aged debilitated patient, who may better tolerate regular fresh foods or baby foods (which seem to offend many people) that are blended for tube feeding because the body has become accustomed to their use over long periods. Furthermore, liquefied natural foods are less costly than oral or intravenous manufactured feeding formulas.

Mechanically blended foods must be carefully strained through a fine mesh strainer to remove bones, seeds, and fibrous material that may plug the tube. Foods can be liquefied via screen or colloid mills for large-scale use. Tube feedings must not be prepared in bulk amounts to last several days, rather, they must be made up each day, dated, and disposed of if not used within twenty-four hours. The use of liquefied natural foods must be supervised carefully due to the increased risk of contamination. If not prepared, bottled, and stored properly and administered within twenty-four hours, a facility formula may serve as a medium for bacterial growth, which may cause diarrhea.

Other Therapeutic Diets

The standard diabetic diet could be based on the regular diet but should eliminate concentrated sweets. For diabetic patients who need to lose weight, the dietitian should develop a diabetic diet with lower caloric content. Overweight patients who are not diabetic must receive a diet that is limited in calories. A fat-restricted diet is prescribed for patients who are concerned with a high cholesterol level, or for patients with gall bladder problems, in which case vegetables are also excluded.

Other frequently prescribed diets that should be included in a diet manual are a bland diet, which eliminates foods that are stimulating or irritating to the stomach, and diets altered in residue, which are used to treat and control symptoms of diverticulitis, diverticulosis, and atonic constipation. Residue, or fiber, refers to carbohydrates that are not digested and absorbed by the body. The low-residue diet requiring the use of specific cooked fruits and vegetables (which may need to be mashed or pureed) and refined breads and cereals was until recently the standard treatment for diverticulitis and diverticulosis. However, some nutritionists now affirm that the high-residue diet, which emphasizes whole grain cereals and bread and high-fiber fruits and vegetables, may be more effective for the control and prevention of these gastrointestinal disorders.

Nourishments

Finally, the diet manual should delineate the nourishments provided regularly or when specially ordered by the attending physician. Nourishments have greater nutritional value than standard between-meal snacks and are offered when a patient's weight is below normal limits or when the patient's intake at meals is insufficient. Nourishments should be prepared in the kitchen daily and dated before being sent to the nursing unit pantries; those not eaten must be removed when replaced by the following day's supply. The nursing staff should maintain a record of nourishment consumption so as to be able to review the patient's food intake thoroughly when examining weight loss or gain.

Special Diet Requirements

The nursing facility will have to determine if the range of diets offered will also satisfy the requirements of certain religious observances and, if so, to what extent. Will additional equipment and facilities be needed? For example, Jewish residents may request kosher service, and if they are not rigidly orthodox, the use of kosher frozen food trays is a viable alternative. To accommodate patients who observe strict dietary laws, a kosher facility with two separate kitchens—one for meat dishes and one for dairy foods—is the only answer. It would be extremely cumbersome for a nursing home without a kosher kitchen to try to prepare several different types of therapeutic diets for kosher patients.

MENU PLANNING

Menu planning must take into account the nutritional requirements for those on the regular diet and those on therapeutic diets. Menus offered may be nonselective or selective for all meals or for some, either of which can be cyclical and repeated after a prearranged period.

A set menu offers almost no choice to the resident except that preferences related to beverages or manner of cooking eggs or special dislikes may be followed in most instances. Nonselective menus purportedly save money and time and mirror the food service of a resident's home, where set meals were customary. Frequently, residents prefer a standardized breakfast; many people like the same kind of cereal or eggs with the same beverage every morning.

However, the importance of food to the institutionalized person raises the issue of not being able to please everyone with a single menu and, therefore, the advisability of adding some choice. The opportunity for personal decision making in one's daily routine should be encouraged among the ill aged, who so often have all decision-making responsibilities taken away from them. Perhaps a compromise would be for the heavier dinner meal to conform to a set menu, with a backup choice for personal dislikes, and for the lighter meal to offer a choice of hot and cold entrees.

By designating the dinner meal to conform to a set menu, residents are ensured of receiving one nutritionally complete meal. Providing choice from a selected menu may not guarantee the same assurance. Also, a choice menu for the dinner meal would not be possible unless the nursing home had the facilities and personnel to cook two or more full meals.

Cycle menus can be planned on a three- or four-week basis, with separate cycles prepared for the different seasons. This system reduces the arduous task of continuous complete meal planning: after the initial menus have been field tested and adapted to the special needs of the nursing home residents, they need only be adjusted according to the availability of foods or changing tastes of residents. This flexible approach will allow the food buyer to take advantage of seasonal good buys, which can be offset by the occasional prearranged use of a more expensive food item. Thus, while a certain amount of standardization is helpful to the dietary staff, resident meals should be flexible.

The dietitian and foodservice supervisor should plan the menus at least one week in advance and post them in the dietary department for kitchen staff to refer to when needed. The upcoming week's menu should also be posted in an area where residents, other staff, and visitors can see it. After their use, menus should remain on file for a minimum of one month.

The question of when to serve dinner—at mid-day or in the evening—should be determined by patient preference. Dietary staff may prefer to have the heavy, more complicated meal at noon when it is easier to recruit personnel. Noninvolved staff may opt for their customary practice of dinner in the evening. Although some residents may concur with that pattern and state that the heavy meal keeps them satisfied until morning, other older people prefer to have their large meal at mid-day because it agrees with their digestive processes.

Some nursing homes use a five-meal-per-day plan, which means that five small meals are served at intervals during the day and evening. Less food is offered more frequently to allow for the smaller appetites of less active older people. Even with the conventional practice and minimal requirement of three meals per day, mid-morning, afternoon, and pre-bedtime snacks must be provided to augment the residents' food intake.

Many persons advocate the use of wine or liquor to enhance the sociability of mealtimes and to stimulate flagging appetites. Perhaps the nursing home can institute a carefully supervised cocktail hour or serve a glass of wine with dinner. Such a practice may keep relatives and friends from secretly bringing liquor to residents, who should not drink without supervision.

RESIDENT MEAL SERVICE

Types of service in a single skilled nursing facility may be diverse—tray service for those who are essentially bedbound, table service for those able to benefit from group dining, and cafeteria service for staff and selected residents.

A foodservice may be centralized or decentralized. In centralized service, all trays or plates are assembled in a central kitchen and are transported via heated trucks or conveyors to dining areas and patient bedrooms and returned to the central area for washing. Decentralized tray or plate service permits the transportation of prepared bulk or portioned items via hot and cold trucks to serving pantries for assembly and delivery to dining areas or patient bedrooms. In this type of service, items such as coffee, toast, and eggs may be prepared in the individual pantries. Dirty dishes may be washed in areas adjacent to pantries or in the central kitchen and returned to pantries in preparation for the next meal.

While centralized kitchen service requires considerable kitchen space but only limited pantry areas, it provides the best check for uniformity in quality and portion control. Furthermore, equipment in a central kitchen does not need to be duplicated elsewhere in the facility, and personnel may be used to the best advantage in one site under direct supervision. In the centralized system, where even toast is prepared in the kitchen, the speedy transportation and distribution of food is an important component of an effective dietary service, for hot and cold dishes must be served at the proper temperature.

Coordination with the nursing staff will be necessary to achieve a smoothly run meal service for residents. Tables must be set when the meal trucks arrive on the unit, although not too far in advance to limit use of the area for other activities. Residents must be made ready for dining and assisted to the dining area, if necessary, before the meal is placed on the table.

It should be predetermined if the food for residents who need to be assisted in eating is sent up before or after the food for self-feeding patients, according to arrangements made by nursing personnel. If the feeders require so much more time to finish their meals, some nursing staff may be assigned to that duty while others distribute dishes to and pour beverages for the self-feeding patients.

Meal supervision is a function of nursing but requires the cooperation of dietary personnel, especially with respect to allowing sufficient time for the residents to eat. Color-coded tray cards identifying the patient's diet, beverage preference, assistive devices used, and other pertinent information should accompany each patient's tray or covered dish to guide the nursing staff.

Seating arrangements in the dining room will require some thought. Perhaps two patients who need maximum assistance and one who needs only encouragement may be placed at the same table with an attendant. The nursing staff will have to decide whether patients receiving modified diets—especially those that are mechanically altered— should be seated at the same table with residents who are not on special diets. For some residents, the sight of chopped or pureed food may be unappetizing and spoil their dinner. Others may find it disagreeable to dine with someone who must be fed. And intellectually impaired residents who eat from their neighbor's plate need close supervision.

Meal service should be scheduled according to the needs of the patients and the total program, with no more than a fourteen-hour lapse between the evening meal and breakfast. The tendency for the evening meal to be served too early must be carefully avoided. An early supper or dinner will guarantee an overly long evening for residents or too early a bedtime.

EMPLOYEE MEAL SERVICE

Meal service for personnel can be offered via vending machines, snack bar, coffee shop, or cafeteria. Vending machines, which can be stocked by the dietary department or by an outside vending service, have the advantage of being accessible twenty-four hours a day—a particular advantage for the night and evening staffs, who are on duty when other foodservice systems generally are not operative. Coffee shops, which serve light meals such as soups, sandwiches, salads, desserts, and beverages, have proved popular in very large institutions. Partial table service with waitresses might be provided in facilities that are large enough to support such a service. Coffee shops or snack bars may be an extension of the dietary department or may be run by volunteers and/or auxiliaries as a convenience and a source of funds. The nursing home must ascertain the need for a separate permit for a coffee shop or snack bar that is not operated from the main kitchen.

The cafeteria is the most typical arrangement for service of food to personnel. Menus may be extensive or limited. Frequently, personnel like to bring their own sandwiches and purchase only items like desserts and beverages in the cafeteria.

The use of the cafeteria may depend on the philosophy of the nursing home concerning the pricing of staff meals. Some institutions prefer to operate on a nonprofit basis and consider the cafeteria a convenience for both employees and management. Others prefer that it be operated as a business, with an allowance for some profit. A third group feels that personnel have meals at the nursing home to accommodate the nursing home schedules and, therefore, that the cafeteria should be subsidized by the institution to provide a benefit to employees.

A break-even position seems to make the most sense, the rationale being that the nursing home should neither profit from personnel meals nor sell them at a loss, which generally is neither appreciated nor understood. An exemplary foodservice can be a great morale booster and poor employee dietary service can be extremely detrimental to effective management–employee relations. Residents' and visitors' attitudes toward management, too, can be influenced undesirably if employee meal service is known to be unsatisfactory.

If both residents and staff are served from the same kitchen and have the same menu, several factors must be borne in mind. Employee serving times should not coincide with the serving time of residents' meals to ensure that food is not delayed in its arrival to the resident units and possibly affect its serving temperature. A separate, earlier cooking of staff meals may be necessary if employees eat before residents. Although dietary staff must follow a set schedule of serving times, flexibility is needed to provide meals to personnel who may have missed their break due to an emergency.

An effective dietary department depends on a combination of qualified and well-motivated personnel, successful operational practices, and good facilities and equipment. The timing of kitchen tasks is important to make certain that no one person or piece of equipment is overloaded at any given time. Complicated meals may require some advance preparation, but in no instance should food be cooked hours ahead so that it will need to be reheated prior to serving.

RECORDS

The diet card is completed by the nurse when the patient is admitted or when there is a change in diet. It notes the patient's name, the diet order, and if there is an altered consistency. A diet card for each patient is maintained in a Kardex in the kitchen for reference by dietary employees.

The supper menu choice form, completed daily, notes patients' selections. It is used to prepare the correct quantity of each food item.

A diet census sheet records the number of each type of diet served for every meal every day and notes the total number of meals served to patients, staff, and guests.

To facilitate guaranteeing that required cleaning procedures assigned to personnel have been completed, a checklist may be developed whereby the assigned employee initials the work he has completed.

The nutritional history form (Exhibit 10–1) must be completed as soon as possible after admission of the patient; the information should be gleaned from the patient in the initial interview. If the patient is unable to offer this material, the responsible relative should be asked to provide it. By learning the patient's dietary habits and food preferences, the dietitian can develop a plan of care designed specifically for the patient.

EXHIBIT 10-1
Nutritional History

NUTRITIONAL HISTORY

Patient's name _____ Admission date _____

Room no. _____

In the interest of providing good nutritional care for your relative, we would appreciate your assistance in completing the following form. Thank you.

1. Typical Daily Food Plan:

    Breakfast   Noon Meal   Evening Meal

2. What foods or beverages does your relative particularly like?

3. What foods or beverages does your relative particularly dislike?

4. Please check the foods in the following list that your relative likes. (These are typical between-meal snacks that are served to residents.)

    fruit juice and fruit punch
    cookies and crackers
    milk
    eggnog
    custard
    milkshakes: vanilla, chocolate, strawberry, coffee
    sandwiches: peanut butter
                 cream cheese and jelly
                 American chesse
                 cold sliced meat
                 egg salad
                 tuna salad
                 chicken salad

The nutrition care plan documents and collates information received from the patient or his relative, disabilities or handicaps affecting the patient's dietary program, nutritional goals for the patient, and the method of implementing those goals.

The dietitian should record the patient's progress in the chart on the nutritional progress note form. Changes in the diet order, a list of medications, and a weight record should be reported on this form for quick reference, along with space for progress notes.

A marketing list should be sent to the kitchen daily by the charge nurse on each unit. This form orders certain staples and the tube feedings required for the day, to be kept in the pantry of each unit.

Standard recipe files should be a part of the records maintained in the kitchen to ensure that meals will be prepared according to standardized recipes. Standardization prevents the loss of nutritional values due to food waste or changes resulting from quantity cooking, such as not needing to cook 50 lbs. of meat twice as long as 25 lbs. Standard recipes preclude cooking more than is needed and guarantee that food will be prepared as intended (and thus appear appetizing).

FACILITIES AND EQUIPMENT

Dietary departments that are arranged efficiently with delivery and storage areas contiguous or close to preparation areas can be managed more easily and economically. However, the kitchen layout must have sound infection control techniques such as having food preparation and storage areas separate from both the dishwashing and garbage disposal areas, distinct sinks for cleaning food and handwashing, carefully laid pipes and drainage systems, proper ventilation, and a floor plan that keeps delivery men and unnecessary personnel from passing through the kitchen.

Good lighting and noise control are as important as the layout of the department. Lighting can make a difference in the safety, sanitation, and maintenance practices of dietary personnel; the use of light colors for walls and ceilings in kitchen areas is suggested for this reason.

Noise control in food preparation and service areas is important for reasons of morale and safety. Proper planning, such as in the separation of dishwashing areas from dining rooms, is basic. Other suggestions for noise reduction include the careful inspection of the noise produced by refrigerators, freezers, and ice machines prior to their selection and purchase. Compression units should be sealed, and motors and compressors should be mounted on bases with vibration isolators. Vibration isolators should also be used on dishwashing equipment. The sheet metal of dishwashers and metal sinks and cabinets should be undercoated for partial noise reduction.

Other considerations in dishwasher purchase are to make sure that the temperature of the wash water reaches 150°F (66°C) and the rinse water 180°F (82°C), and that the washer is equipped with a ventilating fan.

Special attention should be paid to the dishwashing process. For example, speedy handling of dirty dishes and utensils will keep food scraps from hardening. Maintenance of proper water temperature, correct racking and exposure time, and the use of standardized amounts of detergent and water contribute to effective mechanical dishwashing that meets sanitization standards.

If employee meals are prepared in the central kitchen, the staff dining room should be adjacent to the kitchen for accessibility. It should include an adequate number of tables and chairs, a coffee pot, and a small refrigerator for personnel who bring food from home. A bulletin board for posting employee notices would also be convenient in this room.

The dietary staff should investigate whether to use china or plastic plates. China is more attractive and is not subject to staining, but plastic, of course, will not break. The selection could be based on the disabilities of the patient population, with plastic used for confused residents who might be apt to break china. Similar considerations would be appropriate for glass or plastic beverage containers. An inventory of china, glassware, and flatware should be maintained in a locked cabinet in the storeroom.

Staple food items must be stored in a cool, ventilated room that is equipped with rustproof metal shelves arranged at least one foot from the floor. No foods, either canned or packaged, may be stored on the floor, and opened packages of dry items should be placed in carefully labeled stainless steel and/or plastic containers.

Cleaning items must be stored in an area separate from food goods. Paper goods, too, should be in a specially designated section of the storage room.

Other food storage and holding equipment should include a freezer, a walk-in and/or compartment refrigerator, and a salad refrigerator. All these appliances must have an easily readable thermometer. The refrigerators should be maintained at 45°F (7°C) and the freezers at 32°F (0°C).

Major cooking equipment that belongs in an institutional kitchen includes two ranges—one with flat-top heating surface and the other with six individual grated heating surfaces—with ventilating fans and a built-in automatic fire extinguisher, a grill, and an attached oven that

FIGURE 10-1
Off-floor Food Storage

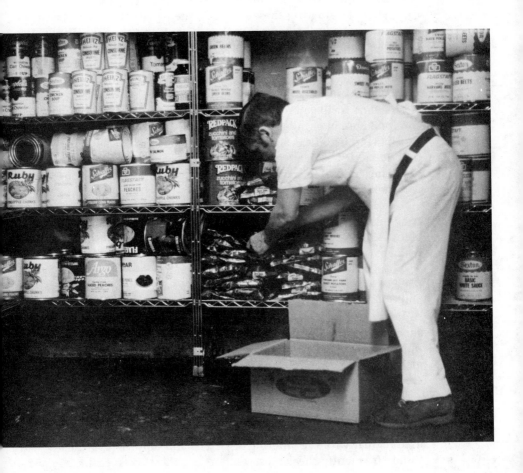

may be used for both roasting and baking. A convection oven might also be provided for more rapid roasting and baking. A steamer, a rotary toaster, two six-gallon coffee makers, two heavy-duty two-quart blenders, a floor-mounted mixer with attachments for grinding, grating, and so on, and a heavy duty food slicer are also needed.

A particularly important concern of the foodservice in skilled nursing facilities is that food temperatures must be properly maintained. A variety of distribution methods may be used for this purpose. Limitations such as the immediate availability of elevators sometimes deter the speedy distribution of food carts and thus mechanical aids are needed to ensure the maintenance of heat. Covered hot plates, preheated pellets with an insulated plate assembly, and preheated sectional heat-resistant, heavy glass plates sealed in an insulated container are methods of choice. All three require thermal containers for soups and beverages.

When considering these methods, the dietary staff must take into account the medical problems of the residents and the durability of the equipment. For residents who are confused, the heated pellet system might prove dangerous. Even metal plate covers may be too hot for nursing home patients to handle. Insulated plastic plate covers are safe for patients but may be spoiled by the heat of the mechanical dishwasher, and insulated compartmentalized plates are not appropriate for continued use over indefinite periods.

Other possibilities are the use of heated carts or trucks for trays or for individual dishes. Such carts are costly, heavier to wheel, and may undergo mechanical breakdown, but they may be the preferable method of food delivery.

To test food temperatures after serving and upon delivery to the resident units, a stem thermometer must be used. Cold foods should be below 45°F (7°C) and hot foods above 140°F (60°C) when placed at the residents' dining tables.

Major dietary equipment should be bought or replaced by a competitive bidding method that takes into account both quality and availability of service. The director of maintenance should always be consulted regarding such purchases. The consulting dietitian, foodservice supervisor, and administrative director should confer and decide on the purchasing of smaller equipment, such as trays, china, silverware, and glassware. The availability of these items in open stock should be considered for replacement purposes.

Food Items

To maintain healthy competitiveness, at least two vendors should be used regularly for the ordering of all food and supplies. The dietary staff should frequently check these vendors' accuracy, costs, quality of goods, reliability in delivery, and willingness to stock items needed by the nursing home. Local vendors should be given preference in order to develop good relationships with community tradespeople for fast, dependable service.

The foodservice supervisor must arrange with the purveyors for specific delivery days during the week so that supplies are on hand when needed. To guard against emergencies when deliveries cannot be made, the facility should have on hand a forty-eight-hour supply of perishable foods and a one-week supply of nonperishables (commercially produced food products). Delivery schedules vary according to the items. Dairy products and bread should be delivered four to five times during the week, meat and fresh produce twice a week, and canned and packaged goods, cleaning supplies, and paper goods once a week. Deliveries of frozen foods can be less frequent—every two to three weeks—if the freezer space is available, as their shelf life is much longer.

The process of receiving foods is as important as ordering good quality and proper quantity. Meat, fish, and poultry should be weighed upon delivery and inspected for freshness. Particular caution is needed in observing for damaged cans and packaged goods, leaks, and broken bottles. Frozen foods must be frozen upon receipt and immediately placed in the freezer. Items should be dated when received, and stock should be rotated so stocked foods are used before new deliveries are.

Convenience Foods

Food items bought in ready-to-use or partially prepared form such as frozen, canned, or dehydrated food, bakery products and other desserts, and individual packets of sugar, cream, and jelly reduce labor hours in the dietary department. When consideration is being given to the purchase of convenience food items, the savings in labor time should be subtracted from the total cost of the particular food. Sometimes new equipment will have to be purchased and additional space found—e.g., additional freezer area—in the kitchen to accommodate such convenience foods. The total equipment cost including repairs, electricity, and depreciation should also be considered when planning the budget. Likewise, the available facilities for resultant increased trash disposal will also require study.

While the use of prepared food is advocated to cut waste and labor and thus overall costs, economy may not result because generally, proportionately little foodservice labor goes into actual cooking. Prepared foods must still be placed in dishes and served; items such as desserts have to be portioned prior to serving. A further consideration in the use of prepared foods is the steadily increasing cost of energy, which might make microwave ovens too costly to operate.

Although convenience foods and disposable serviceware may be acceptable to hospital patients when the hospitalization is brief, nursing home residents may reject such meals and accoutrements as long-term experiences. In the skilled nursing facility, the use of tablecloths, china, and cutlery may add an important homelike dimension to mealtime activities.

RELATIONS WITH FAMILIES AND VISITORS

Problems raised by families and visitors relating to the food service may often be intertwined with other more emotion-laden issues regarding their relative's placement in the nursing home. Therefore these issues are most appropriately discussed by the dietitian with the social service worker, and perhaps best left for his action.

Arrangements must be made for allowing for families and visitors to dine with their friends or relatives. The nursing home should clarify how much notice is required, whom to notify, how much it will cost, and where residents with guests may dine.

Certain regulations should be developed and communicated regarding bringing in food to residents. Visitors should be asked to announce food gifts to the nursing staff to make sure that it is allowed on the patient's diet and to make arrangements for its refrigeration or proper storage. If residents keep candy, cookies, or fruit in their rooms, the nursing staff must be aware of it so that it will not be left there indefinitely with the potential of attracting bugs. The infection control committee may want to address itself to the issue of families bringing in home-canned or jarred foods because of the possible hazards of improper preparation.

SUMMARY

Mealtime is a primary time for socialization and is a focal point of the day in an institution. The majority of nursing home residents are former housewives who feel competent to evaluate the quality of the dietary service due to their decades of cooking experience. The ethnicity and cultural backgrounds of the residents cannot be overlooked when planning menus for long-term residents. By offering choices in menus and meal hours, residents are able to exercise some decision making in their otherwise structured lives in the nursing home.

NOTES

1. U.S. Department of Health, Education and Welfare, Public Health Service, Office of Nursing Home Affairs, *Long Term Care Facility Improvement Study*, Introductory Report (Washington, D.C.: Government Printing Office, July 1975).

GENERAL REFERENCES

American Hospital Association. *Diet and Menu Guide for Extended Care Facilities*. Chicago, 1967.

Housekeeping,

Furnishings, and Laundry

INTRODUCTION

In a health care facility, the quality of the housekeeping department cannot be measured only by the aesthetic appearance of the building, equipment, furniture, and linens, for in a larger sense its quality is reflected in patient health and well-being. The housekeeping service leaves an impression on all who enter the facility. Although lay people may be unable to evaluate the nursing care given patients, they do feel qualified to assess the building's cleanliness and physical condition. The thoroughness of housekeeping is often an indicator of the successful management of the skilled nursing facility to patients, personnel, families, and visitors.

The laundry in an institution with 100 beds should be operated in coordination with the housekeeping department. Other departmental functions include promoting safety by conscientiously reporting potentially hazardous conditions; furthering infection prevention and control techniques; limiting the use of utilities such as heat, electric lights, and water; monitoring of noise produced by department equipment; and working harmoniously intradepartmentally and interdepartmentally. The housekeeping staff should strive to maintain safe, sanitary, orderly, and pleasant surroundings both efficiently and economically.

OUTSIDE MANAGEMENT CONTRACTS

Housekeeping is a nursing home service that is frequently contracted to an outside company. The main advantage is that specially trained and experienced personnel use the latest technology and equipment in a well-planned and well-supervised program. Reservations regarding the employment of an outside cleaning service relate particularly to the integration of housekeeping with the other nursing home departments. The cooperation and flexibility of the housekeeping employees may be sacrificed with the use of non–nursing home workers. With the exception of the use of sophisticated equipment and the savings incurred due to the company's ability to buy in bulk, a 100-bed facility can meet all the advantages and more of an outside service at a comparable, and perhaps even lesser, cost.

Arranging for outside contractors for such services as pest control, window washing, and linen rental is generally more desirable for a 100-bed skilled nursing facility than having these tasks performed in-house by nursing home staff. Although the specific contract may appear more costly, it is important to include in the comparison the expense of fringe benefits, vacations, depreciation of equipment, cost of providing a sufficient inventory of linens, and so on. If the facility is unionized, labor differences may be even more apparent. The providers of outside services are specialists in their fields and thus should have more expertise than nursing home personnel and should be able to work more rapidly.

Each outside service used requires special forethought and planning. For example, if an outside service is used for window washing, the responsibility for cleaning and washing window screens needs to be spelled out clearly in the contract, as does the appropriate time of day to wash patient room windows. The contract with an exterminator must include the routine service and specific arrangements for emergency service. Although city garbage service may be available, the use of a private waste carter may be tailored according to the needs of the skilled nursing facility, with more frequent visits and the use of a dumpster in place of numerous untidy garbage cans.

STAFFING PATTERN

Although the staff complement of the housekeeping and laundry department in a 100-bed skilled nursing facility depends on several factors—such as square footage, finishes, building design, and amount of laundry to be done—all of which will be elaborated on later in the chapter, the department is composed of the standard key positions, such as executive housekeeper, maid, porter, floor custodian, and laundry worker.

An interior designer should be retained and consulted whenever changes are contemplated regarding furniture refinishing or reupholstering, window treatments, bedspreads, painting, and, of course, significant alterations.

Executive Housekeeper

Under the supervision of the administrative director, the executive housekeeper is responsible for the cleanliness of the building and the care of patients' laundry and bed and bath linens. He directs the entire housekeeping and laundry service, coordinates it with other nursing home services, and supervises outside contracted services, including the exterminator, window washer, and garbage collector. On a daily basis, he makes rounds through the entire building to ensure that sanitary standards are being upheld by all personnel.

The executive housekeeper has the final decision in the selection of new housekeeping employees. He develops and conducts a staff training program emphasizing infection control principles. In addition, he establishes standards of performance, work procedures, and the schedule of duties for housekeeping personnel, which must take into consideration the activities of other departments.

The executive housekeeper is responsible for the requisitioning and judicious use of supplies and equipment for the department. He should always be alert to new products on the market and should experiment with them as he sees fit.

The responsibility for supervising housekeeping and laundry services is substantial, as the department's activities reach into all physical areas of the building and therefore have an impact on the entire nursing home community. The housekeeper must be both firm and flexible— firm in abiding by established sanitary and cleanliness standards, and flexible in operating the department around the constraints placed on it by other departments. The executive housekeeper must exercise considerable judgment in regard to intervening in other departments and initiating new procedures to overcome difficulties.

An executive housekeeper should be a high school graduate. Course work in personnel management, infection control, and/or institutional housekeeping is desirable, and substantial housekeeping experience in an institutional setting is mandatory. The housekeeper must be completely knowledgeable regarding the functions of the other nursing home departments as well as their internal housekeeping duties. Finally, he must be aware of government regulations affecting housekeeping and laundry services in health care facilities and be especially attuned to the principles of infection control.

Other Personnel

All other personnel in the housekeeping department—maids, porters, laundry workers, and floor custodians—serve under the direction of the housekeeper who should select and groom one of his staff to serve as assistant and replacement on days off. Housekeeping staff are charged with cleaning and servicing all assigned work areas according to the particular performance requirements as set forth in the master housekeeping plan for the building. During orientation and in-service training, it must be impressed upon housekeeping personnel to perform their tasks as taught in order to enforce good infection prevention and control techniques. They should be advised and supervised in the judicious use of supplies, and in the correct care and storage of equipment.

Housekeeping employees must be individuals who can perform standardized repetitive tasks on a daily basis and understand and follow oral and written instructions. Housekeeping chores may involve some strenuous physical activity, so pre-employment screening should emphasize good health, with no limitations respecting bending, lifting, or reaching. Housekeeping personnel should understand the other nursing home services in order to carry out their duties in a cooperative manner, with as little intrusion as possible. Finally, work should be planned and carried out without unnecessarily disturbing patients.

It is most important to plan work schedules so that the quality of housekeeping is sustained on a daily basis. The master staffing for the department must include one summer porter for seven or eight weeks, and one extra maid for thirteen weeks, to allow for vacations. Cleaning schedules and staffing patterns must also take into consideration seasonal variations, that is, in the warm weather more time will be devoted to cleaning outdoor terraces and porches.

Staffing Alternatives

Housekeeping can be accomplished by the so-called specialist methodology where one individual is assigned a specific task throughout the building, such as all the floor care, rather than assigning one person to complete all the tasks in a specific area. Specialists become expert and fast in their job, but may become bored, as well as difficult to supervise because they function throughout the facility. Certain tasks do require special skills and a 100-bed facility should have one trained floor custodian who will be responsible for all resilient and carpeted floors.

The generalist or area assignment method utilizes one employee who is responsible for all housekeeping tasks in a particular section or unit of the facility. Area assignments give the employee a place for which he is accountable, and good or bad work will be noticed and quickly reflect his understanding of each job to be completed in the unit. Given proper motivation, this area generalist should require less and less supervision and, with only one staff member in the area, there is no question as to who will be held responsible for poor quality work or who will be praised for superior effort. Area assignments also promote a team spirit with nursing personnel in the unit, and this sense of mutual cooperation could benefit the general appearance of the facility and the quality of life for the residents.

Another housekeeping variable concerns whether individuals should work alone or in teams. Single workers are easier to supervise but may be slower. They will be more apt to pause and communicate with residents than would a group who have one another for companionship. Thus the single worker may be preferable when dealing with the ill aged.

FIGURE 11-1
Worker and Patient Communicating

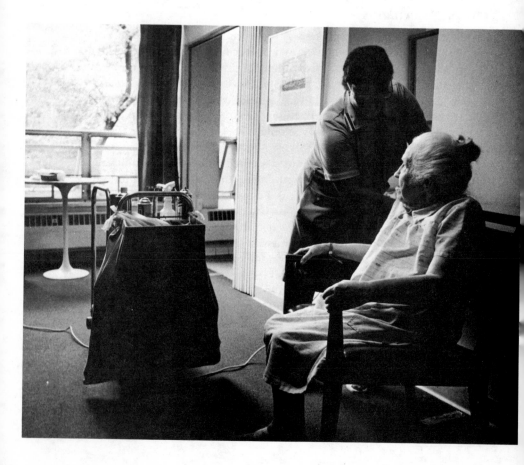

Teams can be efficient for time-limited jobs, such as thorough cleaning upon patient discharge, when personality clashes will not prevail. However, if team members get along well together and develop a sense of camaraderie, they can be very effective and can sustain each other's morale during routine tasks.

Whereas the individual with an area assignment will not have much supervision, the team in a large nursing home may have a team leader or supervisor present with them at all times. Teams can handle absenteeism more easily than can individuals with area assignments. A combination of the area approach and the team approach is probably the most effective plan.

In a busy institution, there is always the temptation to have housekeeping and laundry work done after hours when certain areas are not in use. Less traffic certainly facilitates floor maintenance, but such a program can be successful on a continuing basis only if supervision is provided to prevent uneven work performance. The same is true for hiring a laundry worker for evenings or nights. Such a schedule would promote more effective use of equipment and utilities, but it should be attempted only if someone can oversee the work. Still another consideration is the fact that evening and night cleaning may be noisy and thus may interfere with the residents' relaxation and sleep.

Housekeeping schedules cannot be sacrosanct in a nursing home. Flexibility must be inculcated in the staff training program so that housekeeping personnel meet delays and emergencies with equanimity. Also, housekeeping staff members may be asked to work evenings or extra duty on weekends when special programs are scheduled. For most complete coverage, housekeeping schedules can be staggered. For example, it is helpful if some porters are available to clean floors after the evening meal so that those areas do not remain soiled until the following day.

FURNISHINGS

Furniture and equipment should be selected to meet the physical requirements of the resident population, with particular reference to patient safety, such as the use of rounded edges rather than sharp corners. Chairs should be of a proper height, should facilitate easy rising, should be sufficiently heavy so as not to tip easily, and should have arms and straight legs to keep residents from tripping when moving close to the chairs. Tables, too, must be of adequate weight and should not have aprons. Pedestal tables are desirable for use by wheelchair residents. A minimum of free-standing, easily overturned items like lamps should be part of the decor. To compensate patients for the loss of dexterity or use of hands, push plates or other types of facilitating hardware should be used in place of doorknobs, and indented areas on furniture drawers should replace drawer pulls or latches. Lighting is a vital element in the design of the nursing home and must be appropriately located and sufficiently intense to compensate for visual deficiencies. In corridors, it is especially helpful to use long light fixtures the entire width of the corridor in order to eliminate the creation of shadows.

When selecting outdoor furniture, it is important to keep in mind these same principles, especially since outdoor furniture tends to be lightweight. Garden benches should always have arms and should seat no more than two people. If naturally shaded areas are not available, awnings or umbrella tables may suffice.

The aesthetic and personal needs of the residents, their families, staff, and the community should also be considered when choosing furniture and determining decorating schemes. Bright, gay colors, contemporary furniture, and plants and flowers give a vivid, fresh, and clean appearance. The use of artistic and decorative accessories, including residents' artwork and mirrors will help deinstitutionalize the interior. Changing the color scheme and rotating the artwork will offer variety and stimulation to all who come into the facility.

The nursing home can be personalized for residents if they are encouraged to bring a few favorite possessions with them. Different decor schemes on resident units and in separate rooms, such as bedspreads and window treatments, help identify that area for the resident. Having residents write their own names on door labels is another method of individualizing areas.

Certain administrative needs in terms of trouble-free maintenance and ease of housekeeping should be weighed when selecting furniture and equipment. Fabrics in direct contact with patients should have a plastic finish, and mattresses should have a special coating in consideration of the incontinent patient. Dining chairs should not have crevices in which food can collect. Formica counters should have a suede rather than smooth finish to minimize scratches. Finally, in place of shades, blinds, and/or curtains, narrow slatted blinds should be considered. They can be more than one color and therefore provide their own design, and they do not have to be taken down to be cleaned easily.

Floor Coverings

The selection of surfaces should depend on the anticipated wear and tear, particularly in the case of carpeting or resilient flooring. Carpeting used in nursing homes must comply with specific federal criteria for fire safety, and the cushion and cement used under the carpet must also meet the flamespread requirements. Flamespread tunnel tests for carpet, cushioning, and cement include the rate of flame spread as well as the fuel-contributed and smoke density factors.

FIGURE 11-2
Pedestal Tables Accommodating Wheelchairs

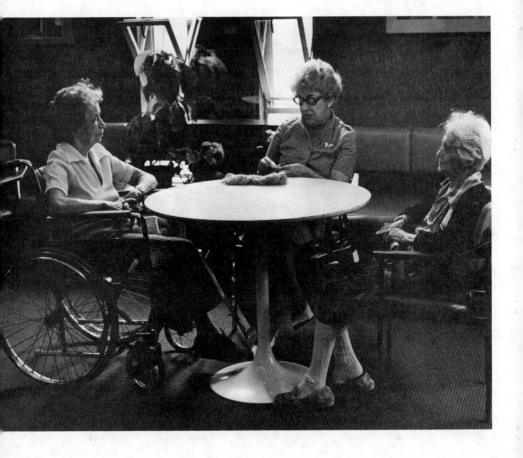

FIGURE 11-3
Resident Art as Interior Decoration

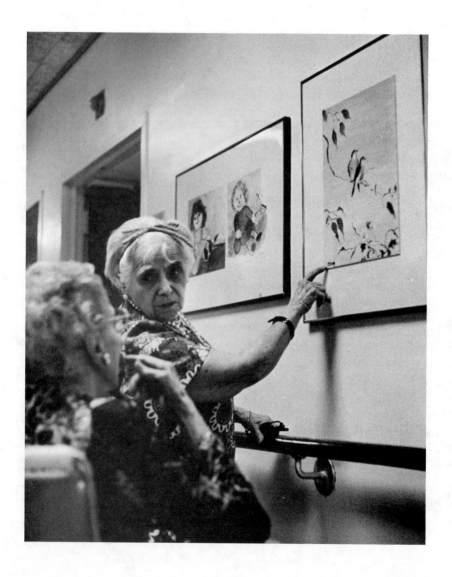

FIGURE 11-4
Room without Personal Belongings

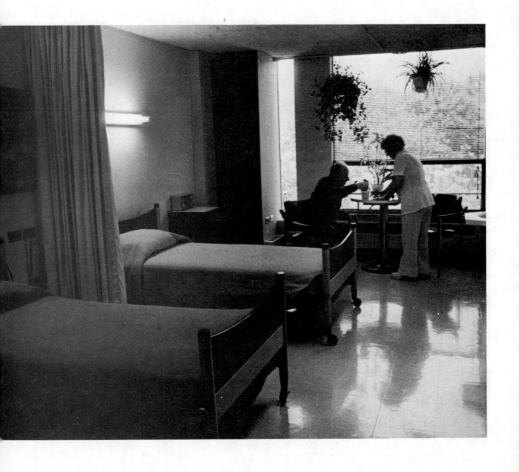

FIGURE 11-5
Room with Personal Belongings

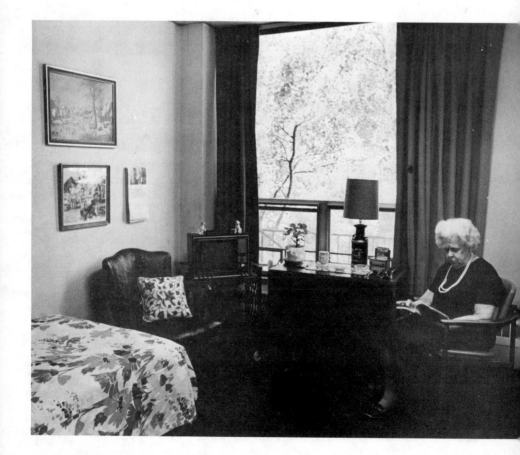

In addition to its attractive appearance, carpeting helps control noise, looks less institutional than resilient flooring, and adds a feeling of warmth and luxury to the environment. Carpet may help reduce patient falls and injury resulting from such falls. It also provides a textural contrast to the smooth finishes of plastic upholstery, metal window blinds, and painted walls.

Conversely, carpeting has certain disadvantages in a long-term-care setting. Obviously, in units where residents are incontinent, carpets are neither sanitary nor practical. They may actually impede the passage of wheelchairs and the ambulation of patients who use crutches and walkers. They may interfere with certain activity programs such as dancing. Obviously, the use of carpeting should be limited to areas appropriate to the nature of patient disability and congruent with area activities.

Resilient flooring such as vinyl, vinyl asbestos, and linoleum can be cleaned easily and thus are good choices for heavy-duty areas. To protect resilient flooring from damage, metal tips on chairs should be removed or replaced with rubber tips. In areas used by incontinent patients, tiles should not be used since it is difficult to clean the crevices between them, and residues are a possible source of odors. A solid-surface vinyl or linoleum would be preferable in such locations.

Hard-surface floors such as quarry tile are best used in nonpatient areas where serviceability and durability are paramount. Terrazzo, ceramic tile, and marble should be treated to provide a nonskid surface for patient safety.

HOUSEKEEPING PROCEDURES

Developing a Work Plan

An effective housekeeping program depends on a good work plan and the efficient use of both personnel and equipment. One method to develop a housekeeping program is to use the architectural plans—which clearly note the square footage and use of each area—to identify, classify, and estimate the work load via color coding. Different colors can be assigned to each type of flooring—e.g., resilient, carpeted, or ceramic tile. The areas may be further identified by filling in the first letter of the descriptive noun, such as H for hall, and a numerical code can be used to identify the precise location of each room or space.

The housekeeper should then proceed to survey the nursing home room by room and space by space to determine tasks required in each, who will do what, when, how often, how long it should take, what equipment and supplies are needed for each job, and how to evaluate completed jobs. Whenever possible, housekeeping procedures should be mechanized to reduce costs and improve performance. After the procedure is written, a time check should be done that takes into account assembling and removing needed materials and equipment, accomplishing the job, and putting all furniture in its correct place (which may not be the way it was found).

Informal time and motion studies, with tasks done at different times of day by different staff members, give a rough idea of a realistic time schedule. The total time required for tasks divided by productive time per housekeeping employee will determine the number of employees needed. This is a more accurate methodology than determining how many rooms a maid can care for each day or how much flooring a porter can maintain each day.

The following guidelines may be used with respect to the timing of housekeeping tasks.[1] The vacuuming of carpet should take from twelve to twenty-four minutes per 1000 square feet, depending on the degree of soil and the amount of congestion in the area. Spot cleaning will take about half an hour, and carpet shampooing will range from three to four hours per 1000 square feet under the same previously mentioned conditions. Sweeping and dust mopping will consume about eight to sixteen minutes per 1000 square feet; the time will vary according to the number of obstructions. These procedures are not recommended for areas used by residents. Damp mopping, a more frequent procedure, will take from sixteen to thirty-two minutes per 1000 square feet, while wet mopping and rinsing will consume twice as much time.

Personnel will spend 75 to 135 minutes per square foot in hand scrubbing with a long brush; hand scrubbing without a long brush will take three times as long. Machine scrubbing saves considerable time: porters should be able to complete 1000 square feet in half to three-quarters of an hour. Machine polishing will take two-thirds the time required for machine scrubbing. Stripping and rewaxing 1000 square feet of floors will take from two to three hours. Of course, the proper sequence followed by personnel in the performance of tasks is crucial with respect to timing. Aimless running takes time but will not produce results. The conservation of housekeeping personnel travel time is essential.

Cleaning Schedules

Routine cleaning and servicing must be provided for patient and staff areas of the facility, with more emphasis given to those areas subject to the heaviest use, such as patient rooms, dining areas, lavatories, bathing areas, hallways, stairs, and elevators. Offices, which should be scheduled for a quick daily cleaning in the early morning, or for thorough cleaning on weekends, will not require painstaking daily cleaning as do other areas. Large activity areas and dining rooms should receive attention early in the day before the patients convene there and may need a quick but effective clean-up and rearrangement of furniture after the completion of programs and meals.

The cleaning of patient rooms is best reserved until residents are not in them, such as during activity programs or meals. Housekeeping and nursing should determine respective responsibilities in caring for a resident's unit and should clarify in advance problems that may arise due to rearranging residents' personal belongings while cleaning the room. Residents may prefer to have the nursing staff handle their belongings, yet that may hinder the work of the housekeeping staff. Furthermore, patients have every right to be present when their personal belongings are put in order. Making beds and tidying bedside stands should be assigned to the nursing staff, while the responsibility for all other cleaning should be given to the housekeeping staff.

Other areas on the nursing units—treatment rooms, utility rooms, nurses stations, lavatories, and bathing areas—will need to be scheduled for housekeeping when they are least in use, perhaps in the afternoon. It should be clear as to which cleaning procedures in these areas will be done by nursing and which will be done by housekeeping.

Corridors, elevators, and stairways must be attended to every day and perhaps more often. For instance, in wet weather when delivery people and visitors track in mud, two moppings a day will be necessary. All entrances should have walk-off mats to catch heavy dirt, grease, and water that is brought in from the street.

Periodic tasks involve a monthly buffing of all resilient floors and a monthly contracted service by the window washer and exterminator. Light fixtures and air and heating ducts should be cleaned and walls should be washed twice a year. On an annual basis, resilient floors will require stripping, finishing, and buffing. Carpets in well-traveled areas should be shampooed at least twice a year.

Before signing out, the housekeeping staff should make a final tour of the building for a last-minute check. Although they may go off duty in the afternoon, the nursing home remains open and fully functional twenty-four hours a day. Both public areas and patient rooms should be checked and ashtrays and wastebaskets emptied, and a final mopping or vacuuming, if necessary, and general tidying up should be performed to leave the facility presentable for the remainder of the day. Dining areas will need a clean-up after the evening meal and before visiting begins.

When a resident changes rooms, is discharged, or dies, his entire room should receive a thorough cleaning and disinfection, including the washing down of the bed and mattress, chairs and tables, and the cleaning of drawers, closets, and medicine cabinets. These same thorough cleaning procedures also should be carried out at least once a year for rooms that remain occupied by the same residents. In addition, the social service department must inform the executive housekeeper when an admission is planned so that the room may be readied for the patient's arrival.

Inspections

The housekeeper must have an inspection program, which may be accomplished via spot checks daily or complete rounds made weekly. On these surveys, the housekeeper should note the need for reupholstering, repainting, furniture repair, and so forth. Of course, inspections concerning safety items, such as the functioning of exit lights, should be performed daily. Indeed, maids and porters should be trained to be good observers—to note when repairs are needed and to report it in writing. The executive housekeeper cannot possibly inspect every single item, but if the rest of the personnel in the department are trained, many eyes will be observing.

The Color Plan

For aesthetic value, it is important that furnishings of the correct colors be replaced according to a coherent plan. Often visitors will move chairs from one area to another and thus mismatch the decor. Likewise, the housekeeping department in a nursing home that tries to provide variety in such items as bedspreads must be alert to see that the nursing department does not use the wrong color spread in a room and thereby detract from the total appearance of the facility.

Safety and Infection Control

Safety is an integral part of housekeeping procedures for patients, staff, and visitors, so the use of "wet floor" signs must be emphasized during personnel training, and prompt response to calls for mopping up spills must be impressed on the staff.

The housekeeping staff should be trained in special procedures to follow up on suspicion or identification of an infectious organism that places residents and staff at risk. Collecting, separating, properly washing, and drying contaminated clothing and bed linen are a primary concern when an infection is present. If a linen rental company is used, the housekeeper must clarify with the company the procedure for handling these linens. The proper method of cleaning and/or disinfecting a contaminated patient's room must be a part of the housekeeping procedure manual.

Clothing Storage

The storage of patients' off-season clothing should be implemented by the executive housekeeper and the housekeeping staff. Depending on the climate, this task would most often take place in early October and early May. With the help of the nursing assistants, each resident's out-of-season clothing should be identified, cleaned, labeled, and stored so that it may be easily located. A record should be kept of what is stored for each patient; it is very important to inform patients and their families of this practice so that no misunderstandings will ensue. Unless the family removes them (which may be preferable), residents' suitcases will need to be labeled and put away in safe storage.

Waste Disposal

Waste disposal is becoming an ever more significant problem in the skilled nursing facility. As more disposables are used, more waste is accumulated. Until recent years, incineration was the most effective way of handling most waste. With the increasing attention being paid to environmental matters, however, incineration has been outlawed in many communities, necessitating more frequent waste pick-up service and introducing the concept of compaction.

Containers for solid waste should have tight-fitting covers and should be easy to clean and small enough for one person to handle when full. Ideally, waste containers should be manufactured of material that does not cause noise and should not have seams or other openings that collect dirt. The collection of waste should not be annoying yet must be frequent enough to preclude attracting vermin, accumulating odors, and prevent the overloading of equipment and facilities. The housekeeping staff needs to be alerted to examine the trash in the nursing units inhabited by brain-damaged patients to ascertain that the patients have not discarded eyeglasses, dentures, or other valuable items in error.

Single-service plastic can liners are preferable to unlined containers, which will require sanitizing or cloth liners, which need laundering. Personnel need to be trained not to overload the plastic bags or they will rupture. Filled liners should be closed with elastic bands or plastic strips. While plastic liners clearly reduce the accumulation of dirt, garbage and trash containers and conveyances used to transport them should be scheduled for frequent washing.

Areas within the building used for the storage of trash should have thorough sprinkler systems. Sometimes refrigerated rooms need to be used to store garbage because of large amounts of trash and/or because of infrequent garbage removal. If garbage or trash has to be stored outside the building, containers should be tightly covered, stored on racks that are at least one foot off the ground, and removed from the immediate building environs.

Biological waste should be separated from routine waste by placing it in specially colored plastic containers and special receptacles. Arrangements for the off-site incineration of biological waste may be made with neighboring hospitals that have such installations, which often are not in continuous use.

ODORS

Odors present major problems in the nursing home because of the nature of the patient population. Irrespective of the attention of the staff and the institution of bowel- and bladder-training programs, incontinent patients will have accidents or will dribble, often immediately after having been cleaned. Thus odors must be present for brief periods. Sometimes the odor of urine will permeate the patient's room in the cracks between floor tiles, in the upholstery, and the draperies, so that even the most vigorous cleaning may not be successful.

The most effective antiodorant is quick clean-up and attentive nursing care. Fresh air, of course, is the best deodorizer, so a plan to air such areas daily and to clean with detergent disinfectant solution is essential. Clothing and linen soiled with urine and fecal matter must be promptly removed. Since confused patients often will roll soiled items and hide them in closets and wardrobes, personnel must search for them.

Lavatories commonly are the site of odors. Unfortunately, many health care facilities have lavatories without windows or natural ventilation. Such lavatories will need more careful attention to control odors.

Likewise, utility areas and custodians' closets are potential breeding grounds for odors. Garbage should always be bagged and removed regularly and cans should be cleaned routinely. Soiled linen should not be permitted to accumulate, as it too will produce unpleasant odors.

Sometimes patients suffering from carcinoma or profuse drainage will have odor problems. Detergents with sanitizers and deodorizing machines may be helpful in maintaining odor-free rooms and clothing.

LAUNDRY

Whether to do laundry on the premises or use a contract service depends on the facility's location, the competence of its personnel, the space available for a laundry, and the cost. An in-house laundry provides complete control over linens in one location, eliminates problems caused by transportation delays, and can fill special rush requests promptly. Smaller financial outlay for inventory results from having less linen in circulation, and more flexibility in weekend usage is possible. The typical nursing home patient generates about five pounds of laundry daily exclusive of personal clothing.

On the other hand, a commercial laundry service specializes in laundry, not in patient care, and thus may have superior equipment and personnel for the job. When an outside laundry is used, it is said that the personnel are more careful in their utilization pattern.

The other alternative to an in-house laundry is to use a linen rental service, which eliminates the need to have funds tied up in inventory.

A nursing home located in a rural area may be forced to do its own laundry, while one in the city will have numerous linen services from which to choose. In a community with a number of health facilities, the development of a cooperative laundry is also a possible solution, but someone must take the leadership in organizing such an installation.

When the decision to use an outside linen rental service has been made, area hospital and other health care facility laundry services should be surveyed. Often a more economical arrangement can be made with a linen rental company that services a neighboring hospital. Since the trucks need to visit the hospital frequently, it may cost the laundry company very little more to include the nursing home in its schedule, which may be of great financial benefit to the nursing home.

If an outside service is used, a minimum of two or three deliveries per week should be planned in order to minimize the accumulation of soiled linen and the need for large storage areas for clean linen. Covered mobile trucks may be provided by the linen rental service or by the nursing home to store dirty linen. Both commercial laundries and linen rental services will need surveillance to assure that linens are mended and/or replaced when needed.

Even if sheets and pillow cases are provided by a linen rental service, the control and issue of linen still remains the responsibility of the housekeeping staff. To prevent costly pilferage, there is really no substitute for counting soiled linen from specified areas to control linen consumption and replacement. Personnel in each area need to be accountable for linen usage and replacement to eliminate theft and misuse.

Laundry service is of much greater interest to nursing home residents than to hospital patients. Whereas the hospital laundry is concerned only with hospital linens and materials, in the skilled nursing facility—where good rehabilitation practices are operative and patients routinely wear street clothing and not bed clothes—the laundry often is concerned only with residents' clothing.

Laundering clothing can be troublesome, as residents will have clothing of different fabrics, both natural and synthetic, in various stages of soil. Sometimes laundry personnel will not exercise judgment and will, say, wash, dry, and thus shrink woolen sweaters. Families need to learn that the nursing home laundry is not geared to do fine hand laundry, so such items should be taken to the homes of relatives for washing or for permanent safekeeping. When patients are incontinent, it is unwise to plan to take their clothing out for servicing as odors will collect rapidly in soiled garments. Such laundering should be done promptly in the facility. When residents' clothing needs to be replenished, families should be requested to provide drip-dry clothing with Velcro or other simple closures.

Provided that clothing is of materials and colors that can be washed together, a systematic method for handling dirty laundry is to provide each resident with a labeled net laundry bag. This bag will be used to collect and to transport soiled things to the laundry and will be inserted into the machine so that the contents will be washed and dried without any possibility of confusion as to ownership. The clean clothing will be folded, replaced in the laundry bag, and returned to the patient's wardrobe or closet.

Soiled linens and clothing should never be placed on bedroom floors or on other furniture. Bed linens should be placed in a covered mobile wagon and promptly removed to the dirty utility room to await transfer to the soiled linen room for pick-up by the linen rental service or to be laundered by the nursing home laundry. This cart should be used only for bed and bath linens.

A separate, smaller truck with a foot-operated cover should be used to collect soiled clothing, and the same storage practice should be followed. It is not desirable to use the same cart for clean and dirty linen transportation and for clothing transportation. If this should become necessary, a thorough cleansing must be done after each use. For returning clean clothing to residents' rooms, it is convenient to use carts with separate baskets for each individual's clothing to minimize the possibility of incorrectly returning patient clothing.

Towels, laboratory coats, and hospital gowns need to be distributed to and collected from the physical therapy, x-ray, and laboratory services regularly. The housekeeper should collect patient clothing weekly to be sent to the dry cleaner. These items must be clearly labeled to prevent loss and to assure proper billing.

Lost and found is a responsibility of housekeeping. Clothes that the staff cannot identify should be placed in a convenient area so that families or residents may search through them. Periodically, a listing of found items might be included in the facility newsletter or posted on appropriate bulletin boards.

One laundry worker should have a part-time responsibility to mend clothing that is in good enough condition to warrant such efforts. Alternatively, a volunteer may be willing to perform this very necessary service for the residents. Certainly, families should be informed when clothing is not worth mending so that they can replace it.

FIGURE 11-6
Separate Baskets for Residents' Laundry

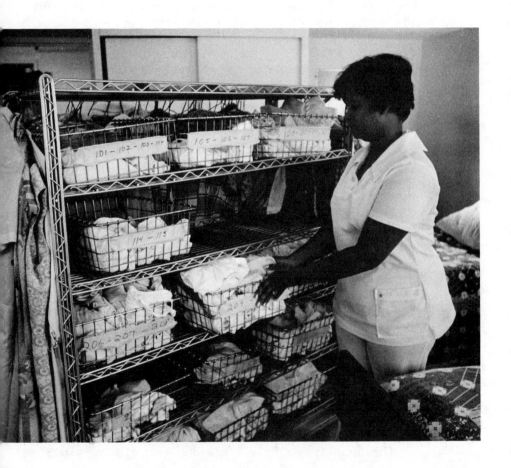

RECORDS

Careful records must be kept if a linen rental or commercial laundry is retained. At the time of each delivery, the housekeeper should note how many of each item were received and how many were sent out to be cleaned. When a discrepancy occurs, the company must be immediately notified.

The executive housekeeper should submit a monthly report to the administrative director, outlining personnel requirements, pounds of laundry—linens and clothing—processed, and unusual trends or problems.

FACILITIES, EQUIPMENT, AND SUPPLIES

Well-designed housekeeping/laundry areas will facilitate the efficient functioning of the department. One room should be designated for the storage of housekeeping equipment and supplies; the nursing units should have housekeeping closets with sinks, pails, mops, and sponges for daily use by housekeeping staff and available to nursing staff when housekeeping personnel are off duty. An office area adjacent to the general housekeeping/laundry area must be provided for the executive housekeeper for desk work and the storage of equipment manuals, inventories, forms, and so on.

Additional safe storage areas must be provided for patients' off-season clothing and suitcases, and the personal effects of deceased residents, which are awaiting pick-up by the family. Containers more dignified than plastic bags should be stocked for this purpose.

Laundry facilities should include a laundry room with washers, dryers, and a folding table. Off the laundry room should be a closet for storing laundry room supplies. A well-ventilated room should be available for storing soiled linens and clothing prior to their laundering or pick-up by the linen rental company. A separate room must be provided for clean linen storage, with sufficient shelving for all the linens and other items such as mattress covers, sheepskin pads, pillows, blankets, and bedspreads.

The executive housekeeper is responsible for the proper and economical use and maintenance of all furnishings in the facility and the equipment of the housekeeping department. All necessary replacements should be requisitioned by the housekeeper. Major purchases should first be approved by the administrative director, and needed repairs should be brought to the attention of the maintenance director in writing.

The administration should keep a control record listing all furniture and equipment and the date of purchase, source, and cost, which the housekeeper can refer to. Furnishings should be listed in the control record according to manufacturer, catalog number, and any other identifying information, and their location in the nursing home should be noted. Vendor catalogs and telephone numbers should be kept for the purpose of reordering.

A reupholstery plan for all furniture should be developed based on a projection of the current upholstery's useful life. The control record of furnishings must contain a detailed record of the upholstery fabric used, to permit reordering of fabrics. If any changes in the upholstery plan are contemplated, the interior designer should be consulted. As with any other outside service, the nursing home should try to use the services of a local upholsterer.

If the facility launders its own bed and bath linens, the inventory of each of these items should be three times the census. Extra blankets, bedspreads, cubicle curtains, shower curtains, pillows, mattress covers, and curtains should always be available if those currently in use are soiled or damaged.

Since suppliers are best informed about new products and equipment, they should be asked to provide consultation, demonstrations, and education to housekeeping staff prior to and after purchase. In selecting equipment, the facility should analyze the pros and cons of using heavy-duty equipment rather than commercial-type equipment. One consideration in the selection of heavy equipment should be whether women as well as husky men can handle the same machine; another is the volume of noise generated by the item.

Where laundry equipment is needed only for patient clothing, heavy-duty machines similar to those found in laundromats are preferable to one very large machine, which is very costly and which, if broken, permits no laundry to be done until it is repaired. If several laundromat-type washers and dryers are available in the nursing home, there is built-in flexibility in case of equipment breakdown.

Laundry equipment also should include a sewing machine and sewing supplies for mending clothing.

Housekeeping materials should be standardized in order to use a minimum number of supplies. Once a week, the executive housekeeper should place an order through the purchasing agent for cleaning and laundry supplies and paper goods. The use of two or three different vendors for the purchase of routine supplies is recommended in order to keep prices, products, and vendor service competitive.

Heavy equipment or large orders of a single item (soap or towel dispensers, lighting fixtures, cubicle curtains) should be purchased through a system of competitive bidding. The administrative director and executive housekeeper should always secure the advice of the maintenance director, and possibly the interior designer, prior to selecting such equipment.

The maids' and porters' carts should contain all needed equipment and supplies for their daily routine so they do not need to retrieve items from the main storage closet continually. Mop buckets and wringers should be mounted on spiders (wheels) in tandems of two or three so that both wash and rinse can be done in one operation. Automatic battery-driven floor machines of nineteen and twenty-one inches are good for open corridors and lobbies; in more congested areas, fourteen-, sixteen-, and seventeen-inch machines are easier to use. Floor machines should be interchangeable for buffing, stripping, and scrubbing. Strap-on vacuums carried on the shoulders are good for cleaning stairwells, air conditioning units, acoustical ceilings, and other places that are hard to clean with wheeled vacuums. A carpet sweeper is useful for a quick clean-up at the end of the day.

RELATIONS WITH PATIENTS AND FAMILIES

The work of the housekeeping department is evident to all who come to the nursing home, and thus it is open for comment. As with dietary, housekeeping and laundry is an area where people feel qualified to pass judgment, and it often may receive the brunt of a family's complaints when their real distress concerns their relative's nursing home placement. When a family is critical of housekeeping, the social service department should be notified so they may acquaint the family with the special housekeeping problems encountered in a skilled nursing facility, such as the control of odors on the unit with incontinent patients, and may pursue the other real emotional conflicts the family is facing.

Housekeeping personnel are especially vulnerable to criticism from residents because of their access to residents' rooms. Misplaced articles can become the focus of improper accusations of housekeeping staff and must be confirmed or negated immediately. It is imperative, therefore, that housekeeping personnel be fully aware of the confusion and paranoia that are frequently associated with the chronically ill aged and that causes such behavior. Repeated problems of this nature with an individual resident will have to be addressed specifically, for both housekeeping personnel and the resident group cannot function effectively with ever-present suspicion. If the accusations seem to be addressed toward one person in particular, it may be necessary to change his unit assignment so that he is no longer open to criticism.

The most common complaint about this department heard from both residents and families will concern residents' clothing being lost or improperly laundered. Families of all new residents must be educated in the absolute necessity of properly labeling clothing; in addition, both nursing and housekeeping personnel must be on the lookout for un-labeled clothing and label it immediately. Second, families should be instructed to supply clothes that can withstand commercial processing, which means hot water washing, hot air drying, and no ironing. The use of Velcro fasteners rather than buttons, zippers, and hooks and eyes will help alleviate other potential problems.

Even with all the precautions of labeling, articles of clothing undoubtedly will be missed. The housekeeper should make sure that the personnel sorting and distributing clean laundry can read English and know resident room assignments. Nursing staff, particularly aides and orderlies, may be asked to help locate missing garments, which ultimately may require a full search of residents' rooms. Once again, however, social service may appropriately intervene to help allay the frustration of families and residents when clothing is missing, and to familiarize them with the problems inherent in an institutional setting, where some confused patients continuously remove clothing from one dresser to another or from one room to another.

SUMMARY

The apparent quality of the housekeeping service affects all who enter the nursing home including patients, staff, family members, volunteers, and community representatives. Everyone feels qualified to evaluate housekeeping, but few comprehend the problems encountered in deal-ing with the inevitable urine odor associated with incontinent patients.

Personal clothing is an important means of identification and ex-pression for residents at a time when they have lost so much of their individuality. Care of clothing, often patients' only remaining posses-sions, is an important concern for residents as well as for their families.

NOTES

1. Richmond Associates, Staten Island, N.Y., *Housekeeping: Floor Main-tenance Procedures.*

GENERAL REFERENCES

U.S. Department of Health, Education and Welfare, Public Health Ser-vices and Mental Health Administration. *Environmental Aspects of the Hospital: Supportive Departments,* Vol. II. Rockville, Md., 1971.

CHAPTER 12

Building Design

and Maintenance

INTRODUCTION

Irrespective of size, the modern nursing home is a most complex structure: a combination residence, hospital, professional building, and office building. In addition to the interior environment, exterior property including the parking lot, the outdoor recreation area, the walks, and the grounds must be managed in both winter and summer. Furthermore, the skilled nursing facility must be functional, comfortable, and safe day and night, 365 days a year. Delegated these responsibilities, therefore, maintenance cannot be a set of crisis-oriented procedures, but rather a continuous, planned orderly process.

SCOPE OF MAINTENANCE

Too little is said about the relationship between building maintenance and patient care. Customarily, nursing and other therapeutic services are considered the determinants of quality care provided by a skilled nursing facility. But it must be remembered that maintenance serves every single department and service in the facility and thus is directly related to patient care. Indeed, when a maintenance department is functioning effectively, it attracts little attention; only when there are problems is its importance apparent.

Examples of the effect of malfunctioning maintenance on the quality of patient care are manifold. When the brake of a wheelchair is inoperative, the safety of patients is in jeopardy. When a bedside rail is broken, a patient may fall out of bed. If the elevator fails to level properly, a resident may trip upon entering. Even such basic amenities as heat, hot water, and window screens reflect on the effectiveness of the maintenance department. The patients' well-being will certainly be affected if kitchen or laundry equipment are not in working order. The increasing use of mechanical equipment and the resultant possibility of breakdown in such items as audiovisual nurses' call system, electric suctioning devices, and electric beds further underscores the importance of maintenance to quality care.

The role that maintenance plays in safety and in emergencies also needs to be emphasized. During utility interruptions, the successful operation of the emergency generator will ensure the continuance of mechanical services. Fire drills, emergency evacuations, and related in-service programs usually are conducted and directed by maintenance personnel.

There are important financial ramifications to the quality of the maintenance program. When the nursing home's accountant determines that particular equipment, such as the elevator or the boiler, should last fifteen or twenty years and accordingly plans a depreciation schedule, he does not take into account the maintenance director's competence, even though his ability may help extend the life of the equipment. A poor maintenance director, on the other hand, may adversely affect the usable life span of the machinery.

In either case, most administrators are not in a position to assess this ability. If the boiler and elevator originally cost $100,000, a depreciation figure of $5000 per year assumes a usable life of twenty years. With poor care, they may last only fifteen years, and thus the actual depreciation factor will rise to almost $7000 per year. While this is not seen as a maintenance cost on the operating budget, obviously a direct relationship exists between the quality of maintenance and the cost of maintenance.

Another hazard related to the financing of maintenance results when the maintenance program is sharply curtailed for reasons of economy. The curtailment may mean deferring all but emergency repairs and hiring low-paid but ill-qualified personnel. Instead of decreasing costs, such efforts may in fact increase expenses due to the more rapid deterioration of inefficiently operated and poorly maintained equipment. The maintenance director must educate the administration and the governing body in the folly of trying to save pennies when dealing with ever-escalating replacement costs of building and equipment.

Besides excessive operating costs, substandard maintenance may result in an increased risk of liability suits. The sharp increase in monetary awards to persons who have proved negligence in the care of buildings, grounds, and equipment underscores the financial importance of maintenance.

STAFFING PATTERN
Maintenance Director

Because of the financial consequences, it is apparent that the chief of the maintenance department is a very critical position; thus ability rather

than salary should be the primary determinant when recruiting someone for the job. Poor judgment could cost the nursing home many thou-
sands of dollars and great inconvenience.

In contrast to the body of knowledge required by the director of
nursing, medical director, or physical therapist, the qualifications needed to cope with the responsibilities inherent in the position of maintenance director are not readily understood by many people in the long-
term-care field. If not a graduate engineer, the candidate should have
had previous hospital, hotel, or nursing home experience; depending on
the location of the nursing home, local regulations may require that the
maintenance director be licensed.

The maintenance director must be completely familiar with all requirements, codes, and laws governing nursing home operation, including the *Life Safety Code;* the National Electrical Code; the Occupational
Safety and Health Act; applicable state licensure, federal criteria, and
Joint Commission accreditation requirements; and city building, plumbing, fire, and electrical codes. (Copies of those materials should be readily
available in the maintenance office for reference after surveys and before
remodeling.) It is particularly important for the maintenance director to
belong to engineering associations to keep informed about new equipment and materials.

In the development and organization of a new facility, it is highly
recommended that the governing body hire the director of maintenance
or chief engineer directly after hiring the administrator, to whom he
reports directly and with whom he confers regularly. It will save much
time, grief, and money after the building has been completed if the
maintenance director is completely familiar with the location of shut-off
valves, access panels, and the like. Indeed, an experienced maintenance
expert can suggest appropriate locations for such crucial items during the
course of constructing the nursing home, for he and his staff will have to
contend with accessibility of valves and access panels when repairs and
servicing are needed.

Similarly, during building rehabilitation or additional construction,
the maintenance director can be extremely helpful in advising or consulting with the architect and administrator regarding the most practical
way to use or adapt existing mechanical elements of the building. He
also can offer advice to the administration on bids received for construction projects.

A nursing home maintenance director will need to understand elec-
tronics, communication systems, elevators, and possibly x-ray equipment. He should be familiar with steam systems and electrical
equipment, including motors and switch gears. He should have a working knowledge of plumbing and be experienced in fitting and replacing

pipes and repairing valves as well as keeping plumbing systems clear and unobstructed. Since lubrication is such an important component of the smooth and economical functioning of machinery, he should be knowledgeable in the use of lubricants.

An effective maintenance director must have an inquisitive mind in view of the rapid changes in techniques, tools, and supplies. He must continue to learn by reading technical publications and be able to articulate clearly and give understandable, well-organized directives to those under his supervision.

Furthermore, the maintenance director also will serve as an educator. He must train the staff in the use and limitations of equipment. For example, he must show the nursing staff how to use the autoclave and the suction apparatus. He must instruct the housekeeping staff on the proper use of the floor machinery. In turn, he will learn from members of the nursing staff how, for example, to install certain equipment for best patient use, or where to affix stall bars to the wall for physical therapy.

Sound judgment and organizational qualities are essential qualifications of the job since the scope of the maintenance department's work is so widespread and often unplanned. The development of priorities will be a never-ending process. The maintenance director will need a memory for details and must be familiar with the routine of other nursing home services so as to arrange both preventive maintenance procedures and emergency repairs. He will need to be a good manager in order to plan and provide for the successful, ongoing operation of the physical plant, requiring the supervision of his own staff and coordination with other facility staff members.

Other Personnel

The number of people required for the auxiliary maintenance staff depends on the size and complexity of the facility and the amount of work to be done by full-time staff members and by outside contractors. In a larger facility where most building and maintenance tasks are completed by the nursing home staff, some specialization in job categories will take place. Even in a 100-bed facility, two workers could spend full time in a continuing painting program; the full-time services of an electrician, a plumber, and a carpenter could be easily justified in a 500-bed institution. A medium-sized nursing home, however, presents a greater challenge because more versatility is expected of the maintenance workers; they may have to paint and repair plumbing as well as plow snow in the winter and care for the lawn in the summer.

It is preferable to recruit for such positions more mature persons, who may be pleased to work in one location after having spent years moving from job to job. A variety of employee skills would be advantageous to the functioning of a well-rounded maintenance department. Even though the nursing home salary may not be on a par with craft union wages, the worker will be guaranteed continuous employment with no layoffs.

A certain amount of physical strength—but more importantly, agility and dexterity—is required of the maintenance personnel, who must work in cumbersome or awkward positions or with hazardous equipment. It would be essential to consider the physical limitations of any maintenance department member and its effects on the individual's ability to carry out his duties safely.

Although set hours may be the usual routine for the department, the maintenance director and his staff must be available for emergency duty. Assigning weekend and holiday coverage duty will also be necessary, perhaps with an abbreviated schedule. With the building operating twenty-four hours a day, the maintenance department's responsibility will not end when they go home for the day.

EXTERNAL ENVIRONMENT

Several considerations should be addressed when choosing the site of the skilled nursing facility if it is not attached to or located on the grounds of a general hospital. Proximity to a general hospital and to professional offices is a primary concern in order to expedite close medical supervision and access to special services, as is accessibility to the cultural, social, and religious activities of the community. The nursing home is best located within easy availability of public transportation for the convenience of staff and volunteers and visitors, particularly elderly friends and relatives of the residents, who may find it difficult to travel.

The plot of land on which the nursing home is situated should be large enough to accommodate several different outdoor areas comfortably. A sufficient area for parking for all those coming to the facility must be allotted, including an appropriately designated area for handicapped visitors and staff. The parking lot should also include a protected area with easy access, such as ramps, to the building. Such access is important to make it easier for—and thus to encourage—residents to go out into the community. Delivery and service areas must be located where they will not interfere with the safety of residents during their outdoor activities.

The grounds of the facility should be designed to foster the free movement of ambulatory patients, as well as to provide proper safeguards for the more physically and intellectually handicapped residents. The garden should be easily accessible from the building via ramps and level ground and sidewalks, and it should have both sunny and shaded areas. Walkways with handrails, wheelchair riding paths, and firmly anchored benches with arms should be planned in any outdoor area for resident use, with specific areas set aside for waist-high gardening for selected residents.

INTERNAL ENVIRONMENT

The physical structure of the nursing home must comply with construction standards promulgated by federal, state, and local authorities, which take into consideration the criteria of the *Life Safety Code.*[1] Ample space should be allocated for daily patient activities: sleeping, bathing and toileting, dining, walking, socializing, recreation, and personal grooming. Areas must be specified for the several services provided in the nursing home, including nursing, medical, dental, pharmaceutical, rehabilitative, social, clinical laboratory, diagnostic x-ray, dietary, housekeeping, laundry, and maintenance services, and business office. Due to the lengthy stay of the nursing home population, storage areas for residents' seasonal clothing must be planned for, as well as sufficient space for keeping equipment, supplies, everyday patient possessions, and records. Accommodations for staff—such as lounges, dining rooms, baths, and lockers—must be included in the physical plant. Volunteers also will need lockers and may share staff or visitors' lavatories.

The architecture of the building can serve as a tool in patient management, beginning with the design of the individual nursing units planned for different levels of care commensurate with varying patient needs. A compact thirty-bed concentrated care unit for the more physically handicapped allows for close supervision by the nursing staff. Thirty-six mobile physically ill residents with associated mental impairment would be placed in a second section, where nursing controls would be readily available. Possibly a third, less controlled unit for thirty-four moderately disabled patients that encourages socialization would be included. Alternatively, a third unit could be used as a hospice for the terminally ill, but the relevance of such a specified unit in a skilled nursing facility may be questioned, given the chronically ill nature of the patient population. Indeed, while many of the patients may be in various stages of dying, the death process can prove very protracted, lasting years rather than months.

The second unit for the mentally impaired should be larger than the other units due to the increasing number of patients presented for admission to skilled nursing facilities who require the specialized care available on that unit.

FIGURE 12-1
Three Levels of Care

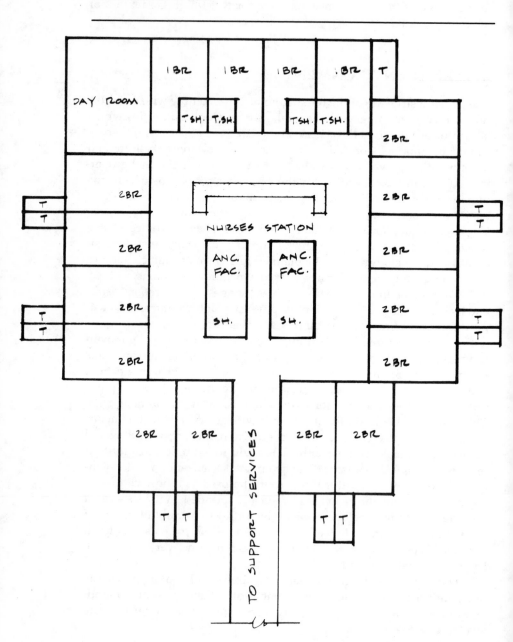

30 BED CONCENTRATED CAF

FIGURE 12-1 (cont.)

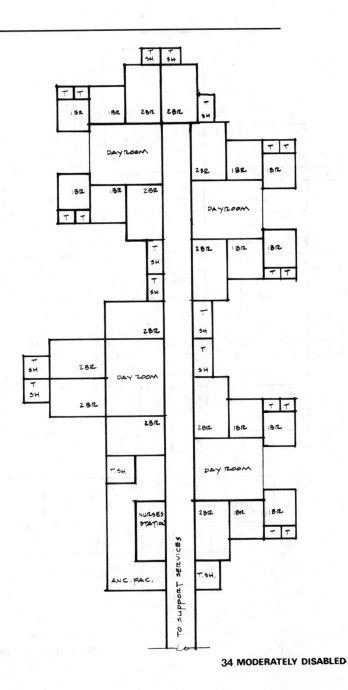

34 MODERATELY DISABLED

FIGURE 12-1 (cont.)

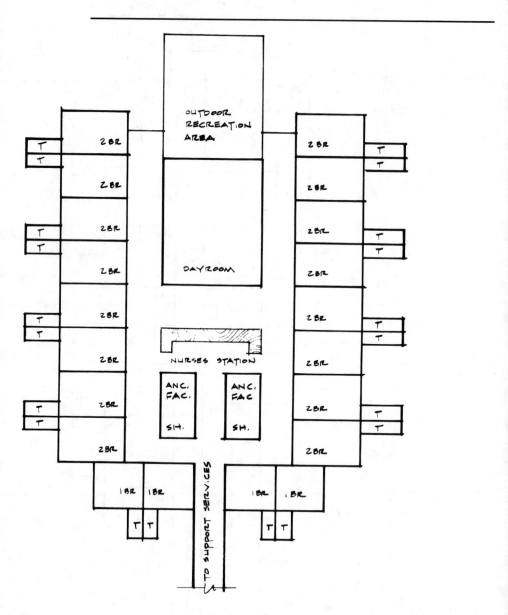

36 BED MOBILE PHYSICALLY ILL
WITH MENTAL IMPAIRMENT

Architectural considerations in the design of the building would also include ensuring that resident bedrooms are sufficiently large to facilitate the movement of handicapped persons who depend on wheelchairs, crutches, walkers, and canes, and locating community and dining areas to encourage residents to socialize. Toilets should be easily accessible to wheelchair patients, and they should be the proper height for the resident to help himself.

As a general rule, nursing homes are designed for eacy accessibility for the handicapped, with ramps, handrails, and grab bars used throughout. Specific items may need particular attention, however. For example, certain equipment may need to be lowered, such as closet rods, light switches, medicine cabinets, and mirrors. Space should be allocated for bedroom wheelchair storage, for 27-inch-deep (57.5-cm-deep) counters, and for fold-down shower seats. To help residents with visual handicaps, raised numerals should be used to identify rooms, and at least one telephone should be modified for use by the hard-of-hearing.

PROGRAM

People get their first impression of the nursing home from its exterior environment. For the sake of aesthetics and for patient, staff, and visitor safety, outdoor areas—including terraces, gardens, and paths—should be kept tidy and trim.

The nursing home structure is subject to extremes in seasonal temperatures, normal deterioration, and slight movement and settling, all of which necessitate continuous attention to the integrity of the building. The semiannual inspection of the building exterior to check its soundness and condition and to perform preventive maintenance when needed must be part of the maintenance department's routine.

Outside Management Contracts

An analysis of the feasibility of the use of outside contract services or in-house labor is particularly pertinent in this department due to the many skills required of the maintenance staff. A general rule of thumb would suggest that maintenance performed inside the building, particularly in patient areas, be done by nursing home staff. For example, contract painters might be preferable in outside work where elaborate scaffolding and dexterity are of paramount importance. However, painting in resident areas—where patients may be confused and disoriented, may move the equipment, and may distract the painters—is more easily accomplished by workers familiar with the patients' behavioral characteristics. In some instances, outside contractors, such as window cleaners, who come to the facility monthly, become sufficiently familiar with the residents to be able to complete their work without undue distraction.

The size of the job and time required of full-time staff to complete it will also be a deciding factor. In determining whether to arrange for an outside contractor for painting, it can be estimated that about 300 square feet of floor, and about 200 square feet of smooth walls, can be painted in an hour. Naturally, enameling and rough or textured walls will take more time.[2]

Cost is frequently a determining factor in deciding whether to hire an outside contractor. The cost of the services should be weighed against the cost of employing full-time personnel, including fringe benefits and insurance coverage for these periodic or seasonal jobs. Also, specialized equipment for jobs such as landscaping and snow removal would have to be purchased and maintained by the nursing home.

When considering equipment service contracts, the complexity of the servicing is a major factor. Sometimes a service contract may be written that excludes routine cleaning and servicing, thereby utilizing the capability of the maintenance department and reducing the cost of the contract. X-ray equipment and elevator repairs may prove too complicated for most maintenance departments to handle. For office equipment such as typewriters, photocopiers, and mimeograph machines, outside service contracts are essential in order to secure the correct replacement parts. Similarly, medical instrumentation like electrocardiograph machines or diathermy units should be serviced by the manufacturer's service agent except for the replacement of simple items such as cords and switches. Movie and slide projectors for the activities department probably will require servicing by the manufacturer service organization except for minor items.

Routine repair on laundry equipment, public address systems, and sterilizers can be handled by the maintenance staff provided that appropriate parts are stocked at the facility.

Even if contractual arrangements are made with outside organizations, however, these functions should be managed and supervised by the director of maintenance to avoid confusion and discoordination. Such arrangements must consider the outside agency's availability, and a clearly defined time frame for their response to emergencies should be agreed upon in advance. It is incumbent on the maintenance director to inform the appropriate staff of an outside service contract so that the service agency may be contacted directly if the maintenance staff is not available in an emergency.

Preventive Maintenance

Only the uninformed or inexperienced believe that maintenance is concerned solely with the repair of equipment and facilities to restore

FIGURE 12-2
Repairing Autoclave

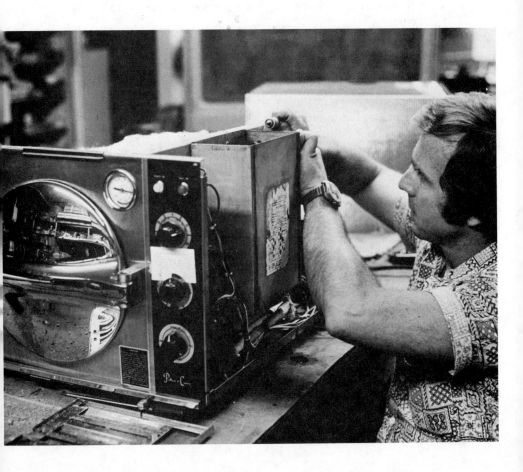

function and appearance. This would mean that the maintenance department responded only to mechanical breakdowns, leaks, and other specific problems, with the goal of efficiently returning the building and equipment to proper service and condition. Rather, the cost of building and equipping a modern skilled nursing facility mandates that the maintenance program be more than a response to mechanical and structural failure. Its primary objective is to maintain function and appearance in order to prevent breakdowns.

Theoretically, a completely successful preventive maintenance program would eliminate the need for any corrective or emergency maintenance. Naturally, as fewer labor hours are spent on emergency repairs, more time will be available for preventive work. On a realistic basis, emergency maintenance should represent only about 20 percent of maintenance labor, while 80 percent of maintenance labor should be spent on scheduled or preventive maintenance. In addition, much time is lost when the mechanic has to stop what he is doing, pack up his tools, and move to another part of the nursing home to do an emergency repair.

Basically, the components of preventive maintenance consist of inspection and related adjustments, minor repairs, and lubrication. The time benefits to be derived from a preventive program include less nonfunctional time for equipment, fewer big repairs, longer time spans between repairs, and longer usable life of equipment. Among the cost benefits are less overtime pay for emergency repairs and better control of spare parts, resulting in less money tied up in inventory. Finally, preventive maintenance may make it possible to identify people who are careless and indifferent in their handling of mechanical equipment and to remedy such problems.

The maintenance director needs to determine the frequency of inspections, giving full consideration to the ages of the structure and equipment and any other special characteristics. There may be several timetables for a given piece of equipment. For example, a gear-driven heating burner with a rotary cup may be cleaned daily, adjusted weekly, and lubricated monthly. To determine the correctness of a particular inspection frequency cycle, it is useful to compare unplanned or emergency maintenance with planned or scheduled maintenance. Whenever possible, equipment maintenance should be scheduled when the equipment is not in use or when usage is at a minimum. For example, the dishwasher should be checked before clean-up time, preferably in the afternoon before the evening dishes need washing.

Inspections must be performed by skilled mechanics who are sufficiently familiar with the equipment to be able to evaluate the performance in order to diagnose problems before the machinery breaks down. Examinations also must include a survey of the building and grounds to learn of any defects in the roof, masonry, parking area, or walkways. It is preferable to have more than one person responsible for inspections. In this way, one may serve as a safety check on the other's performance. Similarly, when one is ill or on vacation, the other inspector will be able to handle this important function easily.

Planning is a basic component of an effective maintenance program. Routine preventive maintenance procedures must be appropriately scheduled to achieve their intended purpose, while the scheduling of nonroutine repairs will depend on several variables. Current staff work assignments may take precedence over the repair requests. A particular part may be needed that will take time to locate, although this situation should be rare since advance planning should guarantee a stock of parts needed for most work. The repair of, say, the boiler may require the services of an outside contractor such as an electrician or a plumber who is not immediately available. After a job has been started, unforeseen factors sometimes arise that mandate rescheduling the repair or a temporary work stoppage.

Work Requests

The department head should make requests for repairs in writing to the maintenance department. Personal and telephone requests should be honored in emergencies but discouraged in the case of routine repairs, for it is virtually impossible for maintenance staff members to remember each verbal request as they proceed through the building with their assigned tasks.

Internal procedures for processing work requests are essential, and it is the duty of the maintenance director to determine the order of repairs. Even after the work order has been given, there must be a method of follow-up to ascertain that the repair was done.

The most important factor in determining tbe priority of repairs is how the scheduling will ultimately affect patient care. For example, nurses' call bell repairs should take precedence over fixing laundry equipment, but an elevator repair should be completed before remedying a faulty patient lifter, as the elevator is needed to transport people and meals.

The maintenance director or his designee must be able to determine whether a repair is vital and must be carried out immediately or whether it should be given a later priority. In the case of certain repairs, such as an elevator breakdown, it is vital to interrupt the present work schedule and to complete the repair immediately. However, although a breakdown in the autoclave should be remedied the day it is reported, the maintenance staff should not halt their present tasks to take care of it immediately.

Careful judgment often is needed to determine the appropriateness of repair or replacement. An item's age, effectiveness, and original and replacement cost must be weighed against the cost of labor, parts, and future utility. Such decisions can be made only by a competent and experienced maintenance director, who will explain the available options to the administration.

Minor construction is also within the purview of the maintenance department. Customarily, it is defined as work that can be completed without consultation with an architect and/or engineer, such as the installation of shelves and partitions, the rehabilitation of a central supply area, and the building of new outdoor pathways. However, the prime purpose of the maintenance department is to maintain and operate the nursing home plant. Thus careful advance planning should precede this kind of in-house work to ensure that the condition of the plant and equipment do not suffer. It may be that an outside contractor will be less costly in the long run.

Major Equipment Systems

Sump pumps, which are sometimes required to raise the water for discharge to waste lines located at a higher level due to special building and terrain considerations, must be checked daily for proper operation. Adequate air gaps or vacuum breaks are the preferable methods of protecting the water supply against contamination.

Several types of heat distribution systems can be used in nursing homes. Hot water or steam may be more desirable for older people, who are sensitive to cold. Either produces a more constant supply of heat than do radiant electric panels or forced air systems. Forced air systems, however, have the advantage of being usable for both heating and cooling.

By law, boilers usually have to be covered by casualty insurance. Such insurance provides a safeguard in that the insurance company performs annual internal and external inspections of boilers and furnaces. Thus an outside expert assures that this essential equipment conforms to acceptable standards of performance. In some communities, the building department also inspects boilers regularly.

Two boilers are mandatory so that one will serve as an auxiliary if the other breaks down. Operating both boilers continuously costs little more and prevents oxidation, which can clog the feedwater lines in the unused boiler. (Alternatively, a deaerating feedwater heater may be installed for this purpose.) Thus if one boiler breaks down, the other is able to pick up immediately and carry the load alone, without the need for maintenance personnel to come in to switch to the auxiliary unit.

All safety-related boiler equipment should be routinely installed in duplicate: one should be in use and one should be regularly tested and ready for emergency use. Feed pumps that introduce the fuel into the boiler are critical to boiler operation and require safety devices due to possible faulty ignition of gas or oil; thus they also must be installed in duplicate.

A stand-by electric generator is necessary to assure the operation of nursing home services if utility service is interrupted. The generator should be diesel or gas driven so it can be activated when electric service is halted. The electric generator must be operated at least thirty minutes per week to guarantee its adequate functioning.

In existing buildings, the director of maintenance often is involved in planning air conditioning. The advantages of window units include low initial cost, no necessary floor space, easy repair and replacement, and capacity for individual control. They do not require special engineers, but they are noisy and unattractive, and they serve no heating purpose in the winter. Through-wall units are better, need little maintenance, and do not require piping, permitting existing radiators to be replaced by the unit.

The ventilation system will be subject to continuous preventive maintenance to ensure its operation. The nursing facility should institute specific requirements for numbers of air changes per hour for different areas to ensure the provision of clean, fresh air, and the exhaust of stale, possibly contaminated air.

ENERGY CONSERVATION

An important responsibility of the maintenance department is to promote energy conservation throughout the facility. In addition, a temperature control training program should be offered to all personnel, emphasizing the effective use of energy. Next to labor costs, utilities (water, fuel, and electricity) represent the next largest expenditure in building maintenance.

For patient areas, a temperature of 75°F (24°C) is recommended. A temperature of 65°F (18°C) should be maintained in nonpatient areas during working hours. When storage and work areas, such as occupational and physical therapy, are not used at night or on weekends, 60°F (16°C) is sufficiently warm. The location of controlled-zone heat should be examined to determine proper placement for fuel economy. Zone heating must be carefully designed so that each area subject to one control is maintained at a suitable temperature. The thermostat controls should be placed properly—not in a drafty spot or in the direct sunshine.

Certain precautionary measures should be taken regarding the heating system. The hot water temperature for heating the building should be kept at the lowest possible level to meet heating needs. Similarly, in the case of steam pressure, the lowest pressure consistent with reasonable heating needs should be sustained. In both instances, the temperature may have to be reset manually each day. Draperies, blinds, and shades should be drawn or closed at night. Heating in indoor garages, foyers, and walkways should be adjusted or eliminated completely.

The proper maintenance of the boilers will affect energy conservation. First and foremost, boilers should be kept clean, as dirty boilers use more fuel. Fuel input and combustion should be checked and adjusted accordingly. The damper controls on the boilers should be regulated to ensure a proper draft. Temperature gauges on flue stacks should verify the temperature of flue gases. The minimum number of boilers consistent with efficiency as well as continuous service should be operated.

Time clocks on ventilation units should be set to function for the shortest acceptable periods. Ventilation units may be operable without outside air when the temperature falls below 25°F (-4°C). Only when areas such as conference rooms and cafeterias are in use should the ventilation system operate, and individual manual controls could be installed in such areas. All filters should be kept clean or replaced when needed. A study should be made to determine air leakage in damper openings with consideration given to partially blocking fresh air damper openings to prevent heat from escaping.

The temperature of hot water heaters should be kept no higher than 110°F (43°C), and hot water used in the laundry and the kitchen should not exceed requirements for proper use. The insulation on hot water, steam, and return lines should be checked for adequacy.

Personnel should be reminded to turn off lights via notices and well-placed signs. Lights in occasionally used rooms should be turned off when the rooms are not occupied. Artificial illumination should be eliminated or reduced when natural light is available. The housekeeping staff in particular should make lighting control a part of their daily routine as they complete their cleaning duties.

SURFACE TRANSPORTATION

The responsibility for planning a transportation program and directing the maintenance of the vehicles required by the nursing home should be assigned to the maintenance director. The institution may decide to embark on a transportation program for staff and patients based on the availability or unavailability of local public transportation. The recruitment of personnel and staff safety and welfare may influence this decision, particularly for evening and night personnel. The transportation plan may involve a standard pick-up and delivery procedure for personnel, perhaps providing regular bus service between the institution and a central point, such as a railroad or bus station. Arrangements for transportation during emergencies—such as strikes, blizzards, and natural disasters—should also be part of the plan. The skilled nursing facility may also determine a need for conveying patients to special medical and/or recreational events.

If the facility decides to have a passenger vehicle for the transporting of residents, it should be appropriate to meet the needs of the disabled patients, affording, for example, easy ingress and egress of patients in wheelchairs through doors of sufficient width. In addition to the requirement of medical orders and family permission to leave the institution, the written family permission should authorize staff members to drive the patient to special activities. Specific personnel should be designated to drive the vehicle. Administrative approval should be obtained when special projects necessitating transportation are planned.

The number and type of vehicles needed will depend on the scope of the transportation program. One basic requirement is a four-wheel-drive pickup truck with a snowplow attachment, to be used by the maintenance department exclusively. If transportation for personnel and patients is anticipated, a van or minibus with a patient lift would be suitable. On a regular basis, it would be used by the maintenance department; however, it could be used by other staff to drive patients or to convey staff members to educational sessions outside the facility.

Whether to acquire vehicles should be a joint decision of the administrative director and the maintenance director. The decision should take into account whether to rent or to purchase the conveyances, what kind of vehicles to select, and how often models should be traded in or changed.

The maintenance director should authorize the scheduling for the use of the vehicles, their proper care and servicing, and the selection of a specific service station for the purchase of fuel and repairs.

INSPECTION BY GOVERNMENT AND INSURANCE AGENCIES

Various agencies will inspect the physical facility throughout the year. The maintenance director should accompany inspectors during their tour of the building to provide helpful information or explanations, to be available for recommendations, and to record each inspection, including the signature of the inspector, his position, and the date in a "Record of Inspections" book.

Prior to the expiration date of insurance coverage for the liability of the building, elevator, and boiler, the insurance carriers will inspect the premises or equipment for any adverse conditions that need correction. To guarantee continued coverage, the maintenance director must follow the directives of the authorized inspector concerning all insured equipment in the nursing home—from the boiler and elevator to the fire extinguishers and outside walkways.

Several government agencies are mandated to conduct surveys of the facility for varying purposes. Municipal agencies will be designated to perform plumbing, multiple residence, boiler, elevator, and air pollution inspections.

Visits by the fire department will be understandably frequent. The fire inspectors will want to know the layout of the building, the range of patient disabilities and the amount of assistance required to evacuate the building, the number of staff on duty over a twenty-four-hour period, and other specifics in order to know the needs of the residents and staff in the event of a fire emergency and to plan accordingly. In addition, the examinations of the facility for fire hazards will be part of their routine schedule. A fire inspector will also attend unannounced fire drills and staff training sessions to provide professional consultation in this very important part of the in-service program.

Surveys to evaluate the physical plant and equipment are made by the state health departments for licensure renewal, and for Medicare and Medicaid certification, and by the Joint Commission for accreditation. Other government agencies who may visit the facility periodically to assess aspects of the physical plant include county departments of health and the Occupational Safety and Health Administration.

PURCHASING

The amount of inventory to be stocked is a major consideration. One of the important factors involved is standardization. If parts and equipment are standardized to the fullest possible extent, inventories will be smaller, less money will be tied up in supplies, and less space will be needed for storage.

The availability of specific parts must be carefully studied. In general, a three- to six-month inventory will assure smooth functioning of the department. If specific parts are known to be in short supply or difficult to locate, a longer time frame may be needed.

To avoid carrying a large stock of noncritical supplies, arrangements may be made with local hardware stores to permit assigned maintenance personnel to purchase (and sign for) certain stipulated items up to a specific monthly budgeted figure. This policy will assure the availability of these parts without utilizing storage space and operating capital.

In addition to such an arrangement, the maintenance director, with the help of the purchasing agent, should still select several area vendors for the purchase of parts, routine supplies, and equipment. Once again, the use of more than one regular supplier is advantageous for the comparison of quality, reliability, and prices.

FIGURE 12-3
Fire Department Verifying Maintenance of Extinguisher

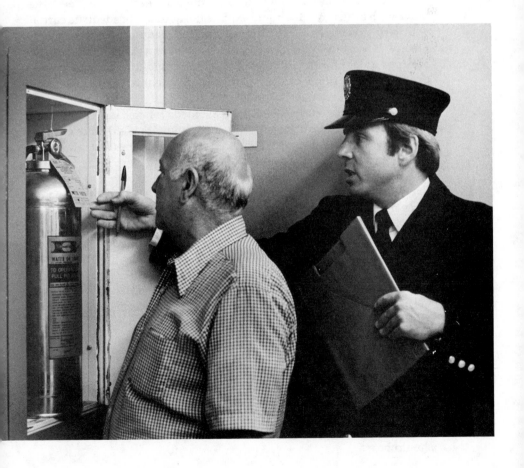

Since fuel represents a major budgetary item in nursing home operation, bids should be secured annually from at least three suppliers. The maintenance director must prepare detailed specifications. Outside contract work—such as lawn care, snow removal, and painting—also should be awarded on the basis of at least three competitive bids based on detailed specifications.

It is imperative that the maintenance director study the specifications of any new equipment prior to its purchase. He will be able to assess the ease or difficulty of installation and repair, and his analysis may save man-hours and money. For example, an autoclave that is superior in its function and reasonable in price may require the installation of utilities that make the equipment prohibitively expensive to operate.

Before giving purchase approval, the maintenance director should ascertain whether safety devices are included. In addition, he should not consider equipment that has sharp edges, crevices, poorly fitted doors and handles, squared rather than rounded corners, and wheels that move with difficulty. He should explore the question of adequate current and wiring as well as ease of repair and the manufacturer's reliability. Finally, it is critical that he determine that all aspects of the equipment are appropriate for the intended use; for example, a motor may be adequate for the periodic use of a piece of equipment but not for frequent stopping and starting or for prolonged use.

Potential difficulties should be avoided; for instance, ventilation should be provided for motors in damp locations to yield more effective operation, and sealed bearings and transistors should be used rather than tubes for reduced maintenance.

Whenever possible, time clocks should be used to activate and deactivate equipment such as outdoor lighting. When such labor-saving devices are used, the maintenance staff must remember to reset the clocks as the days lengthen or shorten.

RECORDS

Work sampling, a management tool to evaluate the utilization of personnel, is particularly desirable in the maintenance department, for workers are spread throughout the building and grounds, often without direct supervision. In work sampling, the director of maintenance randomly observes individuals or groups of maintenance staff to determine what they are doing at a particular time. They may be working, not working, talking, traveling, obtaining supplies, cleaning up, and so forth. After a reasonable number of observations are made over a certain period, the results are analyzed to determine how the workers are spending their time, whether improvements are needed, and what those improvements should be.

Among the most important records for reference are the building blueprints—architectural, mechanical, and structural. The blueprints should be updated as changes are made in the building and mechanical equipment. They should always be stored flat or should be hung.

The maintenance work order (Exhibit 12-1) can serve three purposes. It can be (1) the written request for work ordered, (2) the proposal of the work needed—estimates of cost, labor, new parts, and equipment—and (3) the record of completion. This information will assist in determining the value of continuously repairing equipment or the justification for its replacement. The need for such in-depth consideration will vary according to the size and complexity of the job; however, work order documentation is useful in planning preventive maintenance schedules as well as in evaluating the work of the maintenance department. The nursing home should establish a guideline regarding additional authorization required from the administrative director when planning costly, time-consuming, and/or decorative alteration work.

Maintenance records should be sufficiently detailed to allocate labor and materials needed for repairs to specific departments to produce accurate operating costs for that particular service.

The maintenance director must keep a schedule of all equipment, its date of purchase, and its cost, along with warranties or guarantees.

Three manuals should be provided with each new piece of equipment: two for the maintenance department and one for the department that uses the equipment. Also, abbreviated operating instructions should be attached to or displayed near each piece of equipment.

Manuals should contain instructions, limitations, procedures for repair and maintenance, diagrams, a parts replacement list, and a troubleshooting guide. The new equipment should be carefully and permanently marked with the name of the manufacturer and all identifying and descriptive material about the equipment for ready reference.

The use of checklists, which clearly delineate all items to be inspected, can help the maintenance staff in their routine surveys of the building and grounds. Separate checklists can be developed for daily, weekly, monthly, quarterly, or semiannual surveys. These checklists also can be designed to serve as a record of preventive maintenance performed.

A paint color plan for the entire building—walls, ceilings, doors, floors—must be on file and amended when the interior decorator changes the color scheme. All other finishes—together with the brand names of such items as counter tops, acoustic tiles, resilient flooring, carpeting, and ceramic tile—should be permanently on record in the maintenance department files.

Using the daily log book, which notes the department's activities and expenditures, and the monthly work order records, the maintenance

EXHIBIT 12-1
Maintenance Work Order

```
                         MAINTENANCE WORK ORDER
A.  WORK REQUEST (to be completed by department)

    Dept. _____ Date _____ Requested by _____

    Detail description of work requested:  _____

    _____

    _____


B.  WORK PROPOSAL (to be completed by Director of Maintenance)

    Date received _____ Work order no. _____ Date assigned _____

    Assigned to _____ Projected completion date _____

                                                            Charged to Dept.
                              Description          Cost       (Account No.)
    Parts and         _____  _____  _____
    Supplies
                      _____  _____  _____

                      _____  _____  _____

    Equipment         _____  _____  _____

                      _____  _____  _____

                      _____  _____  _____

    Labor (No. of     _____  _____  _____
    Man-hours)
                      _____  _____  _____

    Contracted        _____  _____  _____
    Service
                      _____  _____  _____

                      _____  _____  _____

    Total Cost                                   _____

    If required, approval by Administrative Director _____

C.  RECORD OF COMPLETION

    Date of completion _____ Actual man-hours worked _____

    Description of work done:  _____

    _____

    _____

    Maintenance worker _____ Date _____

    Approved by _____ Date _____
```

director should prepare a monthly report for the administrator. More than merely a summary of the month's activities, it keeps the administrator informed of work in progress and delays encountered and can help acquaint others with the department's priorities when they become impatient with delays in follow-through on their own requests. It is also a tool to assist the maintenance director in the review of planning and scheduling, and staff capabilities and efficiency.

FACILITIES AND MAJOR EQUIPMENT

Several areas within the nursing home are the responsibility and/or for the use of the maintenance department, including those designated for major systems such as the boiler room, elevator room, electrical room (which also houses the fire alarm system and heat detection unit), incinerator room (where permitted by law), and emergency generator room. Hazardous materials such as paints should be stored in covered metal containers placed in metal cabinets with solid metal doors in sprinklered rooms. One or two large rooms, depending on the amount of work done by in-house staff, must be allocated as workshop space for the department.

Although generally the skilled maintenance director will provide his own tools, the nursing home should provide certain major pieces of equipment to guarantee the smooth functioning of the department. These major tools include the following:

> 12-amp welder
> radial arm Dewalt saw
> tilt Arbor table saw
> joiner
> floor-mounted drill press
> grinder
> oxyacetylene set
> cement mixer
> gasoline-driven compressor
> portable pump
> industrial vacuum cleaner
> dollies
> hand trucks
> stepladders of different heights

In addition, a portable carrying chest with an assortment of frequently used parts and tools should always be fully stocked for prompt response to any need.

A maintenance garage should house all gardening tools and equipment used for exterior work: extension ladders, snowblowers, snow-plow, and so forth. Vehicles owned by the nursing home may also be stored in the garage.

SUMMARY

The building design and its maintenance impinge on everyone and everything that takes place in the nursing home. It affects the aesthetics, safety, control of infections, freedom of patient movement, range of programs, and staff and visitor satisfaction. A preventive maintenance program can contribute to energy conservation, relief from malpractice suits, and cost control. This department must deal with the added challenge of trying to maintain a structure that is in continuous use by many patients who are behaviorally disturbed and unable to follow precautionary directions.

NOTES

1.   National Fire Protection Agency, *Life Safety Code*, No. 101 (Boston, 1967). Subsequent editions not currently applicable to nursing homes.
2.   Richmond Associates, Staten Island, N.Y., *Housekeeping: Floor Maintenance Procedures*.

GENERAL REFERENCES

American Hospital Association. *Hospital Engineering Handbook*. Chicago, 1974.

CHAPTER 13

Safety

INTRODUCTION

Residents in skilled nursing facilities are primary targets for accidents because of their physical and behavioral disabilities: frequent small strokes, which cause falls; slower reaction time in response to danger; diminished visual and auditory abilities; and confusion and disorientation. However, personnel, volunteers, visitors, suppliers, and purveyors also must be protected by a carefully monitored safety program.

The safety program for a skilled nursing facility involves three aspects: accident prevention, buildings and grounds security, and fire safety and emergency plans in the event of fire, natural disasters, utility interruptions, or other anticipated occurrences.

It is the administrator's responsibility to plan for the safety of the nursing home community. Safety is concerned with the proper staffing, equipping, operation, and maintenance of the nursing home and the elimination of hazards. In addition, safety is affected by the actions of patients, staff, visitors, and volunteers. Therefore training in safety measures must be provided to all these groups and must include adequate education to potential hazards.

Accidental injuries are costly in terms of increased costs of workmen's compensation and professional and public liability insurance. Of more critical import is the cost to the skilled nursing facility of a damaged reputation in the community should the facility become known for carelessness and indifference to safety factors.

Since accidents do not just happen, it should be the safety committee's mission to eliminate all possible causes, understanding that they cannot prevent medical problems like strokes, but that they can plan with an understanding of patients' limitations. The safety committee is discussed in more detail in Chapter 16.

Resident education is also an important part of the safety program. Residents who are intellectually intact should be given a thorough indoctrination to the safety rules and regulations for their own well-being and that of their peers. It is paramount that they understand certain procedures, such as using specified exit doors to the garden area that do not activate alarms.

Conversely, the staff must be reminded that residents are participants, albeit indirectly, in all safety practices. For example, during night fire drills, it is important to announce on the public address system when the drill is over; otherwise patients in bed may believe that a real emergency exists, and they may be waiting fearfully for assistance.

As safety is a concern of all who come into the nursing home, initiative and involvement to improve conditions as well as responsibility for maintaining current safety standards should be encouraged. A suggestion box for personnel, residents, volunteers, and visitors to offer ideas on improved safety practices may encourage shy people who wish to remain anonymous. Or a prize and write-up in the facility newsletter may stimulate others who enjoy recognition to participate actively in the safety program.

BUILDING CRITERIA

It must be assumed that the building has been constructed, equipped, and furnished to comply with all applicable building codes, state and/or federal occupational safety and health codes and standards, fire protection codes, and the *Life Safety Code* compiled by the National Fire Protection Association.[1] Where codes differ, it is suggested that the more stringent regulations prevail.

The relevant codes will contain many design specifications to meet the needs of physically handicapped persons for their ease of movement, access to and use of all facilities, and overall safety; the safety committee or officer, however, may recommend additional accommodations. Fire doors, for instance, that are required by law to remain closed may in fact be too heavy and dangerous for wheelchair residents to open. However, if they are held open by an electric magnet that closes upon activation by the fire alarm system, the doors conform to fire regulations yet do not impede the movement of wheelchair residents.

Improved safety features are more easily and economically achieved with amenities rather than structural changes. For instance, the safety committee may suggest the elimination of carpeting in favor of resilient flooring in a patient unit that is heavily populated by wheelchair or walker patients. The use of pedestal tables that do not have an apron for wheelchair patients, or sturdy heavy chairs that will not slide or tip over when residents sit down or get up, may be worthwhile and more feasible.

Such design criteria assure that residents can use the exterior and interior environment freely and easily. Residents are much more likely to be taken or to take themselves outdoors if they do not have to negotiate obstacles such as stairs and steep ramps. Thus proper safety measures actually encourage the social and physical rehabilitation of long-term-care patients.

Although skilled nursing facilities have incorporated into their interior and exterior environment physical features related to safety—such as ramps, handrails, fire-resistant structures, nonslip flooring, grab bars, and nonglare lighting—a continuous surveillance program is necessary to ensure that the equipment, furniture, building, and grounds are free of hazards.

SAFETY INSPECTIONS

Without fail, every area of the skilled nursing facility, even closets and storage areas, should be inspected once a year. Also, surveys at night might unveil precarious situations that go unnoticed during the day. The surveillance team should report its findings to the safety committee for action and recommendations. The committee may wish to develop a checklist to use as a guide during its surveys. The process of preparing such a guide can serve as an interdisciplinary group educational experience.

Routine inspections will reinforce safety concepts for the staff and promote morale, for personnel will recognize that the nursing home values their well-being. The recognition that key staff take time to ensure that safety conditions are proper will further demonstrate that safety is an important aspect of the nursing home program.

ACCIDENT AND INCIDENT PREVENTION

Although prevention relates to both accidents and incidents, the difference between the terms should be clarified. An *incident* is an unexpected event that becomes an *accident* only when there is a casualty. For example, if a patient falls but sustains no injuries, the fall is an incident; if a patient fractures a hip in the fall, the fall is an accident. A prevention program must therefore relate to avoiding incidents and thus to avoiding accidents.

While incidents and accidents affecting residents and personnel are cause for concern, accidents involving visitors and especially family members present special problems. The fact that a relative may trip on an uneven path or may catch a heel on frayed carpet has a more far-reaching effect than the particular incident, for the family member may then ascribe any problem experienced by his relative to unsafe conditions in the nursing home. If a patient falls as a result of a stroke, his family member may mistakenly blame the nursing home as a result of the incident regarding the uneven path. All the family's anxieties will be accentuated by such experiences, and their hostility and suspicion may become apparent. After all, the nursing home is supposed to safeguard the patient. If visitors are subject to avoidable accidents, the credibility of the entire nursing home program is in question.

The first step to accident prevention is good housekeeping by all personnel. Clutter and spills on the floor can be the cause of falls and demand immediate attention. Hallways, fire exits, and stairways must always be clear, especially for emergency use.

Nursing

Each department has its own special safety hazards relating to its personnel and to the residents it services. During the orientation of nursing personnel, it should be noted that patient incidents occur most often at the change of shifts; thus special efforts must be made to keep patients under surveillance during these periods. Patients in restraints must be observed regularly, as sometimes they work themselves into awkward positions that make them accident prone. Since falls from beds occur with some degree of frequency, high–low beds must be in the low position and side rails raised when occupied by residents; cranks must always be carefully returned to their hidden position under the bed to prevent tripping. Where possible, overbed tables should be eliminated, as residents may lean on them for support, only to have them slide away. Catheter tubes must be checked when residents are seated or in bed to make sure that they are not an obstacle to others in the immediate area and that the drainage is uninterrupted.

Safety equipment for patients includes a bedside nurses' call system for each resident and grab bars and call systems in each patient bathing and toilet area. Dusting powder makes for slippery floors, so the nursing staff must exercise caution when using it.

The proper surveillance and storage of portable equipment is an integral part of the safety program. Medication carts should never be left unattended. Furthermore, a procedure should be established in the event of a medication error. Oxygen tanks must be stored in a safe location away from heat.

Crutches, canes, and walkers should be inspected to be sure that their tips have not become smooth from wear. Wheelchair brakes should also be inspected frequently.

Safety also involves protection against the spread of infection. Therefore contaminated wastes must be kept in sealed impervious containers until they are disposed of correctly.

Each resident should have his name indicated on his bedroom door and should wear an identification bracelet to facilitate routine checks at bedtime, while passing medications, and during mealtime to make sure every resident is accounted for. Alarms on exit doors should be checked at each shift change to make certain that they will activate in case a patient should attempt to leave the premises.

Dietary

All but dietary employees are prohibited from entering the kitchen. Wet or greasy floors are always a concern in the kitchen and must be attended to immediately. Needless to say, dietary staff must be trained in the careful use of sharp equipment and hot stoves, ovens, and dishwashers to avoid burns. The kitchen in particular is no place for games or practical joking, as carelessness is the first step to an accident.

Housekeeping

In housekeeping, care must be exercised in handling trash collection and disposal to prevent accidents and the spread of infection and to promote fire safety. When using powerful cleaning chemicals, detergents, and abrasives such as steel wool, personnel should wear rubber gloves. Plastic eye shields should be supplied for those who do high dusting or ceiling cleaning or painting. Only laundry personnel should be allowed to operate washers and dryers, as they are familiar with the equipment and are present during its operation. Lint traps in dryers must be regularly cleaned to prevent fires.

Whenever the work of housekeeping or maintenance personnel poses a precarious situation—such as during floor washing—warning signs should be used to redirect traffic around the area in question. One side of a corridor floor should be washed at a time, allowing traffic to pass safely on the other side. Extreme care should be exercised in the use of electric equipment to see that electric cables do not cross corridors or traffic lanes. Housekeeping carts, buckets, maintenance trucks, and tools should not be left unattended or where they are not easily visible.

Maintenance

There are special areas of concern that the maintenance staff should check during their daily plant inspection. Doors to stairwells and hazardous areas must remain closed. Although a valve is required to regulate the temperature of hot water automatically, its operation must be routinely checked to ensure that hot water to resident areas is no more than 110°F (43°C) and that hot water to the laundry and kitchen meets required temperatures. Outside walkways and parking areas must remain level and free of litter and obstructions to prevent pedestrian accidents.

FIGURE 13-1
Caution Sign Marking Hazardous Area

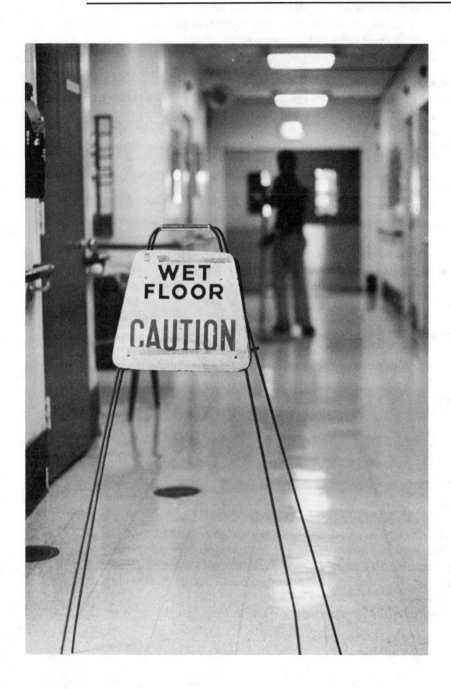

The maintenance department should give first priority to repair jobs of a safety nature. Damaged or broken equipment should be removed from the area, if possible; it should at least be labeled as unusable.

Maintenance staff generally wear skid-proof boots; they should be requested to purchase the nonmarking type so that they will not damage the finish of resilient floors. Of course, wet-wear suits should be provided for outdoor work in foul weather.

When welding, maintenance staff should always wear special head gear, gloves, and protective vests and should use portable welding screens for the protection of others. Tasks such as spray painting, sanding, and boiler cleaning require the use of goggles and respirators to filter out the dust and mist. Hard hats should be part of the maintenance uniform for outside ladder or scaffold work as a protection against dropped hammers and the like. For sewer work, heavy rubber elbow gloves and face shields are necessary protection, and linesman's gloves are essential for electrical repairs.

Policies for All Personnel

All staff members should wear sensible, nonslip shoes. Incidentally, in many instances safety would be well served if patients were to wear lace-up sneakers, which provide better traction than most slip-on styles.

Again training in safety is essential for every employee in every department. All staff should be taught the proper way to lift people, heavy equipment, and supplies, as improper lifting is a major cause of occupational accidents. In all departments, instructions for using equipment should be posted near the item. Employees must be instructed on the use and location of emergency switches and controls.

An emergency first aid kit, maintained and administered by the director of nursing or his designee, must be available for use by personnel.

Government regulations require that all skilled nursing facility employees have pre-employment and annual physicals. In addition to ensuring that staff members are not carriers of disease to a susceptible patient population, this requirement exists for the safety of each individual, to confirm that he can carry out the duties inherent in his job category. With specific federal legislation barring employment discrimination on the basis of handicap, pre-employment physicals gain further significance in assuring the employer that the applicant can perform the job for which he is applying. In conformance with the law, pre-employment medical examinations must be required of all applicants regardless of any handicap.

Physicals also establish a basis for evaluating whether injuries or illnesses suffered subsequent to employment are truly the result of occupational hazards. Again, this information would help determine

FIGURE 13-2
Maintenance Worker Wearing Protective Gear

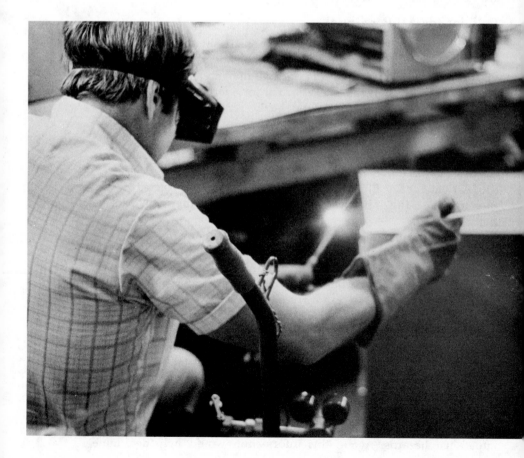

whether the candidate is suited for the job if indeed he has a history of physical problems that would be exacerbated by the type of work he would be doing.

Finally, healthy employees are an asset to the facility's safety program, for they are less tired, more careful in their work, on the job more regularly, and more concerned with and aware of good safety practices.

Personnel safety is fostered by the federal Occupational Safety and Health Administration, which was created as a result of the Occupational Safety and Health Act passed by Congress in 1970 to assure safe working conditions without hazards that might cause death or major injury. Routine unannounced on-site inspections are part of the legislation, and detailed records of occupational injuries and illnesses sustained in the previous calendar year are required to be kept. Penalties are mandatory for each major violation. Since nursing homes must conform to many other codes and regulations that include safety precautions, it is unlikely that federal and state surveyors would have missed major hazards.

Accident/Incident Records

All incidents/accidents involving patients, staff, and visitors must be documented. The accident report is used as a basis for workmen's compensation claims; therefore all incidents and accidents should be recorded, no matter how minor. Unfortunately, staff members frequently think themselves not injured and do not report a back strain after having lifted a heavy patient, when indeed they need medical attention a few days later.

All the advantages of proper maintenance of accident records scarcely need to be elaborated. Among the major advantages are that the records form bases for identifying weaknesses to be remedied in the physical environment and in employee work practices, for nursing home legal records in case of professional or public liability cases, and for focusing employee and volunteer educational programs on safety. The medical director should review patient incident and accident reports for ideas about how to improve patient care procedures.

GROUNDS AND BUILDING SECURITY

The nature of the patient population in a skilled nursing facility mandates an active security program in their behalf. Precautions consistent with the facility's size and geographic location are needed as well for staff members, volunteers, and visitors.

The nursing home will have to evaluate its problems and concerns to verify the need for a specialized security force. The amount and kind of security features that are built into the structure and the surrounding grounds will help determine whether security guards are needed at all and, if so, when and where. Consultation with the local police may be helpful for this purpose. Perhaps only one security officer on duty during the evening and night would suffice, although conditions in the area may call for more officers to cover the entire premises at any given time. The security force requirements of the nursing home will determine whether it should employ its own security department or contract with an outside firm for the service.

The first priority of a security program, as with all safety programs, is the protection of residents. In the case of the chronically ill aged residents in a skilled nursing facility, this means taking precautions to preclude their wandering out of the building or off the premises. In addition to a clearly written wristband with identifying information, all residents should have their photographs taken shortly after admission and affixed to their health record for ease of description in case they are missing. Properly placed mirrors and nursing stations may help keep confused patients from entering stairwells and elevators unattended.

Outdoor areas should be completely enclosed by sturdy, attractive fencing with gates for entering and exiting. Such measures provide one more obstacle for the confused patient to overcome before leaving the grounds.

The building entrance used by visitors should be staffed during visiting hours by a receptionist, who will ascertain that unaccompanied residents do not leave the building unless so permitted by their attending physician. An intercom system connected to the main nursing station could be used by evening and night visitors to announce themselves and gain entrance to the facility. When not directly supervised, all exits and entrances should be controlled by an audio-visual device that would warn the staff of a resident's departure. Staff members must be trained to respond instantly to the alarm system and to institute an immediate search if a patient is missed.

The search for a missing patient should be a clearly defined process so as not to waste time. Once it is determined that the patient is not in the building via a careful search (including the rooftop area) and is not checked out in the off-premises book, the supervisor should contact the administrative director, giving a full description of the patient and incidents leading up to his disappearance. In the meantime, all available nursing home personnel should fan out into the surrounding neighborhood. Should this initial search prove fruitless, the administrative director should contact both the police and the patient's family, keeping them informed at regular intervals until the patient is found.

New personnel and volunteers should be screened carefully and observed during their initial weeks of service. In a large facility, staff identification tags with photos are essential; in a small facility, name tags delineating the employee's name and position may suffice. Volunteers should be required to wear identifying name pins, especially volunteers who do not wear uniforms.

Visitors to the facility should be limited to using the main entrance and should always be asked to identify whom they are visiting or the purpose of their visit. All nursing home personnel should be instructed to question strangers they find in the building or known persons who have no reason for being in a particular area. Those who have no business at the nursing home should be requested to leave. In a large facility, visitors may be given passes as a way of authorizing their presence.

Where permitted by law, people—including families, staff, and volunteers—leaving the building with packages and bags must be able to account for the contents to designated individuals. An effective screening program of new employees and volunteers should preclude pilferage and theft.

Lockers that are not easily accessible to visitors, but are under some kind of ongoing surveillance, should be made available to employees. Personnel should be informed as to what items are acceptable for storage in lockers; for example, coats are appropriate, but money and cameras are strongly discouraged.

Sometimes female staff will request escort service to their cars at the midnight shift change. The security guard, if available, may provide this. If transportation is not easily obtainable, it is wise to provide taxi service at that time to assure the staff's safe arrival and departure. Alternatively, the nursing home may provide its own taxi service to and from a bus depot or other central location to assist personnel commuting to work at odd hours.

The most effective means of securing the interior environment of the nursing home from intruders is to deter entrance to the building. The use of panic bars on all outside doors allows for their immediate use during an emergency, while preventing unauthorized persons access to the building. Employees as well as visitors should be restricted in the entrances and exits they are allowed to use. All exits and entrances should be well lighted, have alarms that sound at the nurses' station if they are opened inappropriately, and be observed by guards or closed-circuit television. Bright lighting in parking areas and generally surrounding the building is a further deterrent to troublemakers.

For the safety of important documents and resident cash and valuables, a fireproof safe should be installed in the business office. An automatically timed alarm system should be attached to the safe to provide added security when the office is closed.

Patients should be requested to give their valuables to their families or to place them in the nursing home safe. Similarly, they should keep only small amounts of cash in their rooms, with the balance of their funds deposited in the nursing home safe. Families also should be apprised of these and other security measures. New clothing or keepsakes brought into the facility should always be shown and/or reported to the nurse in charge so that some personnel will be familiar with the article in case it should be misplaced.

Certain areas of the nursing home should be locked when not attended, such as central, dietary, and linen storage because of their large stocks, and x-ray and laboratory rooms because of costly equipment. Also, office areas with expensive dictating equipment and typewriters and the business office, with its safe, should always be secured when unattended.

The lock security system for the nursing home is a crucial part of the overall security plan. Arrangements for a master, submaster, and individual keying system should be made at the initial design stages in order to allow the proper lock tumblers to be installed on each door. This system would allow certain staff members to have a master key for all locks, others such as department heads to have a key for only those areas to which they routinely need access, and still others to have a key for only one office.

The distribution of keys should be assigned to one person, preferably the director of maintenance, who would be able to duplicate keys when needed. Naturally, if a lost key is cause for concern, the lock must be changed.

FIRE SAFETY PROGRAM

Probably the most important responsibility of the safety committee is to promote and oversee a rigorous fire safety program. Following that charge is their obligation to develop sensible and workable plans for facility operation when faced with reasonably expected emergencies, whether they be man-made or natural.

The various disaster plans should be compiled into one booklet for reference when needed and for use as an educational tool. All personnel should receive a copy during orientation, with instructions to become familiar with the salient points of each plan, especially how it relates to them. A copy of the booklet should also be placed at each nursing station and department office.

Staff training is an essential aspect of each disaster plan. Classroom sessions can be held to review the institution of each plan, the special problems encountered when it is put into effect, individual personnel assignments, the use of fire alarms and extinguishers, and methods of evacuating patients. Attendance at these sessions should be mandatory.

Unannounced fire drills should be held at least once a month, under differing circumstances, and should be distributed among the three nursing shifts. The drills must be supervised closely to ascertain that all personnel respond immediately to their assignments. A minimum of twice a year, during good weather, drills should be expanded to include practice evacuations. The safety director should write a report to evaluate each drill, mentioning how long it took and detailing any special incidents.

The *Life Safety Code* of the National Fire Protection Agency dictates specific requirements to which a skilled nursing facility must conform in order to be considered fire-safe. The requirements mandate specific fire-resistant construction, especially for certain high-hazard areas, stairways and other vertical passageways, and corridors. The *Life Safety Code* also covers interior finishes (curtains, carpeting, ceiling tile, and furnishings) and fire warning and safety equipment, and lists regulations concerning staff education and the development of disaster plans.

Conforming buildings have floor areas with two separate fire sections, each with a means of egress so that the section with the fire can be closed off and the fire contained while people are moved to other floor sections and evacuated. Separating the fire sections must be fire-resistant doors that remain closed or are held open via an electromagnetic device, which releases them when the fire alarm sounds.

Required fire safety equipment includes heat or smoke detection devices, which activate the alarm; manual alarm boxes; sprinklers that operate in the area from which the alarm is sounded; and stationary and portable fire extinguishers.

A fire extinguisher is classified according to the type of fire for which it is effective. The *Life Safety Code* stipulates that the fire hazards in a defined area dictate the type of extinguisher(s) that should be available in that area. Extinguishers must be clearly labeled, in good operating condition, recharged as needed, and checked annually.

The fire safety program is of utmost importance due to the enormous responsibility that the nursing home has in caring for severely disabled residents. Consultation from the local fire department is crucial during the development of the plan. The plan should contain four major parts: an ongoing fire prevention program, a quick fire alert system, an efficient fire control plan, and a well-rehearsed evacuation method. Staff training materials should emphasize smoking regulations and the proper disposal of cigarettes and matches, good housekeeping, the proper storage of supplies, especially combustibles, and the importance of having *all* electrical equipment repaired by knowledgeable persons. The location of alarm boxes, fire extinguishers by specified type, and fire exits must be identified in the disaster plan booklet, and might also be indicated on floor plans posted on individual floors.

Smoking, a major cause of fires, is best controlled and limited to certain areas rather than prohibited. Complete prohibition of smoking among patients, personnel, and visitors is almost impossible to enforce and will lead to surreptitious smoking.

Smoking regulations should be carefully formulated with the recognition that patients may be forgetful and thus should smoke only in public areas where supervision is available and never in bedrooms. Visitors and staff must abide by similar regulations. "No smoking" signs with a notation specifically stating where smoking is permitted should be posted in appropriate areas. As an additional precaution, ashtrays and wastebaskets should be constructed of noncombustible materials such as glass or metal, never plastic. Visitors should be urgently requested not to leave matches with residents.

Prompt response upon the discovery of fire is paramount in the fire alert program. The first concern is to remove patients from immediate danger and, only after that is assured, to take time to sound the alarm. A follow-up phone call to the fire department is recommended to ensure that the alarm did sound at headquarters.

Coding the alarm system to the origin of the fire is mandatory, as it allows personnel to know where the fire is. A specifically assigned staff person, such as the nursing supervisor, would then be able to use the public address system to direct the fire brigade. No other personnel should use the public address system, nor should any pronouncement of "fire" be made. Panic must be avoided.

With those two critical steps completed, personnel should then direct themselves to containing the fire. Personnel in each area should close all doors and windows in their immediate vicinity, turn off all electrical equipment operating in the area threatened by fire, shut off all oxygen tank valves, and keep all doors, especially fire doors, closed except when necessary to pass through to combat fire or to evacuate patients. Wet blankets may be placed under closed doors to confine fire and smoke. A window may be opened to get some fresh air, provided the door is closed. The essential "don'ts" are: do not block stairways, exits, or corridors; do not turn off lights; do not use the elevator; and do not panic.

Residents who are aware of the fire must be reassured that everything is under control and that they are safe. Patients who are ambulatory require special attention to keep them from panicking and trying to flee the building.

Actual fire fighting is undertaken by the fire brigade—specially designated and trained personnel who report to the fire scene with extinguishers to bring the fire under control as much as possible before the fire department arrives. However, during the evening and night shifts when fewer personnel, exclusively nursing, are on duty, staff efforts should be directed to caring for the patients rather than fighting the fire.

The nursing home differs from schools and factories, where the main objective when fire occurs is to clear the premises of all persons as quickly as possible. In the nursing home, leaving the building is the last resort. However, there is always the possibility that it may be necessary to evacuate patients and personnel even though the facility may be well constructed and fire protected.

EVACUATION PLAN

Several plans of evacuation routes should be mapped out according to the location of the fire. In all instances, people should be moved away from the fire, either to an immediate egress from the building or through fire doors to a separate fire-safe area that is accessible to an exit. The extent of evacuation would depend on the severity of the fire and the building construction: modern fire-resistant buildings would not need total evacuation, but, more likely, movement of those patients in danger to a fire-safe area. "Horizontal evacuation" means moving patients to a safe area on the same floor, while "vertical evacuation" means the downward movement of residents to a safe area below or out of the building should the fire get out of control. Staff in-service sessions and training manuals should review the principles involved in evacuation so that they may be properly implemented.

When evacuation of an area is ordered, it should be done under the direction of the ranking officer of the fire department. Charge nurses should present themselves to the fire department officer to tell him which patients need assistance in removal from the area. If evacuation from the building is planned, residents should be wrapped in blankets.

The evacuation of the building under any circumstance requires the assistance of numerous transportation services, ambulances, ambulettes, taxis, buses, and individual volunteers. Prior arrangements for the provision of these services is recommended to ensure their availability when needed.

Ambulatory patients should be moved first and not left unattended, as they are subject to panic. They should be instructed to line up outside their rooms, to form a chain by holding hands, and to follow a lead monitor to a designated point.

Nonambulatory patients in immediate danger should be moved first, then others who might be subject to danger if fire should enter their units. Wheelchair residents could be moved in their wheelchairs if only horizontal evacuation is necessary. Other methods for evacuating non-ambulatory residents include the use of stretchers, back carry, hip carry, chair-seat carry (in which two bearers cross hands to form a seat), or blanket "roll." In the last method, the patient is placed on a blanket on the floor, the top corners of the blanket are rolled in, and the patient is pulled, head foremost, to a safe area. Quick removal by bed or mattress in a fire emergency has proved impractical and often impossible.

After evacuation, rooms and halls should be searched for stragglers, and any open windows and doors should be closed.

Upon arrival in a safe area, a resident count should be made (using the Kardex to check against patient wristlets). After the immediate crisis is over and all patients have been safely evacuated, every effort should be made to secure patients' records for transfer along with them to hospitals or other points of evacuation. The charge nurse should record where patients and their records have been transported. Once residents have been relocated, families should be notified of the situation and their relative's location.

In the event of any patient or staff casualties, the ranking officer of the fire department must be notified to arrange for the swift removal of the injured person.

UTILITY INTERRUPTION

Among the more common emergencies to be anticipated is a utility interruption. Although a utility interruption may not be as immediately life threatening or require the same urgency of action as other disasters, it can cripple the building's operation if there is no alternate plan to institute. As with any other emergency, a coordination of efforts is the key to coping with the situation effectively.

Planning for a minimum of a twenty-four-hour period is recommended; if natural conditions in the area—such as floods or hurricanes—make the nursing home vulnerable to more extensive power shortages, the routine plan must provide for longer periods.

Skilled nursing facilities are required to provide an alternate source of electrical power that at minimum illuminates all means of egress and operates all fire detection, alarm, and extinguishing systems and any life safety support systems. Further requirements may be found in individual state codes, and the nursing home may decide to extend its emergency power to cover additional services it deems necessary.

Planning for a utility interruption should then begin with an understanding of what equipment will be operable when powered by the emergency generator; this information should be in the disaster plan booklet. With that knowledge, steps can then be outlined for the functioning of services that will be affected by a blackout.

Initially, a call to the power company should be made to determine whether the blackout is localized to the nursing home or area-wide. The caller should inform the utility company that the nursing home is affected and that it has a special need for electrical service. Throughout the blackout, calls should be made at specified intervals to determine the progress made on restoring services, for example, if power is not expected to return for twelve hours, more extensive arrangements may be necessary.

Key off-duty personnel should be notified of the situation. The medical director, the administrative director, the director of nursing, and the nursing supervisor on duty should coordinate patient management; the director of maintenance, with the help of the dietary director and the executive housekeeper, should coordinate plant maintenance. Other staff members might be asked to report on duty as needed.

Several flashlights with long-lasting fluorescent bulbs should be stored at each nurses' station and in the kitchen, laundry room, and other locations that may require additional portable lighting. Even if the emergency generator provides general lighting, it is helpful to have these flashlights on hand in case the generator should malfunction. Having at least one battery-operated clock and radio in the building is recommended. A battery-operated portable public address system that is used by activity personnel for amplifying programs can be used when the regular system is not functioning. Walkie-talkies for immediate and constant communication, such as during an evacuation, may be even more helpful.

Patients should be reassured about their safety and that of the building. Assigned personnel should remain with residents in community, activity, or dining rooms. Nursing assistants should make frequent rounds of the unit to reassure residents who are in their rooms. This is especially important if the nurses' call system is inoperable. After a significant length of time, if evacuation of the building is not contemplated due to the extent of the blackout, residents should be encouraged to stay in bed and they should be given extra blankets for warmth. At no time should the patient unit or other areas where patients are congregated be depleted of staff.

The availability and quantity of essential supplies of food, medications, linens, and water should be checked, and rationing should be started if necessary. A sufficient inventory of plastic utensils, paper cups, and paper plates should be maintained for use if the dishwasher is inoperable. If the power shortage is limited to the nursing home and/or its immediate environs, arrangements can be made with fast-food outlets or foodservice companies for an emergency feeding program. The need for such backup services would depend on whether the alternate power source was designed to provide electricity to kitchen equipment.

Naturally, if the elevator is not functioning, staff cooperation will be needed to transport food, supplies, and residents between floors. Again, a plan may be needed for rescuing people trapped in elevators if that is a potential problem.

Nonoperation of the heating system in cold weather is a major concern should the power shortage be prolonged. Renting a mobile steam boiler may offer a temporary solution or evacuation of the building may be a viable alternative. Certainly, if the power shortage is area-wide, evacuating the building is no solution. Evacuation under these circumstances would take on a different tone than evacuation done in the face of fire or explosion, as panic is less likely to occur and more preparation time is available. Swift, efficient removal of residents remains the goal, however.

EXTERNAL DISASTERS

Area-wide external disasters might be natural disasters—blizzards, hurricanes, floods, tornadoes, earthquakes—or nuclear or conventional arms attack. For external disasters that might reasonably be anticipated, the facility should develop a disaster plan to cover an adequate period— three or four days in some instances.

Many of the steps outlined under utility interruption—regarding staff notification, auxiliary power systems, and patient care—would apply in these circumstances. The conservation of food, water, and medical supplies takes on added importance and should be carefully supervised by department heads. In an earthquake, tornado, flood, or hurricane, patients should be away from windows, preferably remaining in inner hallways. Special arrangements need to be made for staff, such as transportation to and from work and/or temporary housing. An assigned person should keep tuned to the local civil defense radio station for instructions, and should keep in contact with the area civil defense coordinator.

The lack of utility operation, especially dead telephones, may pose a serious problem during such times. Personnel with citizen's band radios in their cars could be helpful in relaying information or requests to community agencies. Indeed, it may be necessary to disconnect utilities to avoid further damage to equipment.

BOMB THREATS

Bombs and bomb threats are becoming ever more popular ways to instill fear and terror in a community, and there is no reason to think that nursing homes are excluded from such deranged thinking or action. A procedure for handling bomb threats must be a part of the emergency plan booklet; and special training should be given to the receptionist or switchboard operator, who would most likely receive such calls.

If possible, the person receiving the call should give it to the senior person in charge—if not administrative personnel, then the nursing supervisor. The following guidelines would serve the individual handling the call: (1) Note the time of the call(s); (2) during the conversation, try to ascertain when the bomb will go off, where it is, and what it looks like; (3) be alert to any information the caller gives about his knowledge, or lack of knowledge, of the building or personnel. The incident should be promptly reported to the police, and key off-duty personnel should be notified.

The senior person in charge must immediately decide whether to evacuate the building. He will have to consider the weather, the amount of time allowed for a search according to the phone call, other revealing information from the caller, and the past history of such threats.

If the decision is made to evacuate, an announcement over the loudspeaker should state that the building is being evacuated as part of a staff training procedure and that staff members should open all doors and windows. Patients closest to the suspected bomb should be moved first. Never use the elevator for evacuation unless the location of the bomb is known.

Before the police arrive, floor diagrams should be studied, if possible, to organize a search. Only personnel familiar with an area should be assigned to search, for they are more likely to notice any differences. They will be looking for anything that looks out of the ordinary. If the suspected bomb is found, it must not be touched but reported to the person in charge. After the police arrive, a report of action taken should be given, with a review of whether to evacuate the building if it has not already been done.

CIVIL DISTURBANCE

Civil disturbance is another activity that is occurring with increasing frequency and it may, as in an union strike, or may not be directed to the nursing home in particular. In either case, measures must be taken to protect people and the premises from injury.

Appropriate off-duty personnel should be notified of the activity for their information and for their directives. Police should be immediately contacted and kept current about the disturbance, about any damage incurred, and about the need for assistance. If the situation warrants, department heads may need to notify their staff of plans to ensure their safe arrival at work.

When threatened by a group disturbance, the staff should be directed to lock all doors and windows. Outside gates should be latched and staff automobiles should be moved as close to the building as possible to facilitate their observation. If the disturbance occurs at night, all outside lights should be turned on.

If a facility has the services of a security force, its activity should be appropriately altered. Otherwise, male staff members, if available, should be assigned to patrol outside the building.

The administrative director, with guidance from the governing body and appropriate professional staff, should coordinate the release of information to families, volunteers, and the community at large. Outside purveyors and attending physicians will need to be informed of what steps have been taken to assist them to enter and leave the premises. Nursing supervisors should be authorized to speak to families; the activities director must inform volunteers; and only the administrative director or his designee should address the press.

SUMMARY

In summary, a nursing home must confront the safety problems inherent in myriad organizations. It must meet the demands of a hotel, a restaurant, a laundry, a pharmacy, a gymnasium, a social club, a medical office, a school—all superimposed on a fragile group of physically and/or intellectually impaired elderly persons. Constant awareness on the part of all employees of the scope and components of the safety program is the only guarantee of the program's success.

NOTES

1. National Fire Protection Agency, *Life Safety Code*, No. 101 (Boston, 1967). Subsequent editions not currently applicable to nursing homes.

GENERAL REFERENCES

American Hospital Association and National Safety Council. *Safety Guide for Health Care Institutions*. Chicago, 1972.

Business

INTRODUCTION

The skilled nursing facility represents big business in terms of funds expended and people served. With the anticipated continued growth of the over-sixty-five population and the consequent increase in the number of Medicare and Medicaid beneficiaries, the skilled nursing facility can be expected to become a larger and more important agency in the constellation of health care facilities.

Whether the institution is nonprofit or proprietary, whether it is directed by a private corporation or a government agency, management must be informed about the institution's financial position to aid in the decision-making process and to exercise internal control. Internal control is an organized way of coordinating methods and measures used in the nursing home to safeguard its assets, verify the accuracy and reliability of its accounting data, encourage efficient operation, and adhere to specific administrative policies.

The process of accounting provides meaningful documentation for management control. For example, if head nurses are required to sign for supplies such as catheter trays and plastic gloves, thereby permitting comparisons with other similar nursing units, they will be much more concerned with sloppy usage than they will if no records are kept. The head nurse will probably determine whether one shift in his unit is responsible for the carelessness or whether all tours of duty share the culpability. The workers on the designated shift(s) will be queried and eventually responsibility will be placed. In any case, potentially expensive problems can be avoided by continuous efforts at cost control at every level of each department.

The business department has the responsibility of maintaining complete and current financial records for all patients, employees, and accounts in an orderly and efficient manner, thus contributing to the economical management of the facility in accordance with the operating budget. Its functions include chronicling assets, liabilities, and equities; collecting and recording of income; disbursing and recording expenditures; developing an itemized estimate of income and expenses for the operating budget; purchasing and noting the purchase of supplies and equipment; controlling inventory; accumulating statistical data; protecting patients' personal valuables; and maintaining payroll records.

DEFINITIONS AND PRINCIPLES

Board members and key employees—including department heads, personnel in administration, and so forth—should have no direct or indirect ownership or participation in any outside business organization that services the nursing home. This should be clearly stipulated in the orientation of new members of the governing body and supervisory personnel. Even when such business arrangements are completely competitive and aboveboard, apparent conflicts of interest may encourage poor practices on the part of other personnel.

Statistics

Financial data can be interpreted only if accompanied by baseline statistical information. Accurate statistical data must be obtained for the purposes of administrative control; acquisition of material for budget preparation; computation of costs and proper charges; completion of reports to owners, governing bodies, third-party payers, government agencies, patients, families, and the community; and development of long-range plans with reference to replacement and expansion.

Accrual System

The facility should work by the accrual basis of accounting rather than the cash system. In the accrual system, revenue earned or expenses incurred are recorded in a defined period; the cash system is merely a recording of actual cash receipts and disbursements. Personnel vacations, sick time, holidays, and other fringes must also be accrued to determine actual expenses. A more sophisticated method, accrual takes into account the value of assets and liabilities when determining the facility's financial position; therefore it presents a more accurate picture.

Uniform Accounting System

Adherence to a uniform accounting cycle on a continuing basis is necessary to allow for a comparison of activity and to assist in internal control. The calendar year is suggested as the accounting period, to conform with the requirements of most fiscal intermediaries.

Operating Budget

The operating budget is absolutely essential to the functions of management planning and control, for it is a forecast of operation based on the facility's goals with regard to patients, families, staff, and the community; it is also a forecast of anticipated income based on an assessment of the market for skilled nursing services; the number of patient-days for Medicare, Medicaid, or privately sponsored patients; and fluctuations in reimbursement rates set by third-party payers.

The budget considers the upcoming year's planned program for the nursing home, allowing for the expansion of activities and the development of new services. It must also take into account increases in the cost of living and anticipated increases in nursing home expenditures, especially salaries, which are the major expense of the nursing home. A reasonable amount must be allocated as a reserve to meet unexpected expenditures. Although not a sacred document, the operating budget expedites the proper handling of income and expenditures and serves as an adjunct to good management.

Capital Expenditures Plan

When expansion, improvements, or an equipment purchase of over $100,000 is anticipated, a capital expenditures plan to cover a three-year period must be developed in addition to the operating budget. The plan should identify all sources of financing and the purpose of each planned capital expense. The nursing home must receive approval for such expenditures from the local Health Systems Agency before proceeding.

Operating Capital

Operating capital will be required to provide for the time lag caused by the practice of fiscal intermediaries, public assistance agencies, and other third-party payers in providing reimbursement after the provision of services. To allow for such delays in payment, sufficient operating capital for a two- to three-month period should be available. Institutions using a monthly billing cycle may seek interim financing for Medicare and Medicaid patients, whereby the third-party payer will advance a specified portion of the usual monthly billing at the beginning of the month and make up the difference at the end of the month or will provide a predetermined amount of operating capital.

Assets and Income

Assets are things owned by the nursing home that have value, including cash, accounts receivable, inventory, investments, land, buildings, and equipment. Income or revenue can derive from the care of patients, investment income, grants, legacies, estates, and general contributions. Revenue for patient care can originate from private patient funds, public agency funds (especially Medicaid and Medicare), and private insurance funds.

Contributions

The voluntary nonprofit facility should acknowledge contributions to express appreciation and to give the donor a permanent record for income tax deduction. In addition, the facility should maintain a detailed list of all contributions. It should be clearly understood and stated in writing that contributions cannot be a condition of admission or retention of a resident in the skilled nursing facility, nor may contributions be used for the specific benefit of a resident.

Capitalization

Capitalization refers to consideration of expenditures as an asset in the balance sheet rather than merely an expense. A uniform basis will need to be determined regarding what expenditures justify capitalization. Major expenditures with an extended life span, over three years, should always be capitalized and depreciated. Minor equipment will most often be considered an operating expense. Normal repair and maintenance of depreciable assets should be capitalized only if such repair substantially adds to the life of the asset. Such alterations should be capitalized, but the period of capitalization may not extend longer than the life of the original asset.

Depreciation

The building and equipment—assets—should be considered subject to depreciation. In other words, their value lessens year by year due to wear and tear. Depreciation therefore becomes an operating expense, as it decreases the value of the asset; it must be computed to determine the facility's financial position with respect to the value of its assets. The estimated life of the asset used to compute depreciation should be taken from some recognized authoritative source. The straight-line method of depreciation, whereby the same amount is deducted each year, is recommended over an accelerated depreciation schedule, as most third-party payers will follow this practice.

To have the funds available to purchase new equipment when the old is no longer functional, the nursing facility should bank or set aside the equivalent amount of funds as depreciated. Funding depreciation ensures that sufficient money will be on hand to replace depreciated and deteriorated furnishings and equipment.

Book Value

The book value of an item is the difference between the original cost of the capitalized item minus the accumulated depreciation and including any salvage value. Thus if a building is considered to have a life of forty years, its book value would be its historical cost—that is, its cost forty years ago—minus depreciation.

Special Funds

Some facilities receive funds restricted as to use, which may include endowment funds, building replacement and expansion funds, and specific purpose funds. In pure endowment funds, the principal always remains intact; in term endowments, the principal can be used for special events or after a certain period. Funds may be pooled for investment purposes, with the management of investments the responsibility of the governing body. Income generated by principal can be designated for either general or restricted purposes.

Unrestricted funds come from routine daily activities and unrestricted contributions, which the governing body may designate for special uses.

Liabilities

Liabilities are the direct opposite of assets—that is, they are the amount that is owed by the nursing home. Included in liabilities are salaries, accounts payable, and any moneys held in safekeeping by the nursing home for others. Fixed-cost items normally include long-range items—such as mortgage payments, which remain constant from month to month—and represent items that remain stable irrespective of fluctuations in volume of services rendered. Variable-cost items vary because of volume increases or decreases; examples are food and supplies.

Cost-Finding

It is essential to be able to allocate to each department its actual expenses, and thus the cost of providing that service. This procedure is known as cost-finding, an administrative tool used for rate-setting and management purposes. Cost-finding means, for instance, that if the repair of the parallel bars takes more than four hours of labor, the cost of the repair should be charged to physical therapy and not to maintenance. Naturally, careful records need to be kept on work orders so that proper charges can be attributed to each department and summarized on the Details of Costs and Expenses form (Exhibit 14-1).

The same principle holds true with respect to employee benefits. Health insurance and tuition expenses must be charged to the department where the recipient works and not listed under administrative costs. Depreciation for major movable equipment also is to be reported as an expense of the department that uses the equipment.

EXHIBIT 14-1
Details of Costs and Expenses

```
                    DETAILS OF COSTS AND EXPENSES

From _____  To _____
                              Prior Year|Present Year|Present Year
                                Budget  |  Budget    |Month| Period

NURSING ADMINISTRATION

  Salary - director of nursing
  Salaries - supervisors
  Salary - nursing administrative
    assistant
  Related payroll expenses
  Education - tuition
  Education - travel
  Depreciation - equipment
  Supplies
  Telephone

SKILLED NURSING FACILITY
(Direct nursing service)

  Salaries - head nurses
  Salaries - licensed practical
    nurses
  Salaries - nursing assistants
  Related payroll expenses
  Education - tuition
  Education - travel
  Depreciation - equipment
  Supplies

PLANT OPERATION AND MAINTENANCE

  Salaries
  Related payroll expenses
  Education - tuition
  Education - travel
  Depreciation - equipment
  Oil
  Electricity
  Gas
  Water
  Parts and supplies
  Outside services and repairs

GROUNDS

  Salaries
  Related payroll expenses
  Education - tuition
  Education - travel
  Depreciation - equipment
  Outside service contract

RENT or
DEPRECIATION - building
INTEREST
TAXES
```

EXHIBIT 14-1 (cont.)

DETAILS OF COSTS AND EXPENSES (continued)   -2-

	Prior Year Budget	Present Year Budget	Present Year Month	Period
SECURITY				
Salaries				
Related payroll expenses				
Education - tuition				
Education - travel				
Depreciation - equipment				
Parts and supplies				
TRANSPORTATION				
Auto - expenses				
Auto - depreciation				
ADMINISTRATION				
Salary - administrative director				
Salary - assistant administrator				
Salary - other administrative				
Related payroll expenses				
Education - tuition				
Education - travel				
Depreciation - equipment				
Supplies				
Telephone				
Dues and subscriptions				
Licenses				
Legal fees				
Insurance (general)				
Postage				
Service contracts				
BUSINESS OFFICE				
Salaries				
Related payroll expenses				
Education - tuition				
Education - travel				
Consultant				
Payroll service				
Depreciation - equipment				
Supplies				
IN-SERVICE EDUCATION				
Salary				
Related payroll expenses				
Education - tuition				
Education - travel				
Honoraria for visiting professionals				
Depreciation - equipment				
Supplies				

EXHIBIT 14-1 (cont.)

DETAILS OF COSTS AND EXPENSES (continued)   -3-

	Prior Year Budget	Present Year Budget	Present Year Month	Period
MEDICAL ADMINISTRATION				
Salary - medical director				
Related payroll expenses				
Education - tuition				
Education - travel				
Depreciation - equipment				
Supplies				
MEDICAL CARE EVALUATION AND ASSESSMENT				
Utilization review				
DIETARY				
Salaries				
Consultant dietitian				
Related payroll expenses				
Education - tuition				
Education - travel				
Depreciation - equipment				
Food				
Supplies				
Outside service contracts				
HOUSEKEEPING				
Salaries				
Related payroll expenses				
Education - tuition				
Education - travel				
Depreciation - equipment				
Supplies				
Outside service contracts				
LAUNDRY				
Salaries				
Related payroll expenses				
Education - tuition				
Education - travel				
Depreciation - equipment				
Supplies				
Linen rental				
Outside service contracts				
PHYSICAL THERAPY				
Salaries				
Related payroll expenses				
Education - tuition				
Education - travel				
Depreciation - equipment				
Supplies				

EXHIBIT 14-1 (cont.)

DETAILS OF COSTS AND EXPENSES (continued)   -4-

	Prior Year Budget	Present Year Budget	Present Year Month	Period
OCCUPATIONAL THERAPY[1]				
Consultant				
Education - tuition				
Education - travel				
Depreciation - equipment				
Supplies				
SOCIAL SERVICE				
Salaries				
Consultant				
Related payroll expenses				
Education - tuition				
Education - travel				
Depreciation - equipment				
Supplies				
ACTIVITIES/VOLUNTEERS				
Salaries				
Related payroll expenses				
Education - tuition				
Education - travel				
Depreciation - equipment				
Supplies				
Clergy				
LABORATORY AND EKG				
Salary				
Related payroll expenses				
Education - tuition				
Education - travel				
Outside service				
Depreciation - equipment				
Supplies				
X RAY				
Salary				
Related payroll expenses				
Education - tuition				
Education - travel				
Depreciation - equipment				
Supplies				
PHARMACY[2]				
Consultant				
Supplies				

[1] If the nursing home has an occupational therapist on staff, his salary and related payroll expenses rather than the consultant's fees would be an expense.

[2] If the nursing home has an institutional pharmacy rather than a contract with a community pharmacy, appropriate expenses would be itemized.

EXHIBIT 14-1 (cont.)

```
DETAILS OF COSTS AND EXPENSES (continued)                        -5-

                            Prior Year|Present Year|Present Year
                              Budget   |   Budget   |Month| Period
HEALTH RECORDS

   Salary
   Related payroll expenses
   Education - tuition
   Education - travel
   Consultant
   Depreciation - equipment
   Supplies
```

Note: Speech Pathology and Audiology is not listed because in most instances it would be rendered by a consultant on a fee-for-service basis and charged to the patient or his sponsor. However, if the nursing home has an in-house department of speech pathology and audiology, appropriate expenses would be itemized.

Cost Allocation

The skilled nursing facility has some departments whose service will produce income and other departments that provide support services yet do not create any revenue in and of themselves. Nursing and physical therapy, for example, are patient care services for which charges are incurred, whereas housekeeping, which is essential to room and board, does not bring in any income. To fully understand the true costs of operating a revenue-producing department, the nursing home must apportion the costs of maintaining non-revenue-producing departments among the revenue-producing departments. Cost allocation refers to the concept of apportioning the amount of time (and therefore wages) housekeeping personnel spend maintaining nursing units, the physical therapy room, the occupational therapy room, the dental room, and so forth. By using these statistics, the administration can determine the actual costs of operating those departments.

Functional Accounting

Cost allocation is a process implicit in functional accounting, where records are kept according to functions or activities performed. Functions are the related activities performed by several departments to serve a common end, such as providing nursing care. Thus functional accounting is different from responsibility accounting, in which the accounting structure parallels the facility's organizational chart and responsibility for the results can be identified with specific individuals.

Chart of Accounts

The process of making records of business transactions—bookkeeping—is a clearly defined system. The chart of accounts refers to the listing of account titles used in compiling financial data that must be accumulated for the purposes of proper accounting. It is a systematic arrangement of all the accounts of the skilled nursing facility, with numerical symbols identifying each as an asset, liability, equity, revenue, or expense.

Journal

A journal is a book of original entry to record a financial transaction or a business diary. Each journal entry will note what account was debited and credited due to the transaction. Journal entries are then summarized according to each account in the ledger.

Operating Report

The operating report, sometimes called the statement of income and expense (Exhibit 14-2), shows all revenue received or due, and expenses paid or owing as of a certain date. It is useful to compile it to compare the facility's position at the current time with the same period the previous year, thus showing increased or decreased costs in an area.

Balance Sheet

The most complete overview of the facility's financial status is provided by the balance sheet (Exhibit 14-3). It is a report of the financial position at a given moment of time, including assets, liabilities, and owner's equity as recorded in the accounting system.

Certified Audit

On an annual basis, the nursing home should subject its accounting records to a certified audit by a certified public accountant. The certified audit is a critical review of the facility's underlying internal controls and accounting records. After the audit, the public accountant makes a statement as to the propriety of the facility's financial statement.

Cash Transactions

Whenever possible, cash transactions should be avoided. However, cash will be used in vending machines and for meals in the facility cafeteria and/or coffee shop. It should be carefully recorded and deposited daily in the bank by a specified person so that any irregularities can be easily ascribed to that individual. Personnel who participate in receiving, paying, and handling cash and securities should be bonded and should be required to take their annual vacation time so that their control over and recording of cash transactions are occasionally interrupted.

STAFFING PATTERN

The staffing pattern for the business department depends on the accounting processes used—manual, mechanical, or a combination of both. Manual accounting might require more manpower and personnel trained as bookkeepers, whereas computerized accounting would require staff trained to operate the hardware. After an analysis of the accounting procedures, the nursing home would then be in a position to identify its staffing needs.

Prudent management would use a system in which the accounting records and methods of the nursing home business office are designed so that no part of the accounts or procedures is under the sole control of any one worker. In fact, one employee in the business office should work in a complementary fashion to the other so that, in effect, each one is auditing the details of the other's responsibilities.

EXHIBIT 14-2
Statement of Income and Expenses

STATEMENT OF INCOME AND EXPENSES

From _____ To _____

	Medicaid	Medicare	Private	Total
NUMBER OF PATIENT-DAYS				
INCOME PER DIEM				
INCOME FOR ABOVE PERIOD				
Nursing care				
Special care				
Physical therapy				
Occupational therapy				
Visitors' and personnel meals				
Pharmacy				
Laboratory and X ray				
Personal grooming				
Sundry items				
Equipment rental				
Donations				
Reserve for loss--Medicare				
TOTAL INCOME				

	Prior Year Budget	Present Year Budget	Present Year Month	Period
EXPENSES				
Nursing administration				
Skilled nursing facility				
Plant operation and maintenance				
Grounds				
Rent or depreciation (building), interest, taxes				
Security				
Transportation				
Administration				
Business office				
In-service education				
Medical administration				
Medical care evaluation and assessment				
Dietary				
Housekeeping				
Laundry				
Physical therapy				
Occupational therapy				
Social service				
Activities/volunteers				
Laboratory and EKG				
X ray				
Pharmacy				
Health records				
TOTAL EXPENSES				
NET OPERATING PROFIT (LOSS)				

EXHIBIT 14-3
Balance Sheet

<u>BALANCE SHEET</u>
(Date)

<u>ASSETS</u>

CURRENT ASSETS

    Cash in bank
    Savings bonds
    Cash in escrow fund
    Marketable securities
    Accounts receivable
    Inventory
    Prepaid expenses

PROPERTY, PLANT, AND EQUIPMENT--AT COST

    Land and building
    Equipment, furniture, and fixtures
    Motor vehicles

    Less accumulated depreciation

                             TOTAL ASSETS

<u>LIABILITIES AND CAPITAL</u>

CURRENT LIABILITIES

    Accounts payable
    Accrued payroll and payroll taxes
    Other accrued expenses
    Current portion of long-term debt (mortgage)
    Notes and loans payable
    Patients' advances

                TOTAL CURRENT LIABILITIES

LONG-TERM DEBT (total remaining amount owed)

CAPITAL

    Donated capital (for nonprofit nursing home)
    Earnings or capital (for proprietary nursing home)

             TOTAL LIABILITIES AND CAPITAL

Regardless of the accounting process, a 100-bed skilled nursing facility would require at least two full-time people in the business department in addition to the services of a consultant accountant. Larger facilities should consider hiring a controller, thereby limiting the routine activities of the accountant. The business manager reports to the administrative director, supervises the bookkeeper, and is responsible for the daily operation of the office.

Bookkeeper

The task of recording the business transactions of the nursing home—keeping the individual account cards and accounts payable, receivable, and disbursement journals—is assigned to the bookkeeper. The bookkeeper prepares the monthly patient billing, records all receipts, summarizes all journals on a monthly basis for the business manager and accountant to review, and reconciles all bank statements at the end of the month. Collecting, maintaining, and preparing payroll data is a major responsibility of the bookkeeper. A candidate for this position must be able to work under frequent interruptions and maintain accuracy at the same time. The technology employed by the business office would dictate what business machines the bookkeeper would need to have training in, although a knowledge of basic office bookkeeping procedures is essential.

Business Manager

The business manager plans the office routine, ensuring that patient bills and vendor payments are sent on time, that the payroll is completed and distributed when due, that monthly statistical data are gathered, and that the books are properly summarized and ready for the accountant at the end of the month. It might be well to have the business manager post the ledger at the end of the month to serve as a check on the bookkeeper's work. (Items are listed or posted in the ledger according to prearranged categories.) Completion and submission of the quarterly payroll tax return, the weekly federal and state withholding taxes, questionnaires from workmen's compensation or insurance companies concerning employees, requests for patient financial information from third-party payers, and any other forms or information requested by government, insurance agencies, or sponsors would come under the business manager's purview. The review and upkeep of the facility's own insurance coverage, maintenance of the patients' petty cash accounts and interest-bearing accounts, if any, are added responsibilities. Government or insurance auditors and inspectors are assisted in their work by the business manager.

FIGURE 14-1
Reviewing Bill with Sponsor

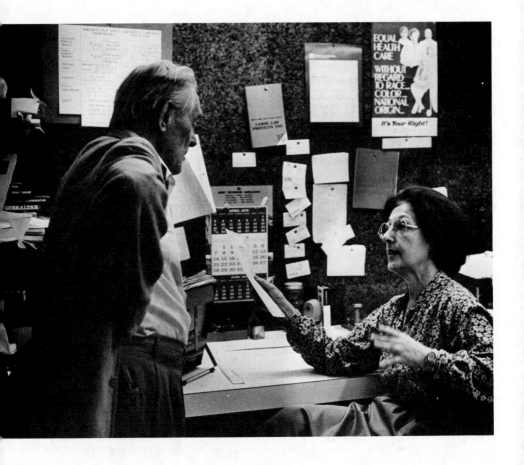

A considerable portion of the business manager's job is devoted to purchasing. In facilities with more than 200 beds, a separate staff position may be required for this duty. All orders would be processed through the purchasing agent, and receipt of goods and invoices verified for accuracy. The business manager must consult with department heads regarding specifications for supplies, equipment, and services, and then seek the best product at the most favorable price. Stores control and issues from the central storage area would also follow as a responsibility.

The business manager must be a person of integrity and initiative with good organizational abilities. An associate's or bachelor's degree in business administration coupled with appropriate length of experience, preferably in a health care setting, would be qualifications for this position. The business manager must also be able to function with frequent interruptions and under pressure. And he must know how to operate the facility's office equipment.

Consultant Accountant

The consultant accountant, who is responsible to the administrative director, is assigned the responsibility of establishing and supervising all accounting functions for the skilled nursing facility. This person should be a certified public accountant. At the end of each month, he should review the books before preparing the monthly financial statements. The accountant interprets accounts and records to the administrative director, assists in formulating budgetary policies and practices, and supervises the preparation of all special financial reports for government and other agencies. He must pay attention to numerous details and be alert to detect errors in correspondence, records, statistics, and clerical procedures.

Also, it has become necessary for nursing home accountants to be familiar with the practices and requirements of third-party payers. Skilled nursing facilities need guidance as to what records to keep, how to interpret reimbursement practices, how to prepare reports to these agencies, what the rate-setting process involves and how it is determined, and how to file appeals. Indeed, knowledge in this area is becoming so specialized that the nursing home may need to retain a separate consultant accountant with that expertise.

RATES

Rates may be structured to be inclusive, partially inclusive, or separate for each unit of service to patients. Inclusive rates mean similar rates for all residents irrespective of their use of services such as physical therapy, medications, and so forth. An inclusive rate encourages the use of all services without regard to the patient's ability to pay, and the attending physician is relieved of the necessity for concern about the additional cost of services he orders for the patient. In addition, sponsors would have a clear idea of the cost of patient care prior to admission, so that complaints regarding extra charges would be avoided.

From a procedural point of view, the obvious advantage of an inclusive rate is simplification of billings and related administrative activities, resulting in lowered costs. Since billings would be easier to understand and cause less questioning, the collection period might be shorter. Inclusive rates should conserve staff time by eliminating the need for preparing charge slips for each service rendered, although it may be difficult to assess the true utilization of services without individual charge slips.

Inclusive rates may incite some patients to complain that they are paying for services rendered to other patients but not to them. For example, some patients will receive physical therapy and some will not, and medication usage will vary from patient to patient. An increase in overall costs is a possibility with an inclusive rate, due to an overutilization of special services. With the simplified rate structure, rate comparisons among facilities is encouraged; the itemization method would make such comparisons more difficult.

Rates should be adjusted when costs change—either after salary increases or after changes in costs of goods. It is preferable to work out the operating budget, compute the rate needed, and have a meeting with residents and/or their sponsors to discuss the proposed increases well in advance of the date of the planned increase. This will afford the opportunity for explaining and discussing the proposed budget and mitigating critical response.

Rates for Third-Party Payers

Rates for patients whose care is covered by third-party payers such as Medicare and Medicaid may be based on actual accepted costs or negotiated costs. A negotiated rate is a rate that the two parties—the provider and the third-party payer—agree to; it is not necessarily based on costs.

Cost-based reimbursement means that the third party will reimburse the nursing home in accordance with what it deems to be usual and proper costs for providing the service. This means, for example, that the amount of reimbursement allowed for a full-time medical director may be considerably below what a nursing home will have to expend in order to attract a qualified physician.

Rates are promulgated on a retrospective or prospective basis. A retrospective rate is set after the fact, while a prospective rate is set prior to the offering of the service. A prospective rate allows the facility to know what its income will be, although subsequent audits by Medicare and Medicaid may disallow certain costs, thereby changing the rate and reimbursement for the period already covered.

PROCEDURES

The business office must have a file containing appropriate financial information about each resident. The completed continuing care contract should be included in this file, since it contains billing information and authorization for special services. Correspondence regarding changes in the patient's financial status, sponsor address changes, and Medicare billings and Medicaid information should be placed in this centrally located file.

Individual account cards must be made out for each patient, identifying the financial sponsor. When the patient's status changes—e.g., from Medicare to private—a new card should be started to separate charges billed to Medicare from those billed privately. If a patient is discharged and later readmitted, a new account card may be needed if the patient is covered by Medicare Part A benefits when he returns. Complete account cards should also be retained in the patient's file.

Incoming mail to the business office should be separated as to bills and checks, with checks stamped for immediate deposit. Outgoing mail should be processed through the business office, where the use of a postage meter is most helpful.

Accounts Receivable

Patient bills should be submitted weekly, biweekly, or monthly, depending on the usual length of stay. The account balances should be maintained on an accrual basis, with the income for services rendered charged to the patient and recorded as gross revenue when earned, not when paid. If the rate is not inclusive, patient billings must identify the separate charges. All patients should be charged for accommodations; other charges might include coinsurance, medications, laboratory tests, x rays, physical therapy, and dry cleaning.

The billing process involves recording the charge on the charges journal sheet and the individual patient account card, and finally preparing the billing statement to be sent to the sponsor. A separate charges journal must be maintained for each of the third-party payers in addition to the journal for private paying patients. If a patient receives a service not covered by the third-party payer or has a coinsurance charge, then the charge is noted in the private charges journal with a bill sent to the responsible party for that amount only.

Third-party payers can be billed only after the services are rendered. A patient is covered by Medicare Part A only when written approval of his eligibility has been received from the fiscal intermediary. A separate billing form for each covered patient must be submitted to the fiscal intermediary for payment.

Patients should be considered Medicaid beneficiaries only after receipt of an identification number, an approved budget, and an effective date of coverage. At the end of the billing cycle, the appropriate Medicaid office is billed once for its beneficiaries in the nursing home.

When checks are received in payment, duplicate deposit tickets should be completed, listing the patient's name(s), for whom the check is made out, the date, and the amount of the check. Separate deposit tickets should be used for Medicare and Medicaid payments. Prudent accounting procedures dictate that two people in the business office be involved with handling checks—one to record and one to make the deposits. The duplicate deposit slip is used to complete the cash receipts journal and to note the credit on the individual patient account card. The provider reimbursement statement that accompanies checks from third-party payers should be used to record payments in their respective receipts journals and accounts receivable cards.

At the end of each billing period, the charges for each type of service rendered should be totaled according to classification of income and then posted, or transferred, from the charges journal to the ledger, which serves as a summary book.

Accounts Payable

All costs and expenses should be recorded on an accrual basis, whereby the liabilities or services and purchases are written as incurred and charged to the operations of the applicable month; the actual date of payment has no bearing on the recording of the expenses. Under this system, the expenses can then be properly matched to the revenue earned for the same period. Finally, expenses should be classified and distributed as an expenditure of the appropriate department.

Using the invoice submitted by the supplier of goods or services, the purchase must be recorded in the purchases journal book and also on the individual vendor account card; if the vendor is not a regular supplier, the expense may be noted on a miscellaneous vendor card. Following the recording of purchases, each purchase must be allocated to the department that uses it. Invoices should be checked against the vendors' monthly statements for accuracy.

All bills should be paid by the tenth or fifteenth of the month except when a discount is afforded by earlier payment. The process for recording payment entails noting it in the cash disbursements journal and on the individual vendor card, or the miscellaneous vendor card, when writing the check.

The paid statements and attached invoices should remain on file until the year's end. At that time, the bills should be categorized according to departments and stored for as long as the consultant accountant thinks necessary.

Summarizing the accounts payable for the month would be followed by posting those transactions in the ledger.

Medicare Part B reimbursement is pursued by the provider of the service. The nursing home seeks Medicare Part B reimbursement for private pay and Medicaid recipients to maximize benefits for Medicaid and for Medicare-eligible private patients. In both instances, the Medicare Part B funds received by the nursing home would be credited to the residents' accounts. Part B billing would be required for certain coverable services such as laboratory, x ray, and physical therapy.

PAYROLL

All personnel should be thoroughly familiar with the payroll procedure at the start of their employment. They, of course, will be asked to complete withholding and other forms to be used in the preparation of the payroll. The following information should be reviewed with them as well as included in the employee handbook: definition of the work week, day and method of payroll distribution, payroll deductions, fringe benefits, system of reporting on and off duty, use of time cards to compute salary, and method of paying personnel who leave before the end of the pay period. The professional nursing staff should understand the difference between staff and per diem salaries.

The preferred payroll period would relate to the needs of the majority of the staff, the nonprofessional workers, who generally can plan their budget more effectively on a weekly basis. Professional staff, however, may be paid less frequently.

Attached to each payroll check must be a statement that duplicates the payroll record maintained by the business department. It should indicate the number of hours worked and the rate of pay, resulting in the gross income earned; deductions, itemized separately, would include federal and state taxes, and possibly insurance premiums, contributions, pension plan payments, and so forth. The net income shown on the pay statement should parallel the payroll check amount.

The use of a mechanical check signer is almost a necessity due to the weekly task of signing large numbers of payroll checks. This equipment should be under the careful control of the business office. A number counter must be part of the equipment to control the number of checks signed. The person or persons who sign checks must be designated by the governing body.

Payroll distribution is no problem in facilities with 100 or fewer employees where all staff are known; in larger facilities that employ hundreds of people, the person(s) charged with the task of distributing paychecks must rely on identification cards or badges.

The total payroll must be distributed to determine each department's expenditure. Payroll summary sheets must be maintained to aid in the preparation of tax returns.

PURCHASING

Effective purchasing can make a substantial contribution to management, patient care, and employee utilization by providing quality material and services at reasonable costs. The nursing home should explore the feasibility of a joint or group purchasing plan with other area institutions for the purpose of effecting savings from enlarged purchasing potential. Within the institution, the question of departmental or centralized purchasing must be considered. Centralized purchasing establishes uniformity and effective controls, whereas departmental purchasing utilizes the department head's expertise. In a 100-bed skilled nursing facility, a combination plan might be instituted where centralized purchasing is the practice except for specialized purchasing by departments, such as dietary and pharmacy.

The purchasing agent must rely on department heads for information about new products on the market. Product price ranges should be discussed, together with specifications for individual items, including such criteria as measurement, shrinkage, weight, thread count, odor, performance, colorfastness, resistance to heat, tensile strength, and visual qualities.

The determination of the quantity of the order must take into account an understanding of the wastefulness of having money tied up in inventory. The amount of storage space available, the rate of usage, possible changing trends in the field that might rapidly outdate the merchandise, and budgetary restraints are all concerns when purchasing in bulk.

Before purchasing costly equipment such as photocopy machines, computers, or automobiles, a careful study should be made to determine whether the equipment should be leased or bought outright. For a voluntary facility, there are no tax benefits to be derived from equipment purchases, so having large sums of money tied up in machinery may be disadvantageous. With a rental, a concern for the obsolescence of equipment is lessened and a new model may simply be leased at the appropriate time. Of course, while rental costs are a bona fide expense, depreciation cannot be deducted. The rental agreement should be carefully analyzed to ascertain that the rental costs are in line with what it would cost to purchase and service the equipment and supplies. For example, the cost per copy via a leased photocopy machine in comparison with the cost per copy via an owned photocopy machine should not be widely disparate.

For ease of operation, the number of vendors for regular business should be kept to a minimum, but their prices should be checked regularly. Preference may be given to local vendors; however, all vendors must be rated and selected according to unit prices, quality of goods, accessibility of parts and service, delivery time, and community relations. Clear policies regarding nonacceptance of presents from vendors must be enunciated to vendors and purchasing staff.

For expensive and/or extensive orders, bids should be sought, and the order should be placed with the lowest bidder who is in conformance with the aforementioned criteria. To support purchasing practices that will hold up under scrutiny by government auditors as demonstrating conformance with the prudent-buyer concept, careful records must be maintained of vendors contacted, the quality of products and/or services, and any other related factors pertinent to the decision making. For some items—such as milk, bread, fuel, linen rental, or equipment or maintenance services—an annual contract should be investigated.

A clear and uniform system of record keeping for purchasing should be used to aid in an effective purchasing program and to help eliminate errors. An up-to-date list of vendors and their catalogs should always be available. Each piece of equipment worth over $50 should be listed on a file card with price, description, vendor, date of purchase, location in the nursing home, cost of maintenance, and estimated period of usefulness.

Purchase requisitions should be processed only through the purchasing agent. A standard purchase requisition form should be used. The price should be noted on the form at the time of the order to verify charges on the invoice. The form should be completed in triplicate for retention by the department personnel, the purchasing agent, and the vendor. Vendors' bills of lading or packing slips should be carefully scrutinized and filed to compare with invoices.

Emergency orders should be placed over the telephone only when necessary, with the purchase order to be mailed as soon as possible. To preclude future exigencies, an investigation should follow to determine the reason for the order.

In a facility with 100 beds, the purchasing agent may also act as the receiving and issuing clerk for central storage supplies. Department heads or other assigned persons may exercise such control over their own specialized departmental inventories. Larger facilities may require additional staff to perform this function.

STORES CONTROL

Whether the storage system is centralized or departmentalized, a stores control system must be developed. The most accurate and efficient system would entail the use of stores requisition slips and the maintenance of a perpetual inventory, which allows for an exact inventory count at all times and avoids overstocking.

If a perpetual inventory system is not used, frequent inventories should be made of all storage areas and studies made of inventory patterns to point up problems. Staff members must be encouraged to maintain a low stock. Inventory usage records always should be kept when more than one department uses the same supplies. Furthermore, there is no need for separate departments to have a back-up supply of the same item, thereby tying up additional money.

Taking inventory refers to determining the quantity and the value of unused supplies, which are considered assets. The cost of unused supplies should be listed at their cost or current market value, whichever is lower. An annual inventorying should be done prior to the completion of the certified audit by someone removed from the usual control of the storage areas.

INSURANCE

With the diverse and unusual circumstances related to insuring health care institutions, a consultant should be hired to assist in the development of the nursing home's insurance program. The purpose of insurance is to protect and preserve the institution's assets, which are subject to risks of destruction, breakdown, legal suit, or theft; to guard against claims for injuries sustained by patients, visitors, and staff; and to provide for losses suffered by personnel both in and out of the course of employment. Careful decisions have to be made about what should be insured, what it should be insured against, and how much insurance coverage is needed. A simple rule of thumb would be to insure whatever the institution cannot afford to replace. The installation of devices to reduce insurance costs such as alarms on safes should be studied prior to the development of a formal insurance program.

Personnel, volunteers, and not the least board members need training in preventive measures to preclude liability of the nursing home. So-called risk management develops a safer environment in the nursing home by anticipating problem areas and remedying them, thereby controlling the cost of insurance via controlling insurance claims and the expense of litigation. Of course, the most effective risk management devolves from good working relationships among residents, families, and staff.

A roster of insurance coverage should be prepared to allow for uninterrupted coverage and quick analysis of present protection, listing policies, due dates, amounts of premiums, and their time of expiration. Descriptions of property insured must be correct, and the name and address of the insured should appear on all policies. Insurance policies should be stored in a safe, fireproof, yet accessible area.

When developing a formal insurance program, the institution should investigate the possibility of group insurance plans with other health and welfare agencies. The purchase of multiperil policies, a package approach for all insurance except automobile and workmen's compensation, should be considered since it would afford a discount in premiums. Regardless of what format the insurance plans take, the facility must carry several basic types of insurance coverage.

Property Insurance

Property insurance should include all-risk physical damage to the building and contents (although this type of policy will not cover the loss of staff or patients' property). In addition to fire, other specific types of risks to be covered include sprinkler leakage or water damage; aircraft damage; earthquake, windstorm, cyclone, flood, lightning, and tornado damage; damage caused by riot and civil commotion; and damage due to vandalism and malicious mischief.

Special attention should be paid to plate glass coverage, which may be unlimited or which may cover only the areas believed to present the greatest potential risk. Also, special coverage will be required for the boiler. Most communities require insurance on pressure vessels, and this dictates regular inspections of the boiler, thereby providing another safeguard.

Workmen's Compensation Insurance

Workmen's compensation insurance covers losses due to statutory liability as a result of personal injury, sickness, or death suffered by employees during the course of their employment. Outside contractors should be required to provide workmen's compensation insurance for their employees. The amount and payment is prescribed by law. Should the Workmen's Compensation Board determine that the employee is entitled to a specific award, it would be an addition to the usual benefits paid. To file for workmen's compensation, an accident form must be completed at the time of the injury.

Comprehensive General Liability Insurance

Comprehensive general liability insurance covers statutory liability because of bodily injury, sickness, or death that occurs at any time subsequent to an accident arising out of the maintenance or use of the premises or property and all operations that are necessary or incidental thereto, such as the use of the elevator. The coverage would also include damages for the care and loss of services to any person as a result of the above. If an accident is caused by an employee during the course of his employment, whether he is on or off the premises, this insurance plan will cover any damage suits filed in addition to mishaps caused by product usage.

A separate liability policy will be needed for automobiles or other vehicles. Protection should be afforded for ownership and nonownership, including leased or hired cars, and for any operator—including volunteers and staff—and for all passengers.

Malpractice Insurance

Malpractice or professional liability insurance is necessary to protect the skilled nursing facility against claims brought as a result of errors of omission or commission in the rendering of or failure to render medical or nursing treatment, including the furnishing of food and beverage, to a patient. The pharmacist should be compelled to carry his own liability insurance.

Malpractice suits demonstrate a loss of the consumer's trust and confidence; thus effective communication among patients, families, and staff is the best antidote to such breakdowns. The increasing number of malpractice claims and the escalating amount of the awards have exceeded actuarial projections for some commercial insurance companies, thereby causing many companies to withdraw from the professional liability market. Those companies continuing to write this type of insurance have raised their premiums considerably.

This state of affairs has encouraged providers to seek coverage from special purpose insurance companies or companies formed by associations or groups of facilities, thus providing greater stability of insurance costs and coverage, better risk management and loss prevention, and lower operating costs. Such organizations operate solely for their own membership so that costs of marketing, brokerage and agency fees, and stockholder profit can be significantly cut back. Very large facilities or chains can undertake self-insurance to circumvent the escalation of liability insurance coverage premiums.

Burglary Insurance

Protection against burglary should be provided for office, medical, and dental equipment. Because it is not covered under property insurance, burglary coverage must also include patients' personal effects, staff belongings, and visitors' property.

Disability Insurance

Disability insurance is required to cover losses resulting from personal injury or illness suffered by employees but not in the course of their employment. Its purpose is to provide a minimal amount of income, determined by the current weekly wages of the employee, to prevent total devastation due to loss of income because of inability to work.

Health Insurance

As an employer, the skilled nursing facility should offer a hospitalization and medical insurance plan to its personnel due to the rising cost of health care and the catastrophic effect that a major illness can have on a family's economic stability, especially with the limited ability of the majority of nursing home employees to afford such protection by themselves. In addition to the usual private insurance plans that are available, the option of membership in a health maintenance organization with its emphasis on preventive medicine may also be offered to the staff. Of course, the nursing home may elect to pay all or a portion of the monthly premium for those who join the plan(s).

BANK ACCOUNTS

The skilled nursing facility may hold a variety of bank accounts for different purposes, according to its needs. If the administrative director is ill or absent for other reasons, at least two members of the staff should be authorized to sign checks, but in no event should the person writing the checks be permitted to act as the signatory.

A general checking account should be established in which all income is deposited; deposits to this account should be made daily, using the double deposit ticket method described earlier. A separate payroll account should be available in which the net amount of the payroll is transferred from the general account to the payroll account on payday; sufficient reserves should be maintained between pay periods. Only one deposit ticket will be necessary to put funds in this account, as it will be only a total sum and not an itemization from several sources.

Other accounts may be opened to serve special purposes. For example, patients who receive and do not spend their monthly allowances may profit from a savings account that will guarantee their earning interest. At holiday time, when families and friends may wish to contribute to a staff holiday fund, a separate account should be opened.

At the end of each month, the bookkeeper should do the bank statement reconciliations before the accountant closes the books.

PROTECTION OF VALUABLES

The responsibility for the protection of all patient valuables should be assigned to the business office. For this purpose, the office should house a locked safe with an alarm.

Each patient's valuables should be placed in a separate envelope labeled with the patient's name, the contents, the date, and the initials of the person inserting the valuable. A signed receipt for the money and/or articles should be given to the patient or his sponsor. As a safeguard against error and as a record in the event of theft, a separate book should be kept recording the same information.

When items are removed from the safe, the patient or his designee should be required to affix his signature, the date, and the amount of money or the name of the article withdrawn on a slip to be placed in the envelope. This transaction should also be recorded in the separate book. The receipt given at the time of deposit should be signed and returned by the recipient.

For any patient funds kept in the safe or held in a separate account, a quarterly accounting must be given to the patient or his sponsor. Upon discharge or death, the valuables or cash should be given to the patient or his sponsor, with the proper written notation made of the delivery. If this is not possible, the items should be sent to the appropriate person via insured, registered mail with return receipt requested.

TECHNOLOGY[1]

Processing methods for accounting have evolved from the manual method—using posting boards, journals, and ledgers with a single-write system—to semiautomatic systems—using bookkeeping machines—to fully computerized systems. The selection of the bookkeeping method depends on the size of the facility, the complexity of the financial data desired, and whether the facility is a free-standing organization or part of a large network. Sometimes the sophistication of the system that is used will reflect corporate rather than individual sponsorship.

It is generally conceded that data processing in the nursing home eventually will service more than the business office and will assist in the overall management and operation, although costs can best be justified in the business office. Certainly the plethora of reports that skilled nursing facilities must make to various agencies demonstrate the advantage of data processing to ease the chore of record keeping and collection. There are software packages—computer programs—to automate the admission and discharge process, the care plan, physician orders and progress notes, medications, laboratory, x ray, restorative services, and so on. An examination of currently available hospital information systems will demonstrate the ultimate possibilities for the long-term-care field.

Computerization is said to produce tighter accounting control, improved speed and processing of paperwork, ease in generating new reports, and a reduction in clerical costs. Of course, clerical costs can be reduced in a large facility only with a large business staff. However, the avoidance of increased labor costs, as requirements for record keeping grow, is a reasonable goal.

Problems to be encountered with computerization might be a lack of flexibility in record keeping and a loss of control over information retained. When reprogramming is necessary to adapt to changing needs, it will be slow and expensive. Finally, turnover of trained staff will be an added concern, as will educating new staff to operate the system.

The alternatives for computerization include an in-house computer or minicomputer, a shared computer system where terminals are located in the nursing home, or the use of an off-the-premises service bureau that processes information, such as the payroll, for a fee. Deciding which system to incorporate will require careful consideration and should be based on a feasibility study that will develop requirements of the nursing home and allow the facility then to seek out the system and vendor that suits its needs. The advice of the consultant accountant should be sought every step of the way.

Questions that require answers in the feasibility study are: What are the institution's short- and long-term needs? What is the current volume of work (size of accounts receivable and payable, the payroll)? What kinds of reports should the computer system produce and what types of information should be included in those reports? What types of calculations should the computer make and how often? What are the current costs of producing this work? What are the staff capabilities for adapting to a new system? What are the priorities in instituting a data processing system (the order of computerizing different procedures)? How fast should the entire system be implemented? What is the initial cost of instituting the system? What are the long-term costs for the system, including maintenance of equipment, cost of supplies, and charges for changes in the software?

After producing the feasibility study, a study of the vendors representing all the possible computerizing alternatives should be conducted. It is important to be definite and firm about what the output of the computer should be: it may require adapting the software package offered by the vendor in order to produce the required information. Adequate provision must be made for the vendor to train the staff. After the system is installed, it is absolutely necessary to run a parallel test, that is, to perform the same work manually and on the new computer system to compare for accuracy, speed, and desired results. The nursing home must provide the quality control, for it alone knows its needs and goals.

Future prospects for data collection to be required of nursing homes are underscored by the increased volume and uncoordinated requests of various government agencies—for example, one form for the federal Medicare program, a different one for the state Medicaid program, yet another for the regional Health Systems Agency, and others for local agencies. More uniformity of data and data systems will be mandated, together with concerns for costs of data processing. These changing requirements emphasize the need for an outside data processing service to purchase hardware and software to meet changing client needs. As the electronic data processing industry begins to address the needs of long-term-care facilities, however, more software packages will be designed to meet those needs.

RECORDS

Numerous records are needed to carry out the major function of the business department in accumulating data for communication to management for its interpretation. To summarize, records will need to be developed and retained for the following information: the annual operating budget, capital expenditures plan, monthly statistical data (Exhibit 14-4), monthly billing statement, and vendor account cards. Journals will need to be maintained for recording charges, receipts, purchases, cash disbursements, payroll, and the distribution of purchases, charges, and/or receipts to different departments, if that information is not noted in other journals, and the general ledger will present the total of all the nursing home's financial transactions for an accounting period. Certain forms will be needed to carry out special procedures, such as the general checking account check and deposit ticket, payroll account check and deposit ticket, payroll check and accompanying statement, and a purchase order form.

Although the business office may not supervise the maintenance of employee records, it will need access to information contained therein, such as the application form and withholding card. The recording of pertinent data gathered from these sources may be transferred to a summary sheet for each employee for easy use and reference by the business office staff. The payroll time cards will be under the business manager's control, as they are supporting evidence for the payroll expended. Copies of any forms completed on behalf of personnel that affect the nursing home's operation—e.g., workmen's compensation, disability, unemployment—must be placed in the employee's file.

EXHIBIT 14-4
Statistical Operational Data

STATISTICAL OPERATIONAL DATA

From _____ To _____

(Year to Date)

	Medicare	Medicaid	Private	Total for Current Month	Cumulative Total for Year
Patients on premises beginning of period					
New admissions					
Patients discharged, transferred, and/or deceased					
Patients on premises at end of period					
Total patient-days					
Number of days in period					
Daily average number of patients					
Patient capacity					
Average patient-days (% of capacity)					

COST PER PATIENT DAY (cumulative total of days for year)____ months to _____

Nursing administration
Skilled nursing facility
Rent or depreciation (building), interest, taxes
Plant operation and maintenance
Grounds
Security
Transportation
Administration
Business office
In-service education
Medical administration
Medical care evaluation and assessment
Dietary
Housekeeping
Laundry
Physical therapy
Occupational therapy
Social service
Activities/volunteers
Laboratory and EKG
X ray
Pharmacy
Health records

EXHIBIT 14-4 (cont.)

STATISTICAL OPERATIONAL DATA (continued)

AVERAGE INCOME PER PATIENT-DAY (year to date)

	Rate	Total days	Income
Medicare			
Medicaid			
Private			

$$\frac{\text{Total income}}{\text{Total days}} = \text{Average income per patient-day}$$

COST PER MEAL

Total cost of dietary for _____ months to _____ $ _____

Patient meals served
Staff meals served
Visitor meals served
Total meals served

$$\frac{\text{Total cost of dietary}}{\text{Total meals served}} = \text{Average cost per meal (food, supplies, and salaries)}$$

Business office records on patients will contain the signed continuing care contract, which stipulates the daily rate; accounts receivable cards; Medicare billing forms; notification from third-party payers as to the eligibility of patients for benefits; and records of charges to patients for services not covered by the daily rate.

The accountant, who is responsible for providing certain information to the administrative director, will need records for the monthly operating report (statement of income, expenses, and net gain or loss), the balance sheet, and comparison of data for the month and cumulative period of months for the present year with data for the same period of the previous year. At the end of each accounting period, an accountant should prepare a certified audit of the facility's accounting process.

FACILITIES, EQUIPMENT, AND SUPPLIES

The bulk of supplies and equipment for the business office will be dictated by the mechanical processes, if any, used by the department and the extent to which the recording of different procedures is automated. For instance, the payroll may be processed by a computer service bureau, with all else done by the single-write system; or payroll, accounts receivable, and accounts payable may all be mechanized by a combination of methods, using a service bureau and a bookkeeping machine.

Irrespective of the hardware used for the bookkeeping procedures, the business office will need two calculating machines (or one for each employee who would use it regularly), one or more electric typewriters, access to a photocopy machine, a safe, a postage scale and postage meter, a checkwriter, and journal and ledger binders (even records produced by a mechanical process will need to be retained in written form). The business office area must be well lighted and have sufficient desk and work areas for all personnel. Filing and storage cabinets will be needed for both records and office supplies. Due to the large amount of telephone communication with in-house and outside people, staff members may need individual telephones.

SUMMARY

The increasing concern on the part of citizens, legislators, and third-party payers about rising health care costs emphasizes the growing importance of nursing home financial management. Uniform systems of cost accounting have been developed to facilitate comparisons among institutions. The growing collection of detailed data will inevitably necessitate the introduction of sophisticated information systems, challenging the financial ability of the small- and medium-sized nursing homes to keep pace with their larger peers.

NOTES

1.   The reference for the bulk of this discussion is George M. Cate, "Data Processing in the Nursing Home," presentation at the 1978 Convocation of the American College of Nursing Home Administrators, Washington, D.C., April 17, 1978.

GENERAL REFERENCES

American Hospital Association. *Accounting Manual for Long Term Care Institutions.* Chicago: American Hospital Association, 1968.
Hospital Planning and Review Council and New York State Department of Health. *New York State Residential Health Care Facility Accounting and Reporting Manual.* Albany: New York State Department of Health, Office of Health Systems Management, November 1977.
Austin, Charles J. "Planning and Selecting an Information System." *Hospitals* 51, no. 20 (October 16, 1977).

CHAPTER 15

Records

INTRODUCTION

The skilled nursing facility is an increasingly complex organization having numerous departments, employing a successive stream of personnel, serving many residents, and conducting business with more and more vendors. With the incessant activity of a modern health care facility, it is virtually impossible for anyone to trust to memory relevant material concerning the operation of the institution. Furthermore, government and surveying agencies continually request documentation of many aspects of the nursing home's operation to substantiate its compliance with the law. To preclude unnecessary effort and expense at some future date, it is imperative that a systematic plan for the organization and coordination of all institutional records be achieved.

Providers must maintain a system for the use, transcription, retrieval, storage, and disposal of all patient health records. Indexes, abstracts, and biostatistics will be produced from these records for use by nursing home management, fiscal intermediaries, researchers, and physicians.

Departmental records are under the supervision of the department head, while patient health records are the responsibility of the records coordinator.

STAFFING PATTERN
Records Coordinator

One full-time records coordinator should adequately meet the needs of a 100-bed nursing home. Facilities with 200 beds or more may justify two full-time people: one would be a registered record administrator and the second would serve as an assistant. Although responsible to the administrative director, the records coordinator should consult with the medical director on proper recording of medical information on the health record, especially in light of frequent physician absence from the nursing home.

The records coordinator ensures an orderly control of all nursing home records, forms, and files by helping staff members to systematize and simplify record-keeping procedures. He aids administration in the completion of reports to outside agencies that require statistical patient information and participates in gathering data for research activities. Responsibilities may include maintaining reprints of all staff professional articles and answering requests for same.

The records coordinator performs a variety of tasks to aid professional and paraprofessional staff members in remaining current in their time-limited reports, assessments, and orders on patients. He answers all requests for patient medical information from third-party payers and others, and he prepares, files, and oversees patient discharge records and the disease indexes.

This staff member must be organized and able to work under minimal supervision. Considerable initiative and judgment is required in collecting and analyzing medical information, in recognizing the need for improvement of existing systems, and in effecting changes. A good working relationship with other staff is necessary to obtain desired results.

An accredited records technician, who has an associate degree or the equivalent, is preferable for this position. Or a high school graduate with some college and a health background, especially in medical terminology derived from classroom courses or experience in a patient care setting, would present suitable credentials. The records coordinator must be familiar with the documentation responsibilities of all professional services in order to be able to determine their adequacy. Remaining current on the regulations governing health records in skilled nursing facilities, particularly with respect to Medicare- and Medicaid-sponsored residents, is essential. It is also helpful for the records coordinator to be a notary public. Finally, he must be able to type and operate other essential office machines.

Medical Records Administrator

If the facility does not employ a full-time medical records administrator (registered records administrator), consultation should be provided regularly by a qualified medical records administrator who would report to the administrative director. As a consultant, this person would guide the records coordinator in establishing the clinical record file and indexes. He would assist in adapting the principles and practices of medical record library science to the nursing home setting and would keep the nursing home abreast of the requirements of government and accrediting agencies. At least semiannually, the medical records administrator should review and analyze a sample of records to determine their accuracy, completeness, consistency, and confidentiality.

GENERAL RECORDS AND FORMS

With the huge volume of forms, correspondence, reports, contracts, minutes, and meetings required and relegated to departmental personnel, the practice of offering a simple, understandable, and systemized plan as the standard procedure for record keeping and for facilitating information retrieval should be operable. Consideration should be given to separate department files or a centralized system, depending on the layout of the building and the frequency of record use. Standardized form sizes should be established to expedite handling and storage. The selection of filing captions according to subject matter or specific name/title should be determined, with the addition of a second filing caption for the purpose of developing a cross-reference file. Once the files have been arranged, personnel must be trained to index and file according to the system.

Meaningful criteria for the retention of records must be developed to ensure that all records retained are useful. Records should be kept to the limit of their potential usefulness and then destroyed (see Exhibit 15-1). Care must be taken not to be hasty in disposing records such as financial reports that are mandated by regulatory or accrediting agencies or are supportive of facility practices that are subject to scrutiny by outside agencies. When in doubt, the facility may abide by the state's statute of limitations.

Microfilm or microfiche should be investigated as alternatives to keeping records in their original form, particularly as they are admissible in a court of law. Microfilm is less expensive because it utilizes roll film, which also makes retrieval of information more difficult. This problem is eliminated with the use of microfiche, which records information on separate film cards. Perhaps material that would be less likely to be needed in the future should be put on microfilm, while records referred to frequently should be converted to microfiche.

Benefits to be derived from these processes include the ability to dispose of the original cumbersome record and the consequent saving of file space; the longer preservation of records afforded by microfilm; and the reduction of filing errors through the elimination of the need for refiling after use. On the other hand, a microfilm and/or microfiche installation is costly and may require the development of a new filing and indexing system. The use of these sophisticated processes is more difficult and time-consuming and as a result, the professional staff may study the records of discharged patients less often.

All forms must be carefully scrutinized to ensure that each achieves its intended purpose, is clear and concise, is used correctly, and does not duplicate information retained elsewhere. The records coordinator

EXHIBIT 15-1
Suggested Periods of Record Retention

SUGGESTED PERIODS OF RECORD RETENTION

Length of Time to be Kept	Type of Record
One Year	Information desk file Telephone index
Two years	Departmental reports Purchasing records
Five years beyond expiration	Insurance policies
Five years	Budget reports Record of food costs and meals served Tax statements
Statute of limitations	Employee records Patient records*
Ten years	Cost statements Medical audits
Until revised	Admission policies Personnel policies
Until new approval received	Joint Commission on Accreditation of Hospitals report
As long as useful	Publications and reports of other agencies
As long as active	Committee reports
Until superseded	Codes Emergency and utility interruption plans Rules for visitors
Indefinite	Annual reports Audit reports Balance sheets Bank records Income and expense statements Legal suits License numbers of personnel Licenses and permits Minutes of meetings Organizational charts Rates and charges
Permanent	Specifications and plans Certificate of doing business Certificate of incorporation Certificate of occupancy Constitution and bylaws History of the institution Medical staff appointments Medical staff bylaws

*May be kept permanently for research purposes

should maintain a master book with copies of all forms used in each department—from administrative and departmental records to patient care records. Whenever changes are contemplated, the records coordinator should be consulted to review these for appropriateness. If the changes are approved, the records coordinator can easily record the revisions by simply noting the revision date on the form.

Due to the large number of different forms and quantities used, the nursing home should consider the use of a mimeograph or a newer type of offset printing machine to reproduce its own forms. In this way, the facility can design nursing forms for its own special needs and can reproduce them without delay at a reduced cost. Colored paper can be used to differentiate forms for different departments. Letters, flyers, or newsletters may also be printed with this equipment. Of course, mimeographing or in-house offset will have a certain inflexibility in the type, size, and color of printing that can be done, compared with the offset printing process used by professionals. But for the majority of the nursing home's needs, it will suffice.

The master control book should contain ordering information about all forms produced by professional printing companies. For retrieving the master stencils (if a mimeograph system is used) of forms reproduced on the premises, the stencil file number should be noted on the form. The master control book is only as useful as it is accurate; therefore it should be updated whenever necessary.

HEALTH RECORDS

The patient health record serves a number of purposes for the patient, the professional, and the skilled nursing facility. Most importantly, it is a basis on which to plan for and to evaluate the care given, and to communicate the results of that care to all treatment team members. At the same time, it satisfies legal requirements regarding the provision and documentation of treatment. While a major function of the health record is to provide data for research, it also assists the facility in evaluating its own services.

The content of health records will be facts, opinions, conclusions, observations, and hearsay; each comment must be worded to indicate its essence.

The Nature of Long-Term Health Records

The skilled nursing facility cares for people who have health and health-related chronic, recurrent, and often incurable problems whose care represents the combined activities of many disciplines; as such, its records are characterized by objectives that differ considerably from the acute and episodic care rendered in the general hospital. Objectives are not to cure but to help residents cope with impairments, to decrease their dependence on others, to diminish their disability, and to help them function at the highest level. Objectives also relate to the quality of the person's life, which presents a challenge with respect to documentation.

A major obstacle noted in nursing home charts as compared with charts in the acute hospital is the lack of correlation between medical diagnosis and length of stay, anticipated outcome, or appropriateness of placement, and services or treatments.[1] Contrary to suggestions of hospital-oriented planners that the nursing home length of stay be equated with specific diagnostic entities, that simply is often not the case and not a viable comparison. The patient with the diagnosis of a fractured hip may be motivated to learn to walk again and subsequently be able to return to his own home, he may require some assistance to ambulate and engage in the activities of daily living in a lesser care protective setting, or he may break down completely, develop decubitus ulcers, refuse to eat, and require major nursing care and related services for survival.

Many experts concerned with developing proper long-term-care records underscore the deficiencies and dangers of applying a medical model based on acute episodic care to long-term care.[2] F. D. Zeman commented on the "multiplicity, chronicity and duplicity" of the medical and social problems of long-term geriatric patients where there is seldom one medical diagnosis and where patients with similar diagnoses react differently to their impairments due to their personal, social, economic, and support resources.[3]

Developing a basic data set for health records helps patient care by serving as a guide for an adequate record and offers a concise profile of the client, which can be used by care givers periodically to assess the patient, measure progress or deterioration, and modify treatment programs. It consists of three areas: demographic information, description of the individual patient, and a record of services and treatments.

In the demographic section of the health record, it is urgent to record the last residence(s) of the patient correctly, as this may provide crucial information for future determinations of eligibility for Medicaid assistance. It is also an important element for health planners to examine. Certificates of need for new long-term-care facilities often depend on the number of elderly people living in a specific area. The fact is that people admitted to skilled nursing facilities frequently are not residents of the particular area; rather, their relatives live there and wish to have the elderly ill person in a facility close to them. Information about the responsible relative and former living arrangements is also useful in longitudinal research studies.

Demographic information also entails instituting a system whereby the patient is identified with his health record for future reference. The serial method of numbering health records where numbers are assigned in order on admission of the patient is the most common numbering method. With this system, a resident who has been admitted, transferred to the hospital, and readmitted may be assigned several numbers, as each new admission will mean a new admitting number.

In the interest of continuity of care, all records concerning one patient should be integrated under one unit or number for easy availability to physicians and other professional staff. This type of filing is called the unit system. New admissions to the skilled nursing facility are assigned the next number in the series as their health record number, but readmitted patients are always given the number they received upon the initial admission.

The records need to describe individual attributes of the resident—the etiology of his illness, and clinical and behavioral manifestations. Although most skilled nursing facility residents are admitted from the general hospital with an interagency referral form, incomplete and inaccurate information is not unusual. The reasons for record deficiencies are manifold. Older patients generally are admitted to the hospital for a particular problem involving a single organ, for example, a fracture of the hip. Thus the accompanying information from the hospital will relate to the hip, excluding the fact that the patient is confused and disoriented, unable to follow directions, and hard of hearing. The orthopedist who serves the patient in the hospital is regrettably unaware of the patient's additional problems when he completes the transfer form to the skilled nursing facility. The skilled nursing facility, on the other hand, must deal both with the functioning of the whole individual and with multiple organ disabilities.

To classify residents according to their ability to perform the activities of daily living, many instruments have been developed to measure this information for clinical records. Likewise, scales have been constructed to reflect the mental functioning of residents. And both types of indexes are needed to delineate the individual attributes of long-term-care residents.

Following the demographic and individual attribute data on the health form is the record of what has been done for the resident. This record will include care plans, orders, and progress notes. A significant portion of the record coordinator's time will be spent determining that the treatment ordered has been rendered, with both steps documented properly.

Problem areas related to this section of the chart will include recording deficiencies of attending physicians, such as failure to countersign telephone orders or sign the accident/incident report within twenty-four hours. This and other similar details tend to occur when physicians visit the nursing home at odd hours without communicating with the unit charge nurse or supervisor, who in all likelihood would have reminded the physician of these omissions.

A more important deficiency is the almost uniform absence of discharge summaries on medical records. When nursing home patients are transferred to the hospital via a telephone order and expire in the hospital, the physician may not have the occasion to visit the nursing home again for a considerable period and thus will not complete a discharge summary. One solution is to institute a procedure whereby the records coordinator assembles the data for the discharge summary, which is cosigned by the medical director.

Nursing records require special attention, and the records coordinator may need to educate nurses to use their valuable time well by writing meaningful notes. Descriptive note writing is a necessity, especially when fiscal intermediaries frequently request copies of nurses' notes, which may be used to determine the patient's eligibility for insurance coverage. For example, a description of a decubitus ulcer must include how deep it is, how much it discharges, whether it is necrotic, whether it can be probed, what the exact treatment has been, and so forth. Similarly, if the nurse noted that the patient had an elevated temperature on Monday, on Tuesday he must note what happened to the fever. Sometimes nurses mention the temperature but do not follow its course in subsequent notes.

Source- Versus Problem-Oriented Records

Health records are either source or problem oriented. In keeping source-oriented records, which are the more traditional format, each person on the health care treatment team uses separate forms. This method of documentation can become unwieldy when the number of professionals who write records increases to such an extent that it becomes too time-consuming to read every record in order to get the whole picture of the individual patient. All the necessary information is recorded on the various forms, but in such a way that it is difficult to use.

The streamlined problem-oriented record reduces the size of the record and the amount of paperwork required of nursing personnel. As a management tool, it plans and organizes productive work activity based on the patients' needs by encouraging the use of logic. These records readily permit the physician to transmit his ideas to other professional patient care staff, add an educational component, and introduce all professionals to the concepts behind data processing.

The problem-oriented record is truly an integrated patient care plan containing four basic components: the data base, the problem list, the initial care plan, and progress notes.

The data base includes the patient's social and medical history, results of his physical examination and laboratory tests, and his functional ability and chief complaints. Each service can evaluate newly admitted patients and add its assessment to the data base.

At a subsequent patient care conference or interdisciplinary meeting, the patient is seen, the data base reviewed, and a list of problems developed. The problems must coordinate with the information available in the data base. The list may include such diverse items as a known diagnosis, abnormal diagnostic or physical findings or symptoms with unknown etiology, and behavioral, social, and mental problems.

Each problem is assigned an index number, which helps ensure that progress notes relate to specific problems and thus that they are meaningful. A date of onset is recorded, and each problem is classified as active or inactive. The period following surgery for a fractured hip may be labeled inactive, but it should be noted in case of future falls and resultant problems. The date when an active problem becomes inactive must be recorded.

Initial treatment plans are then written for each problem, with time-related goals. They may detail the need for more diagnostic workup, for management of the problems, and/or for educating the patient and his family concerning each problem.

Progress notes describe the patient's status with respect to each problem and include narrative notes and flow sheets. On a flow sheet, dates are recorded in the left margin of the page and observations and treatments are written across the page, thereby producing a graphic picture of the care that the patient received. It may also be designed to indicate progress with each specific problem.

Confidentiality of Health Records

Implicit in the formulation and retention of all health records is the confidentiality of the information contained therein, so special caution must be taken to prevent such information from being released to unauthorized persons. Formerly, this also restricted the patient from knowing the content of his record, but increased attention is now being focused on the patient's right to see the record.

Nursing home minutes and committee reports should avoid identifying specific patients by name. During surveys by licensing, certifying, and accrediting groups, the review of health records to determine conformity to standards is permissible as long as names of patients or record numbers are not mentioned in official survey reports. Disclosures to third-party payers should be carefully monitored so that only specific information is released.

Use and Release of Health Records

The health record is the property of the skilled nursing facility; consequently, its proper use and release to individuals is the facility's responsibility. In addition to institution staff, health planners, policy makers, third-party payers, researchers, and monitors of health services will request access to records. It is essential that the authority for releasing health record information be given to someone who thoroughly understands the purpose, content, and limitations of the recorded information.

It is not necessary to obtain patient consent for the release of certain nonconfidential identification data and/or of medical information for the purposes of research and interchange of information between providers of care to achieve continuity of care. Other than the above, the majority of requests for medical information about nursing home patients will come from Medicare and Medicaid. The provider services contract with the Medicaid agency allows for the provision of necessary data in order to substantiate a patient's eligibility for or receipt of services. Requests from fiscal intermediaries, attorneys, or private insurance companies should be granted only with proper authorization.

Responding to inquiries regarding medical information from Medicare, Medicaid, and private insurance companies will involve expert judgment in determining what information should be released and assuring that the information is sufficiently descriptive of the patient's problems, needs, and course of treatment.

Certain administrative staff—including members of the governing body, the facility attorney, insurance agents, the records coordinator, the social worker, the chief nurse, the business office manager (to process accounts or insurance claims), and the medical director—must have access to patient health records, subject to the approval of the administrator, for the performance of their duties. Government surveyors will review charts to verify conformance with regulation standards. Auditors of fiscal intermediaries may have to view certain parts of the health record to verify claims. And quality assurance efforts by the Joint Commission surveyors will necessitate examination of the skilled nursing facility's records.

Guidelines should be developed for the records coordinator, delineating who may have access to health records for research and study and under what conditions. Both the researchers and the nursing home are obliged to protect the residents' privacy in published studies. In most instances, the written permission of patients or patients' relatives for their participation in research studies will be needed.

People who are not on the facility's professional staff must obtain administrative permission to use health records for purposes of research. Such investigators may include nonstaff physicians engaged in research or writing professional articles, public health personnel involved in the collection of demographic data, government workers engaged in epidemiological studies, health planners concerned with patterns of utilization of skilled nursing facilities, or graduate students in health administration, nursing, or social work gathering material for theses.

Among the factors to be considered before approving or denying permission to use the records are: the purpose of the research with respect to improved patient care; the potential liability in making the records available; the qualifications of the researcher, indicating his ability to comprehend the content of the records; the need for the nursing home staff to participate in the study and, if so, to what extent; safeguards for preservation of confidentiality and the possibility that the study might interfere with patient care or staff activity.

It is critically important to use a charge-out system so that records can be located quickly when needed. Records removed from the file should be so noted by the use of an out-guide showing the date removed, and the person removing it should so indicate in a notebook located next to the file cabinets. Records may not be removed from the premises. The nursing home will need to determine a fee structure in response to bona fide requests for transcripts, abstracts, and authenticated copies of records.

INDEXES

The patient index usually refers to an alphabetical file with a card—perhaps the admission card—for each patient. Current inpatients may be filed together, with a separate file designated for discharged patients. The patient index is useful as a cross reference to the admission and discharge registers and may also be used for demographic research projects.

The nursing home may also use disease or treatment indexes. A treatment index shows the types of treatment carried out, such as the administration of particular drugs or therapies. Disease, or diagnosis, indexes are fashioned after the hospital model, which is compiled after the patient's discharge. However, diagnoses may be indexed while the patient is still in residence if a diagnostic history form is maintained for each resident. This record can be particularly helpful, as the diagnoses of the nursing home resident may change considerably throughout the period of residence. The patient may come from the hospital with a diagnosis of a fractured hip and subsequently suffer a stroke in the nursing home, followed by a bout of pneumonia, so that the original hip fracture diagnosis no longer constitutes the working diagnosis.

To record the significant diagnoses, the unit nurse should list each diagnosis on the diagnostic history form with pertinent identifying material for verification by the attending physician. Nurses will need thorough education in this endeavor, as many will have difficulty determining which episodes to record. For example, is an ailment such as an upper respiratory infection worthy of inclusion if the patient has no fever?

Indexing is accomplished by making a card for the first diagnosis or treatment, recording the diagnosis or treatment at the top of the card, and listing the various cases with the same diagnosis or treatment below. As new cards for the same diagnosis or treatment are made, they should be numbered consecutively. The index cards are then alphabetically filed according to the disease or treatment term. In all indexing, it is critical that standard nomenclature be used; otherwise a variety of terms will be used to denote the same diagnosis.

A second method of indexing diseases uses the *International Classification of Diseases, 9th Revision, Clinical Modification (ICD-9-CM)* as its basis.[4] It must be used by all facilities certified for Medicare and Medicaid. The *ICD-9-CM* is a statistical classification of diseases, accidents, poisonings, violence, symptoms, ill-defined conditions, and so on. Although its main purpose is to provide statistical data regarding groups of cases, it can be used for indexing health records as a nomenclature of diseases. It is organized by topics (such as diseases of the skeletal system) by etiology (such as infectious diseases), or by events (such as complications of pregnancy). Such an accepted classification of diseases permits comparison of data between individuals, institutions, and even countries. Of course, such a taxonomy and disease classification is only as valuable as it is correct, and physicians have little training in medical school in the principles of scientific classification.

In long-term taxonomy, additional needs to be met are the following: characteristics of care as well as of disease, classification by individuals rather than diseases, notation of disease outcome by nonmedical personnel, and reliability and validity of criteria.[5] The latest revision of the *ICD-9-CM* includes the classification of impairments and handicaps, which is very valuable in improving skilled nursing facility health records.

PROCEDURES

Upon admission of a patient, the records coordinator should receive a copy of the completed admission card to file. Using the admission information, the records coordinator then develops a list of the utilization review dates for all patients. Two weeks prior to the utilization review committee meetings, a list of all patients to be reviewed should be sent to the director of nursing, the unit head nurses, and the coordinator of social services so that they may have an opportunity to examine each patient's chart to ensure proper documentation. By virtue of the receipt of the list, the head nurses will know that a new nursing assessment form must be completed before the meeting for those patients listed. Patients' anniversary admission dates should also be indicated, alerting the nursing staff of the need for annual physicals.

The records coordinator should spot check inpatient charts regularly to ascertain their completeness and to determine that they are indicative of each patient's current health status. The need for any additional documentation should be brought to the attention of the attending physician, nursing staff, medical director, and allied health professionals. The records coordinator may then convey the overall findings of these chart reviews to the nursing staff and other professional staff in the form of an in-service program to help improve the content of health records.

Selected statistical reports for government agencies may be the records coordinator's responsibility. It is said that the easiest report is generally the most accurate; and the fewer data collected at any given time, the less chance there is for error. Thus daily tabulations of data will provide the most accurate reports and will cause the least pressure at the end of the year when the annual report is needed.

Compiling and supervising discharged patients' records are main duties of the records coordinator. Upon discharge of a patient, all records pertaining to the patient kept by nursing, social service, and the business office should be forwarded to the records coordinator. The records coordinator then carefully examines the material to ensure that all entries are properly signed, that a discharge summary has been written, and that there are no missing sheets, and then he organizes the information so that it is easy to follow and reflects the clinical course of the patient. If the patient has been discharged and readmitted a number of times, the most recent stay should be on top in the discharge file. Business records and privileged information known to the social workers should be segregated from the clinical records, such as on the opposite inside flap of the file folder.

FACILITIES AND EQUIPMENT

A well-lighted and ventilated office with sufficient desk and table space is the main requisite for the records coordinator. If this room is the repository for health records, it must be secure from unwanted intrusion. File cabinets for discharged patient files, reprints of staff articles, and supplies of forms will be needed and will most likely require expansion over a period of time. An electric typewriter, photocopy machine, elec-

FIGURE 15-1
Ample Space Needed for Records Coordinator

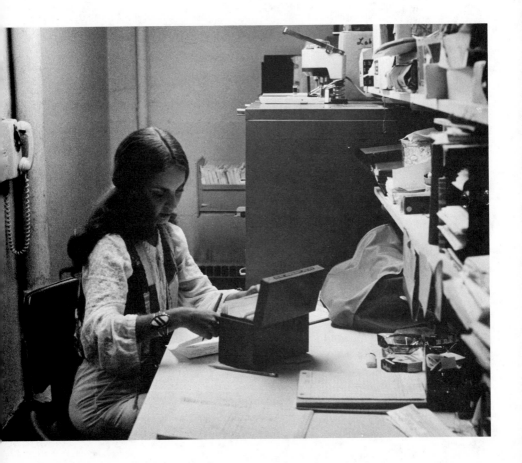

tric hole puncher, and duplicating machine constitute necessary office equipment, along with a medical dictionary and a current copy of the *ICD-9-CM*.

SUMMARY

The escalating number of malpractice claims related to the quality of health care, as well as to the general operation of the nursing home, emphasizes the importance of clinical and business records. Record-keeping requirements have increased drastically and will continue to do so with growing government involvement. Hence, the development of an orderly record-keeping system and well-designed forms for documentation is mandatory.

NOTES

1.   Jane H. Murnaghan, "Review of the Conference Proceedings," *Medical Care* 14, no. 5, Supplement (May 1976): 8.
2.   Ibid., p. 5.
3.   F. D. Zeman, "Myth and Stereotype in the Classical Medicine of Old Age," *New England Journal of Medicine* 272 (1965): 1104.
4.   Commission on Professional and Hospital Activities, *International Classification of Diseases, 9th Revision, Clinical Modification* (Ann Arbor, Mich., 1978).
5.   Norman Sartorius, "Modifications and New Approaches to Taxonomy in Long Term Care: Advantages and Disadvantages of the ICD," *Medical Care* 14, no. 5, Supplement (May 1976): 111.

CHAPTER 16

The Therapeutic

Organization

INTRODUCTION

Traditional systems of delivering health care, in which professionals function as individual practitioners, are deficient in dealing with the complex problems of the institutionalized ill aged. Caring for the chronically ill elderly whose problems involve multiple organ involvement and frequent behavioral disability, superimposed on familial struggles and social dislocation, is too complicated for one individual, irrespective of his abilities. A collaborative professional effort is needed to address all the problems.

In the therapeutic organization, two and two may equal five. When physician, nurse, physical therapist, occupational therapist, social worker, activity coordinator, administrator, and dietitian work together as a team, the totality of their efforts is greater than the sum of each individual effort.

An effective organization is characterized by interdependence. For example, when the doctor orders the physical therapist to work with the stroke patient, it is called a treatment. However, when the patient is encouraged by nurses and activity personnel to walk to the dining room, to the lavatory, to activities, the treatment becomes a comprehensive rehabilitation program. A treatment takes place at a particular time, but rehabilitation permeates all aspects of the patient's daily life.

TEAM ORGANIZATION

Some teams are composed of individuals with professional backgrounds, be they medical, nursing, etc., such as the interdisciplinary team. Other teams represent the cooperative efforts of people who work in the same service and whose backgrounds differ according to their education. For example, the nursing department includes professionally trained nurses and untrained nursing aides.

Irrespective of its makeup, an organization's personal and interpersonal characteristics are of primary importance to its ultimate effectiveness. A sense of mutual trust must be pervasive and this trust must extend to forthright and constructive communication as the group evaluates its needs and its tasks. The members must be able to agree on goals and objectives and the order of priorities. The totality of the individual representatives' experience, knowledge, competencies, ideas, attitudes, and values must be used to reach consensus in group decision making. At meetings, disagreements and conflicts may precede problem solving. The group must, of course, be able to identify problems and plan, schedule, implement, and finally evaluate its own activities.[1]

The team leader may be a physician, social worker, nurse, or other professional. If one person is not designated as the permanent leader, an organized schedule for group leadership may be developed to afford all professionals the opportunity to function in this capacity, or the team leader may change according to the particular situation. For example, when a family problem is addressed, the social worker may function as the leader. However, the health team traditionally has been led by the physician; when interested and informed physicians are available, medical involvement and leadership are helpful.

It is the leader's responsibility to assure the participation of those attending the meeting. He must also ascertain that one or two individuals do not control the discussion. His role is to encourage the group to discuss each patient's plan of care—to bring out negative aspects until a positive approach is developed. This responsibility helps the leader mature and develop and attracts people who want to grow personally as well as professionally. Leaders must want to lead.

Staff organization helps eliminate competition for power, integrates planning, and eliminates barriers. Professionals are not taught in school to work as a team with other professionals; however, therapeutically useful information may come from many sources.

For the administrative personnel to be able to take their proper place in the therapeutic organization, they must be well versed in the clinical aspects of the nursing home operation, with a clear understanding of the current familial and patient issues.

INTERDEPARTMENTAL COOPERATION

Interdepartmental cooperation facilitates the development of the therapeutic organization. The successful operation of the nursing home depends on cooperative relationships, which foster the spirit and purpose of the therapeutic milieu and are necessary for the accomplishment of specific responsibilities of the departments.

Administration

The administration sets the tone for interdepartmental cooperation by encouraging communication among the disciplines. Administrative and/or personnel staff are consulted when one department is experiencing difficulty in working with another department, or if duties need to be defined as the responsibility of one department or another. Consultation may be sought, too, concerning intradepartmental personnel issues, particularly in regard to the interpretation of personnel policies or staffing patterns.

The administration would correctly be consulted on issues pertaining to the use of or condition of the nursing home facilities and grounds. Major equipment or supply purchases should be discussed with and receive the approval of the administrative director.

Direction may be sought from the administration regarding dealings with the outside community—vendors, community organizations, health and welfare agencies—and families.

Medicine

As the initiator of the treatment plan, the attending physician must be accessible to all disciplines and provide directives for their respective roles in the patient care plan.

Coordinating the efforts of all professionals involved in the care of the patient devolves to the medical director, who reviews the overall program and goals of the clinical services. A specific treatment plan may be thoroughly gone over with the medical director for his advice in adapting it to the patient's mental and functional status.

To ensure the delivery of quality care in the skilled nursing facility, the medical director, attending medical staff, and allied health professionals have a responsibility to assist in planning staff in-service programs. Weekly clinical rounds, incorporating the introduction of new residents and the presentation of patients with special problems, should be conducted by the medical director with the welcome attendance of attending physicians.

Nursing

The nursing department is the hub of all activities that take place in the facility and, as such, must maintain good working relationships with all departments. The nursing staff members must coordinate patient care schedules with other treating and facility services. With some assistance from volunteers, they prepare and transport patients to activities or rehabilitation treatments. Larger facilities may have a transportation department.

As the primary care givers, nursing staff members should be informed of all that is being done for the patient so that they may carry through with treatment goals during their work with the patient. They must observe patient response to treatment and report it to the involved disciplines. And they must communicate special patient care procedures, such as the institution of isolation, to appropriate personnel.

Ongoing rapport with the dietary department is particularly necessary because the nursing staff has responsibility for the feeding process. Requesting seconds and substitutes, ensuring that meals are served neither late nor early, and informing the foodservice supervisor of patient likes and dislikes are part of the cooperation between the departments.

The nursing staff must notify housekeeping about an admission or discharge so that rooms may be thoroughly cleaned and prepared for the new patient. The two departments must decide who will clean beds and bedside units and who will put away clothing. Even the scheduling of room cleaning is best developed collaboratively so as not to interfere with patient care.

Housekeeping or laundry provides clean linens to the floors and cares for patients' washable clothing. The nursing staff must cooperate by rinsing linens and clothing that have been soiled by fecal matter. Together, the two departments should watch for clothing that is not properly labeled and label it.

In the area of skilled nursing rehabilitation, unlike the hospital where the departments of occupational therapy and physical therapy take over, nursing is actively concerned with rehabilitation, with the activities of daily living, and with turning and ambulating patients. The nursing staff should seek consultation with the occupational or physical therapist for advice about techniques to incorporate into routine daily patient care.

Nurses, nursing aides, and orderlies need to encourage patient participation in the activities program. Nursing home patients often require continuing stimulation to prevent them from isolating themselves in their rooms. This is augmented by ensuring that the patients are dressed nicely and are comfortable, and by accompanying them to the activity area. One attendant from each unit should be assigned to assist in the program and to be available to take patients to and from the lavatory when needed, and so forth. It is important for volunteers to understand the nature of the patient population; nurses should offer such information when needed and participate in organized orientation and in-service programs for volunteers.

The nursing and social service departments work closely together both before and after patient admission. From the time that a patient becomes a candidate for admission, nursing and social service jointly assess the patient's medical and psychosocial problems and needs, the availability of appropriate services within the facility, and the expectations for family involvement. Together the director of nursing and social worker should visit the patient prior to admission, either in the hospital or at home, to be fully cognizant of the patient's medical and functional status.

Each must keep the other informed about the latest developments in patient and family management in order to establish a unified and consistent approach. The social service staff can be especially helpful to nursing in working through problems related to dining room seating arrangements, patient-peer relationships, acquisition of appropriate and adequate clothing for a patient, informing the patient's sponsor of the need for additional services, discussing both on- and off-premises visiting regulations, arranging patient appointments out of the nursing home, and, of course, issues pertaining to patient–staff–family relationships.

The director of nursing and the coordinator of social services should make rounds together to observe patient function and performance within the therapeutic community, to discuss the most effective and useful manner of providing patient services, and to observe patient response to treatment. Together they may conduct patient and family interviews, perhaps with the medical director and social service consultant, to offer input from their respective areas of expertise and to understand the concerns of the patient and family fully and mutually.

Social Service

The social service department has a special assignment in the skilled nursing facility to assist in making the patient's stay comfortable and successful for the patient, his family, and the nursing home staff. To achieve this end, the social service staff acts as the link between the three parties—relaying facility policy to patients and/or families, assisting staff to understand and deal with a difficult family, and counseling patients and their relatives on the need for skilled nursing care. The social worker is often the one person who can deal effectively with families on delicate issues due to the trusting relationship that has developed between them.

Communication between non–nursing facility staff (particularly part-time consultants) and families frequently is achieved via the social worker. For example, the dietitian may request the social worker to solicit information from the family regarding the patient's past eating patterns, or the social worker may describe patient progress in speech therapy to the family. The social worker may function as the intermediary because he is better known to the family than the dietitian or the part-time speech therapist.

FIGURE 16-1
Nursing and Social Service Planning Patient Admission

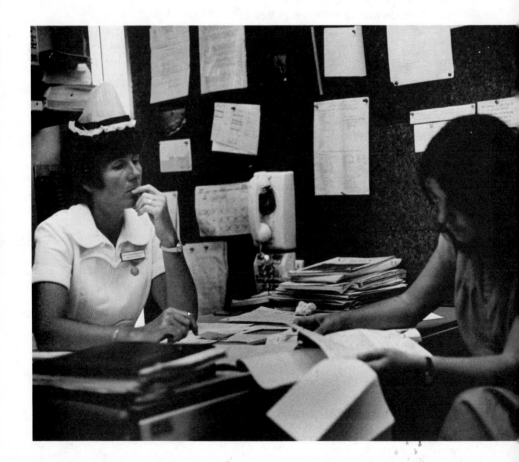

The social service department helps ensure the development and maintenance of a therapeutic community. Staff members must impart the special skills of social work to the rest of the nursing home personnel, and in order to do so, they must be familiar with all nursing home departments with particular reference to patient care and family contacts. The social worker should be ready for, and even anticipate, providing suggestions to other nursing home staff members to assist them in their work related to patient and family management.

Social work staff members inform the business office of an admission by forwarding the signed contract form that notes the patient's financial sponsorship, daily rate, and special services to be billed. If changes in patient financial sponsorship are anticipated, the social worker should inform the business office staff.

Rehabilitation Therapies

Upon admission of a patient who is a candidate for treatment by one of the rehabilitation therapists, the director of nursing and coordinator of social services should meet with the therapist(s) to discuss the patient's medical, psychosocial, and functional status. The physical and occupational therapists and speech pathologist/audiologist must transmit information regarding patient progress to all staff to integrate their care plans into their comprehensive therapeutic programs. Patients who require both physical and occupational therapy intervention should be discussed jointly to note patient progress in each area in order to provide continuity of care.

Working together and with other departments to improve the rehabilitative aspects of the nursing home's program should be one of the therapists' goals. This is especially true with nursing, where the physical therapist and occupational therapist should be closely involved with the nursing attendants' in-service program and the activities of daily living retraining program. The activities coordinator should also benefit from input from the therapists, thereby making the program both more interesting and integral to the comprehensive plan of care for each patient.

Staff members must remember that when the occupational therapist or any other consultant works part-time, his time in the facility is precious and must be organized efficiently to accomplish all that must be done. Educating other direct care personnel is an important aspect of a consultant's position, as he is not always on the premises to assist in patient care problems as they arise. The best alternative is to impress on staff the concepts and techniques of the specialty in relation to routine patient care so they may apply it themselves in their daily work.

The limited presence of the speech pathologist/audiologist necessitates good communication with nursing home personnel, particularly with the nursing and social service staffs. It is important to incorporate the speech pathologist/audiologist into the treatment team via attendance at medical rounds and participation in in-service to foster the concept of the therapeutic community for both the therapist and the other staff.

Activities and Volunteers

An active department of activities and volunteers will aid in the creation and maintenance of an atmosphere of harmony, stimulation, and optimism throughout the facility and thus be advantageous to both residents and staff. Additionally, an activities department that has a sound volunteer program and incorporates other community resources will provide a positive link between the nursing home and the community.

Staff members must be helpful in supporting the activities program by being enthusiastic and encouraging patient attendance. Administrative interest and backing is essential for the program to be successful. The publication of events through all possible means—meetings, announcements, newsletters—is necessary to attain that goal.

As food provides the focus or is an important complement to many programs, the activities staff must frequently confer with the foodservice supervisor to plan menus and refreshments for special events, allowing as much advance notice as possible. Informing the executive housekeeper of special events and needs must also be done sufficiently in advance to allow him to arrange schedules.

Assisting activities staff in arranging furniture for programs and straightening the room at the conclusion of programs is a responsibility of the housekeeping staff.

Volunteers benefit all staff members by providing socialization and additional service for residents. Selective jobs such as mending patients' clothing or accompanying residents on outings may be requested of volunteers, thereby freeing staff for direct patient care concerns.

Dietary

The dietitian often depends on feedback from nursing staff regarding patient eating habits. In turn, the dietitian should be helpful in suggesting alternatives for patient dietary problems. Communication with physicians concerning patient dietary needs is another of the dietitian's responsibilities.

Food costs should be closely supervised through the combined efforts of the business manager, dietitian, and foodservice supervisor, who should keep one another informed of price fluctuations.

Housekeeping and Maintenance

Special cleaning problems, such as incontinent patients soiling carpeting or upholstery or patients hoarding food, require close supervision by both housekeeping and nursing personnel. In addition, both staffs must work together to identify and locate missing patient clothing.

The maintenance and housekeeping departments should decide who will do certain jobs—wall washing, moving furniture, minor repairs, window washing—if an outside service is not used, and how to schedule them.

Irrespective of size, the complexity of modern equipment in a skilled nursing facility necessitates communication and cooperation among all personnel to maintain maximum mechanical efficiency. The establishment of a well-understood and simplified system of written communication for maintenance work orders is the first step toward that end. Every department depends on the maintenance staff to keep its work area and specialized equipment in safe working condition; conversely, the maintenance department expects all personnel to handle equipment correctly and carefully and to report any malfunctioning promptly.

The bookkeeping staff must keep careful records of purchases made and repairs done by the maintenance department. To assist in that duty, the maintenance director must clarify invoices with the bookkeeper and allocate costs to the proper department if it is other than general building maintenance. Maintenance personnel who are authorized to make purchases should be familiar with any established procedures.

Since nursing is the only department staffing the facility at certain times, maintenance personnel must inform the nursing staff regarding who is assigned emergency coverage each night and on holidays and weekends. Also, appropriate nursing personnel must know the location of the listing of outside service agencies and emergency telephone numbers.

The maintenance staff may be asked for assistance in constructing or devising special self-help equipment for residents or in building customized items for programs, such as display racks or booths for a fair.

Records

The records coordinator must remain in close contact with the nursing, social service, and business departments regarding admissions, discharges, internal movement and financial sponsorship changes of residents in order to keep the patient index and related information about current residents up to date. Significant changes in the health status of Medicare patients must be communicated to the records coordinator, who will relay such information to the fiscal intermediary in order to determine the patient's eligibility for benefits. In turn, the records coordinator will offer certain guidelines or directives to the treating staff regarding required documentation for fiscal intermediaries or Medicaid.

The key to the records coordinator's effectiveness is good relationships with all personnel, as his position will involve dealing with all departments. Guidance from the records coordinator in the organization of files and the use and revision of forms or record-keeping books will aid in the efficient operation of all departments. For patient care departments, the records coordinator's advice and suggestions will be even more crucial as a measure to promote the continuity of care and to demonstrate the provision of quality care.

Business Office

All department heads and the personnel director will need to keep the business office up to date on the status of employees—new staff hired; personnel terminated or resigned; vacation, holiday, and sick time due; overtime to be paid; salary increments; deduction changes; and any other pertinent information. Also, department chiefs will be in frequent contact with the business manager regarding purchases planned or made, and requisitioning issues from the central storage area.

Information regarding services to patients is obtained from the social services department. Admissions, changes in the account, additional charges, and discharges must be communicated to the business office promptly. The social worker will also need to ascertain whether the responsible family member or agency will authorize payment for the bed to be held during the patient's absence, and so inform the business office.

COMMITTEES AND MEETINGS

Interdepartmental cooperation is augmented as well as exemplified by committee activity. Some committees are regularly scheduled, standing committees and others—ad hoc committees—meet according to need. A time limit should be followed and an agenda developed prior to each meeting so that the discussions remain pertinent and interesting to the participants. When a particular problem is to be addressed that requires prior consideration, appropriate material should be distributed for individual study before the meeting. Although a designated committee member may record meeting minutes, the administration remains responsible for ensuring their proper recording and maintenance.

Administrative participation in staff committees should be extensive, thereby supporting the team approach to patient care and the therapeutic community. Committees that are essentially concerned with administrative affairs should be planned and organized by the administrative director or a designee.

The administrative director should plan both a weekly meeting of department heads to discuss general and interdepartmental problems and an annual meeting of the governing body. This meeting of the governing body (and, where appropriate, members of the corporation or shareholders) may be opened to interested members of the lay and professional communities to stimulate involvement in the skilled nursing facility.

Joint Conference Committee

The joint conference committee, generally found in institutions with organized medical staffs, is an intrainstitutional committee comprising the medical director and/or member of the medical staff and representatives of the governing body, with the president of the governing body serving as committee head and the administrative director as an ex-officio member. This committee discusses matters of mutual and general interest prior to the regular governing body meeting.

Budget Committee

The budget committee should be composed of a representative or representatives from the governing body, the medical, nursing, and business departments, and the administration. Other departments may also be invited to participate, but a large committee may be unwieldy. The consulting accountant may assist in the budget process by advising the committee on anticipated trends in the economy that will affect costs and revenue. Since charges are based on costs, a market survey of rates in area facilities provides useful information prior to budget preparation.

This committee should meet sometime after the ten-month reports have been completed; on the basis of the first ten months' experience, a proposed budget should be prepared for the coming year. The participation of the various departments assures the credibility of the budget and emphasizes to those involved the importance of abiding by budgeted amounts in the operation of their services.

The completed budget should then be presented to the governing body for approval and to the personnel committee for discussion. Since personnel costs represent 50 to 60 percent of the operating costs in a skilled nursing facility, personnel increments are the single most important budgetary influence. In the case of unionized facilities, this practice will have to be worked out with the union.

Interdisciplinary Clinical Conference

The weekly interdisciplinary clinical conference serves as an educational and informational experience for all concerned staff, as well as a vehicle for the rehabilitation team to explore, plan, and coordinate effective treatment programs and to assess current patient care plans for needed revision. The meetings themselves furnish an opportunity for department heads and others to communicate the progress of each department's phase of treatment with the patient. Discharge planning for appropriate patients is discussed at this meeting. The conference is an opportunity for staff members to become familiar with the medical and psychosocial histories of newly admitted patients and to discuss the current functional status of and the treatment goals for each.

The conference should be arranged by the coordinator of social services and chaired by the medical director. Others in attendance should include the administrative director, director of nursing, social work coordinator, coordinator of activities and volunteers, rehabilitation therapists, dietitian, administrative assistant, attending physicians (when available), and head nurse of the unit to be reviewed. The interdisciplinary committee meeting is especially useful to part-time consultants because it is a succinct way for them to obtain information about patients and to interchange ideas with the staff.

In a three-unit, 100-bed facility, one unit per week should be scheduled for in-depth review, thereby leaving the fourth week of the month open. In this manner, every patient is assessed by the interdisciplinary team on a monthly basis.

Personnel Committee

The personnel committee could be regularly elected by the various constituencies and could meet on a scheduled or ad hoc basis, depending on need. Both management and staff should have the prerogative to call such meetings, and committee members should have the responsibility to report back and forth to their groups to transmit information and to seek solutions to problems. If staff members are rotated for service on this committee, two-way communication can become a reality.

Matters as diverse as the development and review of new personnel policies; wage increases; grievances of staff, administration, patients, or families; and the purchase of new types of equipment or supplies are appropriate for discussion.

The question of reimbursement for service on the personnel committee is valid and should be determined by the committee. Various methods have been used, including reimbursement for time, reimbursement for transportation expenses, or equivalent time off the job.

Patient Care Policy Committee

The patient care policy committee has responsibility to formulate, evaluate, and review policies concerning patient care. The medical director is charged with implementing those policies. Committee meetings should be held, at a minimum, annually and more often if necessary. Members of this committee are the medical director, the director of nursing, social

FIGURE 16-2
Interdisciplinary Clinical Conference

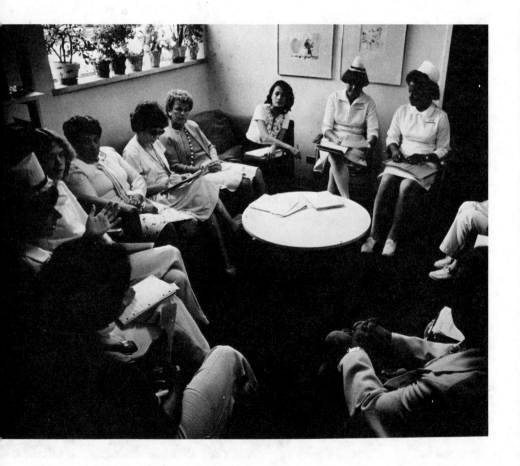

FIGURE 16-3
Personnel Committee Meeting

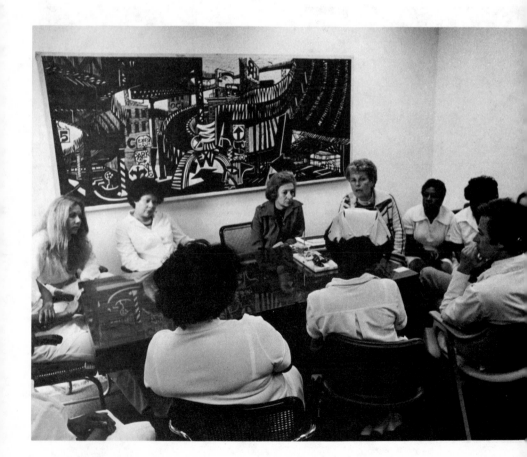

workers, and the administrative director, with other professional and paramedical disciplines serving as resource personnel. Certainly, attending physicians and others who treat patients in the skilled nursing facility should be encouraged to attend meetings to help formulate policy pertinent to their services.

Utilization Review Committee

Utilization review is a federally mandated program emphasizing cost efficiency. The utilization review committee is charged with reviewing the medical course of every patient in the skilled nursing facility to ensure that services received are consonant with skilled nursing care. Anything more or less would qualify a patient for transfer elsewhere to receive the level of care for which he is eligible. Other than the responsibility to review extended-duration cases for appropriateness of stay, the utilization review committee must conduct medical care evaluation studies to ensure the quality of care practiced in the nursing home. The results of such clinical research studies, which do not have to be performed by utilization review committee members but are merely under their supervision, may be used to improve services and programs in skilled nursing facilities.

Members of the utilization review committee in a skilled nursing facility cannot be employed by or have an interest in any nursing home. A minimum of two physicians is required; other professionals may participate as desired. The presence of a certified social worker or professional nurse is desirable for matters other than the medical determination of continued stay. Facility personnel—the medical director (if an employee), the director of nursing, social workers, the administrative director, the records coordinator, and the physical therapist—should plan to attend utilization review committee meetings as resource persons.

The utilization review committee can be organized in various ways. The preferred method would be for the committee to be appointed by the nursing home itself. In this way the nursing home can be certain that committee members have some expertise in long-term care. The only drawback to this arrangement is that it may be difficult to recruit outside interested physicians to serve on a continuing basis.

An alternative to appointing individuals to serve on the utilization review committee is to engage a group to perform the function. Such arrangements could be made with the utilization review committee of the hospital with which the nursing home maintains a transfer agreement or with a designated group such as the county medical society. As a final option, the skilled nursing facility could contract with a profit-oriented company organized to provide this service to area nursing homes.

While the existence of the utilization review committee in free-standing facilities may be terminated, its function will continue. It is problematic whether responsibility for review will be delegated to Professional Standards Review Organizations (except for hospital skilled nursing facilities) or to other outside reviewing agencies.

It is imperative that all attending physicians understand the importance of complying with all requirements for documentation of a patient's condition and treatment program on the chart, as well as the required certification and recertification for continued skilled nursing care. Proper documentation is required by the utilization review committee to make an accurate professional decision and for the fiscal intermediary to make an accurate reimbursement decision. If, in the judgment of the utilization review committee, a change in the quality of medical care is warranted, the attending physician will be notified immediately and arrangements will be made between the committee and the physician.

Either the records coordinator or the social service staff may serve as coordinators for the utilization review committee, meaning that they would plan for and notify members of meetings, work with the nursing staff to assure the completion of the appropriate forms on each patient to be reviewed, and record and maintain minutes of the meetings. Correspondence and additional reports resulting from the actions of the utilization review committee would also be the coordinator's responsibility.

Pharmacy Committee

All policies and procedures relating to prescribing, administering, and dispensing medications are developed and approved by the pharmacy committee, which meets quarterly to fulfill its obligations. Members of the pharmacy committee are the medical director, the administrative director, the director of nursing, the dispensing pharmacist, and the consultant pharmacist (if appointed).

Infection Control Committee

Infection prevention and control is a responsibility of all facility personnel; therefore representation on the infection control committee should be interdisciplinary, including all facility departments and services. Quarterly meetings of the committee are suggested to carry out its duties, and special meetings should be called if needed.

The committee is responsible for developing policies and procedures to accomplish its goal and to ensure that facility personnel observe those directives. Topics for discussion should include patient admission and retention criteria with respect to infection control, environmental controls in all departments to reduce the number of organisms present, aseptic and isolation techniques, pest control, staff in-service, staff performance, resident education, visitor regulations, employee health, and conformance with regulations regarding the external reporting of the presence of communicable and/or nosocomial infections.

Safety Committee

The organization of a safety committee is necessary to monitor the facility's safety program and to provide an interdepartmental overview of the safety problems. The safety committee is responsible for developing written policies and procedures to enhance and ensure safety inside and outside the facility, and to emphasize the former by assuring the development of specific departmental safety policies and procedures.

The administrative director should appoint a safety director, probably the assistant administrator or the director of maintenance, to chair the meetings. The medical director and representatives of the larger departments such as nursing, dietary, housekeeping, maintenance, and administration should form the safety committee. The skilled nursing facility may hire an outside contractor to supervise an aspect of its safety program, such as running the fire drills, in which case this person also would serve as a consultant to the safety committee.

The safety committee should hold quarterly meetings and circulate written decisions and recommendations to the governing body, administration, and appropriate departments and services.

Security problems such as instituting staff parking permits to prevent unauthorized persons from using the facility parking area, particularly at evening or night, may correctly come to the attention of the safety committee. The committee may also regulate the distribution of the building master key to selected personnel. Another responsibility would be to develop an emergency plan for institution during a civil disorder or union strike, which implicitly contains measures for building security.

The committee is also responsible for fire prevention and safety, augmented by routine fire drills. Other emergency plans must be formalized in writing: how to evacuate the nursing home and what steps to take in the event of an utility interruption, a civil disturbance, a natural disaster such as a flood, extreme weather conditions if they are common in the area, a bomb threat, or a missing patient.

Without question, the safety committee must be completely familiar with applicable local, state, and federal safety regulations and should obtain copies of all relevant codes. The committee should be aware of safety organizations and should request appropriate literature from them for use in the in-service program and as library references and bulletin board display material.

The committee should direct a periodic hazard surveillance program and a review of the quality and usefulness of the entire safety program. The organization and implementation of a system of reporting, investigating, evaluating, documenting, and reviewing all incidents and actions taken is a charge of the committee. Finally, the safety committee should provide the content of the material for the orientation and in-service education of staff members, volunteers, and residents.

Intradepartmental Meetings

In addition to interdepartmental committees, intradepartmental meetings should be held when necessary, but at least annually. Reviewing and revising the department's policy and procedure manual should be one activity of such meetings, along with discussion of staffing patterns, equipment needs, and educational issues.

SUMMARY

Whether it is called an organization, committee, group, task force, or team, it is critical that the concern of the team always remain relevant to the residents' needs. The concerted action of the organization or team helps promote the triad of patient, family, and staff in the development of the therapeutic community.

NOTES

1. E. J. Durnall, "A Team Approach to Restorative Care," *First North American Symposium on Long Term Care Proceedings* (Washington, D.C.: American College of Nursing Home Administrators, 1975), 112.

GENERAL REFERENCES

Kramer, C., and J. Kramer. *Basic Principles of Long-Term Patient Care.* Springfield, Ill.: Charles C. Thomas, 1976.

Education and Research

INTRODUCTION

Education and research should play a prominent role in the operation of a skilled nursing facility and the services provided by every department. The nursing home is a therapeutic milieu—a total environment—with structural and human qualities that are subject to improvement when a need for change has been established.

The nursing home is committed to the pursuit and provision of educational programs for numerous reasons. Orientation and staff development are mandated and, in fact, should be offered to all personnel. Because it is part of the health service network in the community, the public should be informed of the skilled nursing facility's purpose and limitations. Students in the medical, nursing, and allied health professions should have an opportunity to augment their professional training with exposure to long-term care. And, finally, the desire to investigate, to change, and ultimately to improve itself is a necessary concomitant to any progressive and vital organization.

Education is not the answer to every problem. Before determining the appropriateness of educational programs to remedy a situation, an assessment must be made to identify the problem and to determine who or what affects or is affected by it. For example, the finest education program cannot change a six-foot corridor into an eight-foot corridor.

Education cannot correct staff shortages, but it can make working in the nursing home a more satisfying experience and, in that way, assist in recruiting and keeping staff. And as personnel grow and develop, the ambience of the whole facility becomes more positive and optimistic. Thus education is bound to affect the quality of patient care as members of the treating staff become more knowledgeable, skillful, and intellectually curious.

In general, continuing education can improve manpower utilization and personnel relations and encourage career development. Training can reduce accidents and carelessness and, it is hoped, costs while improving services.

EDUCATION FOR PROFESSIONALS

Professional staff members can no longer feel secure because of past educational attainment, for the quest for new knowledge quickly makes former learning obsolete. Indeed, the higher the level of educational achievement, the more quickly obsolescence occurs, so that professionals are more threatened by change than most less educated workers. Continuing education is currently required for relicensure of nursing home administrators in many states, and it is beginning to be expected for nurses, pharmacists, and physicians; more professionals may be affected in the future. In some instances, professional associations are mandating continuing education in order to maintain membership in their organizations.

In the past, continuing education was considered an individual responsibility, but today it is the responsibility of the institution to make certain that continuous learning takes place among the leadership staff. Thus the skilled nursing facility educational program must aggressively encourage professional staff to maintain their expertise by increasing their knowledge base.

ADMINISTRATIVE SUPPORT

A comprehensive educational program must have the support and involvement of the governing body and administration to be successful. The administrator must allocate staff time, authorize funds, and make available proper physical and technical amenities. Liberal staffing patterns enable personnel to be free to participate in educational programs.

The administration can also encourage active staff involvement in educational endeavors within and outside the facility. The administrator must acknowledge that education is really a management tool. Although education is costly in terms of time away from the job, eventually it will help staff members perform more effectively and thus save time.

STAFFING PATTERN

Someone must be designated to coordinate the educational programs. A 100-bed institution can easily use the services of a full-time director of education, who is responsible for planning, organizing, implementing, documenting, and evaluating programs conducted in the facility. Achieving this will require both a continuing assessment of the needs of workers, residents, families, and volunteers, and coordination with department heads. The director of education must recruit faculty from inside and outside the facility and tactfully explore with them the most effective methods for teaching their subject matter to adults with various levels of education and experience. The responsibility of supervising field trips to the nursing home made by visiting groups is within the parameters of the director of education's job.

Outside educational activities are also a responsibility of the director of education. He should remain informed of continuing education classes offered by educational or health institutions or professional organizations within the area and encourage attendance by nursing home staff when appropriate. In addition, he should coordinate plans for seminars or symposia cosponsored by the nursing home and local health or welfare agencies.

The development and supervision of the nursing home's professional reference library is also assigned to the director of education. He should review new instructional equipment and material for its potential usefulness in the long-term-care teaching program. The selection of and subscription to professional journals and periodicals and the purchase of books to enhance the scope of the library are facets of library management.

Because much of the educational activity is clinically oriented and directed to treatment personnel, a registered professional nurse is usually selected for this position. A baccalaureate degree is recommended, and clinical exposure to the problems of the ill aged in nursing homes is mandatory. As this is a key position in the progressive improvement of the nursing home, the director of education should demonstrate the creativity and imagination needed to initiate new programs and to stimulate the staff in furthering their own professional potential. He must have leadership qualities, an aptitude for teaching, an understanding of human relations, and the ability to function as a positive and democratic change agent.

PROGRAMS FOR STAFF WITHIN THE FACILITY

Training programs in the skilled nursing facility face some very real challenges. Staff members come from various educational, ethnic, and cultural backgrounds. Some may experience difficulty in reading and writing due to limited education or to language barriers. Reaching personnel on all shifts, developing a sense of pride in such diverse jobs as portering and dishwashing, and making learning interesting for school dropouts are challenges to the nursing home educational program.

Education for adults poses some special constraints and conditions over and above those found in general education. Adult education in the skilled nursing facility is designed to effect changes in the knowledge system of the students as well as in what they understand and feel.

Adults will learn better and will put forth more effort when they derive inner satisfaction from what they are learning. For best results, the educational program should be problem oriented rather than theoretical, and it should center around the experience of the participants.

Developing a Curriculum

The curricula of in-house educational programs should not be merely a routine listing of items required by regulatory agencies—such as patients' rights, safety, infection control, and emergency procedures—and lectures by department heads. Rather, it should be based on the needs of the staff and volunteers at particular times and related to the nature of the resident population and their families. Study topics may be suggested by medical care evaluation studies, departmental analysis, and observation of employee performance, or by conversations with residents, families, staff, volunteers, and physicians.

Once problem areas have been identified, the education director should attempt to develop programs to meet those needs. Education objectives or desired outcomes, which are characterized as being behavior or performance oriented, must be constructed at the outset of the educational planning. Objectives give focus to each program and help determine its success. Objectives should be attainable via acceptable stated performance levels, although constraints for performance are also noted. Behavioral objectives should be measurable and achievable within a prescribed period.

Certain in-service subject areas may be appropriate for interdepartmental education sessions, while others may be specialized for particular services. Training in reality orientation, grief therapy, behavior modification, and remotivation is particularly appropriate for treating staff, including nursing, social service, activities, and physical and occupational therapy personnel. Other more technical subjects such as bowel and bladder training may relate specifically to nursing tasks, but in fact they need to be explained to activities and rehabilitation personnel to assure their cooperation. On the other hand, giving enemas is clearly appropriate only for nursing and possibly the medical staff.

Personnel should be given exposure to the various services provided to patients and families. Consultants such as the dentist and speech pathologist and audiologist can encourage an interest in their fields and thereby improve patient care and assure better communication between staff and residents.

Sensitizing Staff

For the skilled nursing facility to become a humanistic, people-centered organization, all staff—treating and nontreating, technical and nontechnical, professional and nonprofessional—should be sensitized to the processes of aging. Caretakers must learn that older people suffer from multiple losses—loss of home, spouse, health, role, income, and sensory abilities. If staff members and volunteers understand aging, a positive attitude may be generated on the part of those dealing with patients.

There are many ways to demonstrate to personnel how patients feel when staff members tower over their beds or wheelchairs, when they struggle to open doors or to dress themselves, and so on. Perhaps the most unforgettable experience results from role playing, in which staff members assume the roles of patients presented with a variety of disabilities and/or sensory losses. For example, to illustrate visual changes that may plague the ill aged, staff members may be asked to wear goggles adapted with dark strips or spots. Similarly, wearing ear plugs may illustrate deafness. Tactile loss caused by arthritis can be demonstrated by having employees tie shoelaces while wearing gloves. They can learn about taste and smell changes by attempting to distinguish, while blindfolded, between whole wheat and rye bread in the presence of another strong odor. Loss of balance can be shown by having them carry several packages while using a walker to ambulate.

Visual difficulties experienced by patients can be ameliorated by uncluttering spaces, such as by removing unnecessary items on bulletin boards to emphasize important notices, or by using color coding. For persons with hearing disabilities, in-service training could alert staff to the use of gestures and objects to reinforce speaking.

It is more than twice as difficult for blind and deaf persons to function than it is for those who are blind *or* deaf. In-service training must help staff members deal with residents who have lost sensory acuity in several dimensions by impressing on them the value of using touch and the need for infinite patience.

Program Components

The components of in-service are orientation, skill training, staff development, and leadership development. Orientation is routinely offered to new staff to reinforce the facility's purpose and practices, with certain topics explored among all personnel irrespective of their training and service affiliation in the facility. It is directed to the facility's goals, philosophy, organization, and history, and a detailed description of the patient population. A tour of the building—including a discussion of the efficacious use of the equipment and structure in the interest of patient care—is part of the orientation process. Every employee should have the benefit of a review of the personnel policies, and instruction in safety and emergency procedures, infection control, and the principles of patients' rights. Communication skills needed to relate to residents, fami-

FIGURE 17-1
Sensitizing Staff to Patient Disability

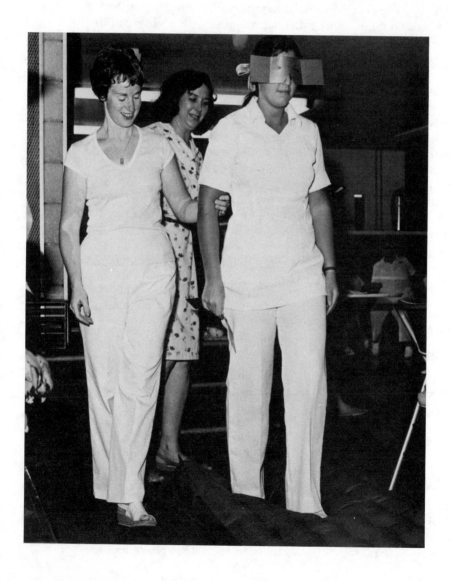

lies, other personnel, and visitors should be explored and reinforced. A department head should orient each new employee to the particular department or service and conduct in-depth discussion of the job description and related expectations.

Staff development is a systematic, continuing process of providing job-related learning experiences for all personnel responsible for direct and indirect services to residents. Increased proficiency in the performance of all levels of staff will improve patient services. Such education encompasses formal and informal exchanges of information and a continuing evaluation of the results of these activities.

Skill training relates to sharpening competencies that impinge on the needs of residents: nursing care, rehabilitation services, activities of daily living, and so forth. Staff members must be initially trained and then periodically reinforced in the proper technique of carrying out certain procedures. The need for a review may be precipitated by a supervisor's or department head's observation of an incorrectly implemented technique or by the admission of a patient who has a special requirement related to the procedure. As with any training program, the purpose for the procedure should be thoroughly explained to the students, thereby enhancing their desire to maintain a high level of performance.

Leadership and management development are reserved for those particularly talented personnel who demonstrate potential for assuming positions of responsibility and authority, or for those currently in such posts who need reinforcement in these areas. Most have had specific professional training without instruction in the skills needed to lead, to plan, to organize, to implement, and to communicate. Thus technically able bedside nurses and engineers still need guidance in the area of human skills—in the art of getting the job done through other people.

Teaching Methodologies

Training is available in a variety of forms. Adults can teach themselves by reading books, periodicals, and journals in the facility library or other health care library. They can learn through programmed instruction; by listening to lectures from experts; by observing demonstrations and asking questions; through discussions; by attending symposia, workshops, and seminars; by participating in role playing and simulation games; through buzz sessions; and even by going on structured field trips, or attending formal courses, conventions, or institutes. Diversification in the nursing home educational program can be achieved by the use of different methodologies, certain of which will be more effective with some groups than with others.

For the benefit of personnel with limited educational backgrounds, a basic word list for reading levels one through eight may be used as a guide for simple and clear written materials. It can be anticipated that many nursing attendants and housekeeping and dietary aides may function between the second and sixth adult basic education reading levels.

Health professional continuing education often follows the model of preprofessional schooling, which is not necessarily the most effective way of disseminating knowledge to adults. Actually, any method that can be described as a systematic learning activity meets the definition of continuing education. While didactic lectures have some value, guided demonstrations affording first-hand experience and conferences are thought to be the most fruitful methodologies for teaching health professionals. In a lecture, nothing is required of the individual but physical presence, while lack of participation is quite obvious in a conference. Sometimes the least informed feel uncomfortable about participating in case conferences and may be reluctant to attend such sessions, making a combination of straight lectures and conferences a good mix.

Regularly scheduled clinical rounds led by the medical director introduce the interdisciplinary staff (including the administration) to the physical, social, and emotional problems and needs of the skilled nursing facility patient. Rounds may be as informal and unstructured as walking from room to room and randomly seeing patients. Such walking rounds have the advantage of being spontaneous and generating a certain amount of intellectual excitement. Alternatively, recently admitted residents or residents with newly apparent problems may be selected for presentation to the group in a central area. These "grand rounds" are preplanned, since preparation time is needed to add to the comprehensiveness of the experience for participating staff.

While much expertise is available within the facility, it can be particularly stimulating to staff members to invite authorities in gerontology and long-term-care to participate in an all-day conference at the facility, where the experts interview patients and families to afford a new perspective for the nursing home staff. Discussions between the staff and the guests can suggest new areas of exploration for improved patient care or alternatives to present procedures. Suggestions from an objective unrelated professional may be more favorably received than in-house ideas and thus may facilitate changes in the program.

Interdisciplinary meetings illustrate another form of education, in which the professional team reviews patients in each unit monthly to determine changes that need to be made in their care plans. At these meetings, the patient care plan is generally used as the focal point for the discussion, although in some instances the patient may be asked to attend the meeting.

FIGURE 17-2
Walking Rounds

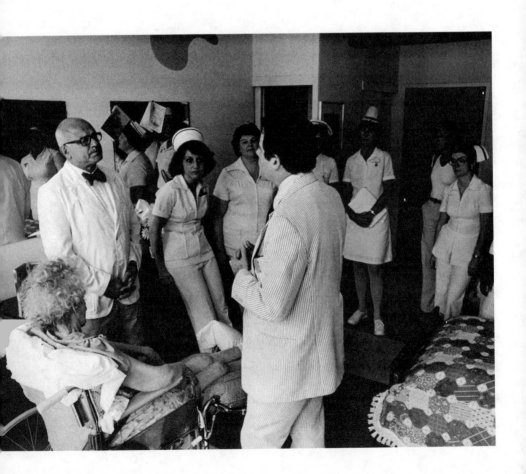

FIGURE 17-3
Grand Rounds

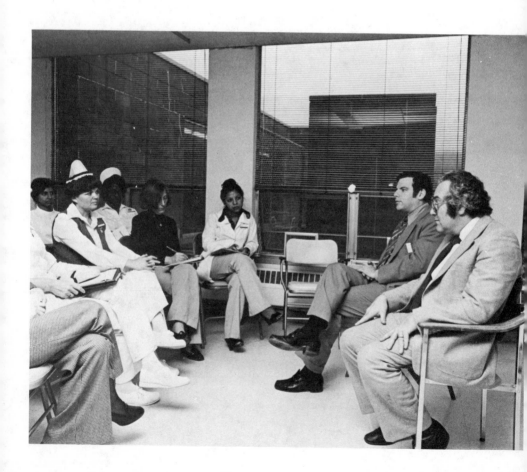

Simulation methods of instruction, particularly with experienced adult groups, are becoming an important way to reach supervisory-level personnel. Simulation methods include management games during which participants make decisions for the nursing home, or in-basket exercises, which are really a combination of a case study and role playing.

An in-basket exercise requires the participant to select a management role and prepare letters, memos, and other written communications normally received by supervisory personnel. The participant must review and organize the materials into a logical whole within a prescribed period, prior to taking action. Thus in-basket exercises illustrate how actions in one department affect others and demonstrate the importance of interdepartmental cooperation.

Many other teaching methods can be used for orientation and in-service education. Filmstrips accompanied by pertinent discussion can be useful in explaining procedures and tasks. Many facilities have learned the value of producing their own video tapes for use in educational programs. The visual portrayal of pertinent material about families, patients, and the surroundings makes video tape a particularly useful training tool.

If the nursing home does not own equipment for video taping, the use of a tape deck to record interdisciplinary meetings and clinical rounds would be worthwhile. Naturally, these tapes may be replayed for the benefit of evening and night personnel, which will help improve communication among shifts. It is important to have an informed discussion leader present at these sessions to relate the films and tapes to the residents' specific needs.

Bulletin boards can be another aid to education in the nursing home. Posters, photographs, and other visual display material can be presented and thus integrated with the formal educational program for residents, staff, visitors, and volunteers.

PROGRAMS FOR STAFF OUTSIDE THE FACILITY

Even the best nursing home with superior educational programs cannot completely rely on inside educational endeavors. It is stimulating for staff to attend meetings, seminars, and courses outside the facility to broaden their perspective or simply to help them appreciate the quality of their own institutional training.

The administration should encourage staff participation on committees and boards of other health, educational, or service organizations. In this way, they will be furthering their own education and that of other community representatives. Upon receipt of notices for educational programs, the director of education should determine whether the program would benefit any personnel. If it might, he should then review the decision with the administrative director, the department head, and the personnel selected. Staff members may also initiate a request when the program announcement comes directly to their attention.

When it is determined that staff will attend an outside educational program, it is suggested that two persons be selected to participate, if possible. When two attend the same course, there is a better chance for feedback and change in the nursing home program, as one individual will reinforce the other. Everyone who attends outside events should be asked to submit a written report of the experience or to report to a particular staff meeting to share his experiences.

Institutional policies should be formulated regarding outside professional affiliations and programs for key staff. Membership in one professional organization, and permission and funding to attend a certain number of educational events per annum should depend on job category and length of service.

Some organizations plan annual retreats for management staff and department heads so that they can study in an environment more conducive to learning. The leadership of such retreats may be rotated among the key staff, or an outside educational consultant may be invited to conduct this self-appraisal and yearly renewal.

In some instances, correspondence courses can meet a particular need for special information, for example, courses designed for medical records technicians or for housekeepers, for whom no substantive training can be provided in the nursing home. Obviously, only individuals who have a high degree of motivation should be encouraged to pursue correspondence courses, although recognition upon completion of the program may help maintain their motivation.

EVALUATION

Since improved patient care is the major goal of all skilled nursing facility education programs, it is important to evaluate the usefulness of each program. Clearly, conceptualized objectives are needed to provide criteria in order to measure results, and the specific programs must be limited to the stated objectives.

Most evaluations are subjective and are in the form of a questionnaire or a rating scale distributed after the program. Personal interviews before and after sessions may be helpful in eliciting frank comments about the quality of the presentation.

Objective evaluations usually use a pretest and a post-test. While this method measures the acquisition of information, it does not measure change in practice. And new knowledge without changed performance does not benefit patient care.

RECORDS

Careful documentation must be maintained of the orientation and in-service programs provided to staff, for regulatory agencies require such information. Also, as an indication of the employee's progress in job development, it can be useful in assessing an individual's growth or in supporting disciplinary actions.

With the help of the department heads, the director of education should develop an orientation plan with accompanying checklists for each department, which would include the general information provided to new employees and information specific to the positions that they are assuming (see Exhibit 17-1). The use of a checklist assures that all aspects of the plan have been reviewed and simplifies the process of recording the completion of each step. When orientation has been completed, the forms can be placed in the employee's file as a permanent record.

The schedule for in-service should be available in a planned, organized fashion, such as on a master calendar. In this manner, program topics, the involved personnel (both leader and students), and the date and time can be seen readily. Medical rounds, seminars, and guest symposia should also be marked on the calendar. The director of education may or may not elect to place programs conducted by department heads or consultants for their personnel alone on the master calendar, but he must have a record of them.

In conjunction with the listings on the master calendar, a more complete description of each program planned—including its objectives, content, methodology, and method of evaluation—should be formulated. Such a course curriculum or lesson plan may be kept on file for future use. Exhibit 17-2 is an example.

Each in-service program conducted, regardless of by whom, for whom, or when, must be properly recorded. The use of a form to complement the program description form would accomplish this by noting the attendance, evaluation results, and any interesting comments or suggestions for improvement.

Finally, a record for each employee must be kept indicating attendance at in-service programs and at outside continuing education programs. To assure documentation at all sessions, a loose-leaf notebook containing a sheet for each employee should be brought to every program for all attendees to sign. Completed sheets may then be placed in the employee's file.

EXHIBIT 17-1
Nurses' Orientation Checklist

NURSES' ORIENTATION CHECKLIST

Name _____ Date employed _____

R.N. _____ L.P.N. _____ Shift _____ Position _____

First Day A.M.	Method	Instructor	Evaluation
Philosophy of long-term care			
Organizational chart			
Administrative policies			
Personnel policies			
Job description			
Department scheduling			
First Day P.M.			
Tour and introduction to staff and patients			
Emergency alarms			
Telephones			
Nurses' call system			
Nurse-family relations			
Nursing policy and procedures manual			
Second Day A.M.			
Special patient services			
Special equipment			
Familiarization with meal serving			
Second Day P.M.			
Admission and discharge procedure			
Physicians' order book and sheets			
Transcribing orders			
Kardexes			
Daily ward report			
Third Day A.M.			
Narcotics records and inventory			
Stop-order book			
Ordering medications			
Observe med. dispensation and administration			
Organization of chart material			
Third Day P.M.			
Nurses' notes			
Clysis			
Nasogastric tube feeding			
Foley catheter (male)			
Foley catheter (female)			
Bladder irrigation			
Restraints			
Decubitus prevention and care			
Fourth Day A.M.			
Rounds on assigned unit			
Med. dispensation and administration			
Fourth Day P.M.			
Study of patients' charts			
Study of care plans and Kardexes			
Participation in narcotic inventory			
Participation in shift change			
Fifth Day A.M.			
How, when, and what to report to physicians			
Specific shift responsibilities			
Fifth Day P.M.			
Review and overall evaluation			

Please use reverse side for comments

Employee _____ Dir. of Education _____ Date _____

EXHIBIT 17-2
Lesson Plan Number Two: Temperature-Pulse-
Respiration

```
            Lesson Plan No. Two:  TEMPERATURE-PULSE-RESPIRATION

Date:  October 23 and 30, 1979       Instructor(s):  Director of Education
                                                     Shift supervisors

Time:   1:30-2:30 P.M               Students:        All nursing aides and
        8:30-9:30 P.M.                               orderlies
       12:00-1:00 A.M.

Purpose:        1.  To describe the circulatory and respiratory systems.
                2.  To teach aides to take temperature, pulse, and respirations.

Objectives:     The aides will be able to:

                1.  State the primary function of the circulatory system.
                2.  Identify the main organs of the circulatory system.
                3.  State the primary function of the respiratory system.
                4.  Identify the main organs of the respiratory system.
                5.  Read a thermometer (both glass and electronic) accurately.
                6.  Take oral, rectal, and axillary temperatures.
                7.  Locate and count radial pulses.
                8.  Count respirations.
                9.  List reasons for the necessity of accurate measurements.
               10.  Recognize and report variations from the normal.
               11.  Handle and care for both types of thermometers.
               12.  Record results accurately.

Materials:      1.  Diagram of circulatory and respiratory systems.
                2.  Filmstrip and projector.
                3.  Electronic and glass thermometers.
                4.  Watch with second hand.
                5.  TPR book or blank Kardex.
                6.  Pencils and copies of quiz.

Methods and     1.  Exhibit and explain diagrams of circulatory and respiratory
Activities:         systems.
                2.  Discuss importance of temperature-pulse-respiration (TPR).
                3.  Show filmstrip
                4.  Aides practice reading thermometers.
                5.  Aides practice taking temperatures with both types of
                    equipment.
                6.  Aides practice locating and taking pulse.
                7.  Aides practice counting respirations.

Summary:        1.  What information does the TPR measurement give?
                2.  Why is it important to be certain of the readings obtained?
                3.  How does this information help the patient?  the doctor?

Evaluation:     1.  Return demonstration performing the TPR as one procedure.
                2.  Completion of quiz.

Follow-up       1.  Observation of aides while performing TPR on patients.
Evaluation:     2.  Review records of TPR.
                3.  Request charge nurse to notify the Director of Education of
                    those aides whose performance is poor in taking TPR.
                4.  Make notation of each aide's performance in record book by
                    November 7.

References:     1.  Aides' Manual, pp. 103-104, 110-111, 113-115.
                2.  Filmstrip "Basic Care of the Long Term Patient" by Trinex Corp.
                3.  C.M. Jarvis, "Vital Signs," Nursing '76, April 1, 1976,
                    pp. 31-36.
```

Maintaining all this material in one area under the director of education's supervision will provide comprehensive files and simplify their retrieval.

PROGRAMS FOR FAMILIES

Families informally begin their education experience with their first visit to the nursing home, when they discuss the possible admission of their relative with the social worker. Naturally, all new families should receive descriptive material outlining the organization and programs of the nursing home and patients' rights, and they should become familiar with the nursing home's practices as put forth in the continuing care contract.

Orienting families to the facility's organization and programs is not nearly as challenging as helping families deal with their feelings about placing a relative in an institution. Each family member may experience unfamiliar emotions in struggling with the reality of decision making in behalf of, for example, a recently widowed, severely confused relative.

Families of newly admitted patients should be invited to attend a series of small-group orientation sessions. To accommodate working members, Saturday or evening sessions are preferable. Led by a social worker skilled in group dynamics, with special staff invited to attend specific meetings or portions thereof, the subjects discussed might range from basic facts about life in the nursing home to the feelings family members are experiencing after their relative's admission.

The benefits of the group sessions are practical and therapeutic—practical because orienting families by group saves time, and therapeutic because family members often can work out their problems together on a feeling level.

At periodic intervals during the residence of their friend or relative, families and/or sponsors should be requested to meet with several members of the interdisciplinary team to review and assess the resident's progress. It is essential that the family, the staff, and the patient (if he is aware) share the same view of the patient's abilities and disabilities and prognosis.

At subsequent intervals, requested by the family member or by the nursing home, information should be shared and plans formulated with respect to discharge, continued stay in the same unit, or transfer to a different unit. At such assessment sessions, it is desirable for family members, the resident, the medical director, the director of nursing, the social work consultant, and other specialized staff who have had specific involvement with the patient to be present.

When family members really become involved at the nursing home, such as through volunteering, they benefit from a unique form of education. They have the opportunity to participate in the daily happenings of the nursing home and to observe the staff's commitment to care for chronically ill, disabled, and dependent persons. Such an experience may help family members be more understanding, have more patience, and develop respect for nursing home personnel.

PROGRAMS FOR VOLUNTEERS

Board members of voluntary agencies clearly represent volunteering at a professional level. Board members are selected for their particular expertise in such areas as finance, construction, marketing, law, and so on, but they often have limited or no knowledge about long-term-care institutions. Trustees have a time problem, so education programs will have to be planned to dovetail with their schedules.

The format for the board orientation and continuing education programs may vary. Sometimes new members can be oriented at a special meeting immediately prior to the regular board meeting held by the director of education, by the director of volunteers, or by a designated well-informed board member.

The first subjects for discussion with new board members are the nursing home's philosophy, mission, and short- and long-term goals, followed by an orientation session devoted to the nature of the patient population, the program, and the staff needed to effect the nursing home program, and concluded by an in-depth tour of the facility. Orientation may be augmented by a review of the bylaws; charter; table of organization; handbooks for patients, families, and personnel; a recent annual report; copies of minutes of the previous year; medical staff bylaws (if appropriate); and reprints of staff articles.

As an ongoing effort, continuing education may be provided to the board by allocating time at specified meetings for department heads or professional staff to describe the activities under their jurisdiction. Board members should also be on the invitation list to appropriate in-service programs and should receive copies of the facility newsletter and reprints of currently published staff articles.

Individual volunteers need to know much of the same general information but require less material related to planning and finance than do board members. The pattern of simultaneous orientation for several new volunteers rather than separate instruction for each is more effective, as group experiences encourage discussion. In some facilities, adult and junior volunteers have separate orientation classes but attend joint in-service programs. This is a highly individualistic decision and depends on the people concerned.

In-service is particularly important for volunteers, as their resident and staff contacts will precipitate inquiries about medical, psychological, and familial problems. At appropriate times during the year, formal in-service may be planned, in which professional staff give patient presentations and didactic talks, and other key staff members may participate. Health career goals for young people and for more mature volunteers is a natural outgrowth when the clinical and educational experience is successful.

People who volunteer at the nursing home regularly have numerous structured and unstructured educational opportunities. However, most long-term-care facilities are blessed with groups of volunteers who visit on a one-time basis or at irregular intervals, sometimes merely at Christmas to sing carols or monthly to conduct birthday parties for residents. Such groups have the fewest opportunities to become familiar with the facility's patients, programs, and staff, but they do need some special educational preparation prior to their volunteer activity. A brief orientation is mandatory before the appointed time of the activity; it should include a frank discussion of the nature of the resident population so that the volunteers will not be disappointed or offended if some residents appear disinterested during their presentation.

PROGRAMS FOR STUDENTS

The nursing home is a repository of information about the chronically ill elderly, providing an exposure for students in medicine, nursing, administration, and the allied health professions. Such exposure may be short term or long term for individuals or groups of students. Brief experiences should be avoided, as the impact of the chronically ill aged may be too great to be absorbed in a short period.

Groups of students may visit the nursing home for a day, for several days, or for an academic term of clinical experience. Even day-long field trips to the nursing home should be more than an examination of the architecture. When possible, case presentations by the interdisciplinary staff are a good introduction to the nursing home's patients and personnel.

Depending on the purpose of the visit, other appropriate staff members should assist the director of education to plan the program. Certain guidelines for visitors should be followed to assure some uniformity of training.

The nursing home may be approached by a nursing school with a request for an entire class to spend four to six months in clinical training. When collaborating with other institutions in education projects, the nursing home must continue to have complete control over patient care.

The program's educational goals should relate to the needs of the nursing home as well as to the needs of the nursing school. The curriculum should have the approval of both organizations and should be designed to ensure the acquisition of the competencies needed by nurses in long-term-care settings.

Other elements to be considered are the ratio of students to instructors, the number of students to be assigned to a particular unit, the facilities to be used by students, the level of performance expected of the students, and the training of the instructor in the clinical aspects of nursing in a long-term-care setting. Such instructors should be thoroughly oriented to the nursing home patient and program before they begin to supervise. If the instructor is not sympathetic to the needs of the institutionalized aged, the entire experience will be unfavorably colored for the students.

The small number of personnel truly interested in working with the ill aged underscores the importance of training and educating. Therefore skilled nursing facilities that possess the capability have a special obligation to serve as training sites for medical, nursing, and social work students. Students in physical, occupational, and speech therapy and therapeutic recreation should also be encouraged to utilize the skilled nursing facility as a placement during their academic program. Individual graduate or undergraduate students placed in the nursing home for a practicum or residency may spend as little as a month or as long as a year.

Field placements are an opportunity to influence preprofessionals during their formative period. Even if they do not remain in the long-term-care field, residency experiences may develop a lasting concern for the problems of the institutionalized ill aged. Probably the most important lesson to be learned during field placement is the need for the team approach in working with the ill aged and their families.

Administrative residents who will be working in the acute or long-term-care field also can benefit from the wide variety of experience available in the skilled nursing facility. Indeed, future hospital administrators would have a much clearer understanding of the meaning of continuity of care following a nursing home residency.

In all instances, before individual students are accepted for residencies, an in-depth interview and an exposure to the nursing home patient population are essential. When field placements at the nursing home are considered, it is imperative that sufficient staff time be available for thorough supervision and guidance.

Unless the student has had previous practical experience, the first several months will be primarily a learning period. Only in the second part of his residency will the trainee be able to carry out responsible tasks. Because of the time input involved with residents, their value as working staff members is hard to measure. While students add a certain positive quality to the nursing home program, there is an associated cost.

PROGRAMS FOR THE COMMUNITY

The nursing home is a particularly valuable health teaching resource because the patients remain there long enough to be observed and studied. Professionals such as nurses, social workers, clergy, and physicians working in other settings can benefit from clinical demonstrations, interdisciplinary case presentations, and homogeneous or heterogeneous symposia conducted by the skilled nursing facility staff. Particularly enlightening for participants is exposure to families and their problems.

With the increasing emphasis on shared services among health care agencies, it is surprising that more effort has not been expended in sharing educational opportunities. There is general agreement on the cost savings implicit in sharing highly technical expensive machinery, but educational programs for nurses proliferate in the hospital, in the skilled nursing facility, and in the visiting nurse service, at great cost to all parties.

To maximize the continuity of care and to eliminate duplication of effort, joint educational endeavors should be developed to permit each agency to explore areas of greatest familiarity; appropriate staff from all facilities would be invited. Thus, for example, nurses in all settings would become familiar with the care of the intellectually impaired ill elderly. And greater understanding would tend to improve the care of confused nursing home patients when they are transferred to the general hospital for surgery.

Key facility staff have an obligation and should be encouraged to disseminate specialized information concerning nursing home patients and their families outside the facility via papers, lectures, and panel discussions. Speaking engagements should be accepted with the understanding that the speech or discussion notes should be written out in advance to make certain that the presentation is studied and thoughtful. The speech or talk need not be read, but it must be carefully planned in a professional and scholarly manner to do credit to the speaker and to the institution he represents. The submission of such presentations or papers for publication should be explored with the approval of the department head or the administrator.

The lay community needs to have first-hand contact with the concerns and needs of long-term-care patients, for too often consumers are well meaning but poorly informed about nursing homes and their patients. Clearly it is a responsibility of the nursing home to educate the general public by drawing them into the nursing home and by encouraging staff to carry their message into the community. Invitations should be extended to civic and cultural organizations to visit the nursing home to learn more about its services, or to use the facility's community rooms for meetings, conferences, or special events.

Volunteering in the nursing home is the most direct and successful form of education that can be offered to the lay community. Volunteers gain first-hand knowledge of life in the nursing home. When such an experience is complemented by a thorough educational program for volunteers, they too become ambassadors for the facility and spread its message among friends. The director of volunteers, then, has a large role to play in communicating to the lay community and must be active in contacting schools, churches, businesses, and other organizations to educate, and incidentally to recruit volunteers.

BUDGETING FOR EDUCATIONAL PROGRAMS

The director of education formulates an overall budget for education, keeping in mind that the costs applicable specifically to certain departmental personnel must be included in that department's budget as an expense. The director of education, the department heads, and the administrative director should carefully review the departmental budgets for education so that each is reasonable, comprehensive, and conforms to the institution's educational policies.

A major item will be the salary of the director of education. Other education departmental expenses will include the purchase or rental of audiovisual equipment and supplies, honoraria and travel expenses for visiting experts, and promotion and arrangement costs of sponsoring programs open to the community. Other factors that need to be considered when budgeting for educational programs are subscriptions to professional journals, staff memberships in professional organizations, and the purchase of books and training manuals. When off-duty staff are requested to attend programs, they should be reimbursed for transportation and provided wages for their time. Another expense occurs when replacement staff are needed for personnel who attend educational programs during their normal working hours. Finally, the budget must include the cost of attendance at outside programs plus incidentals such as meals, lodging, and transportation.

In an effort to encourage career development, the facility may appoint or elect a scholarship committee whose function would be selecting a predetermined number of staff members from different categories for scholarship aid to further their health career status. In some instances, aid could be tuition and books, while for heads of household it might also include stipends for living expenses.

The nursing home will have to determine its policy regarding stipends for residents and students. There are advantages and disadvantages in offering stipends or work-study programs to students. Some institutions with willing and highly qualified professional staff may not have funds available for such educational activities, so the training experiences they could provide would be denied to potential students.

In many instances, however, students in training who seek placement in long-term-care institutions tend to be mature individuals with familial responsibilities. They may need some financial support and may be able to offer more to the agency than the inexperienced graduate student fresh out of college, and thus merit a stipend or modest salary. In some cases, the nursing home may assist an individual who shows aptitude in a particular area to seek professional training, with the understanding that he will work in the nursing home for a certain period once he has completed schooling.

REFERENCE MATERIAL

To encourage and facilitate educational endeavors on all levels, an in-house library under the director of education's direction is a valuable resource. Reference material must be easily accessible to foster its use by all staff.

The director of education and all department heads should be encouraged to select a list of appropriate periodicals and journals to which the nursing home should subscribe. At the end of the year—or less often, depending on the frequency of the publication—issues should be bound for permanent retention in the library. Likewise, books and audiovisual materials should be purchased regularly to provide a broad-based library. A special information file of articles and reprints topically filed for easy reference should be assembled on a continuing basis.

Besides material directed to the specific disciplines of nursing, nutrition, activities, social work, and so forth, an assortment of books and magazines concerned with gerontology, geriatrics, and long-term care should form the nucleus of a skilled nursing facility's reference library. Pertinent government publications concerned with such subjects as Medicare, Medicaid, Occupational Safety and Health Administration, and Equal Employment Opportunity should also be included.

One of the benefits of membership in a professional association—either group or individual membership—is the use of its library resources. Copies of pertinent reprints in the organization's files are usually forwarded upon request.

Another advantage of membership in such organizations is that their newsletters and journals will contain notices, and possibly reviews, of recently published studies or texts. Thus the director of education, administrative director, or department head can remain informed about the latest information available and can assess its value for inclusion in the facility library.

RESEARCH

For any organization to remain viable, growing, and productive, it must always look to what it is doing and how it could do it better. This is especially true in the case of the skilled nursing facility, where the clinical course of the patient must be examined with respect to his physical, social, and emotional status. A knowledge and understanding of family reaction and adaptation to the institutionalization of an elderly relative is critical to the patient's achievement of rehabilitation potential. The nursing home must survey its role in the health care community, how it can improve within that context, and what the community—professional and lay—can do to help it accomplish its objectives. The nursing home must conduct a concentrated examination of services, the building and equipment, and staff on a personal and professional level in order to be aware of the problems and needs in providing care. Most importantly, research can often point the way to needed change.

When residents, staff, families, or volunteers participate in research studies, they must be so informed and must give their consent. This is known as informed consent.

Two ways to conduct a research study are (1) to analyze the data on a particular date (cross-sectional research), and (2) to study the data for an extended period (longitudinal research). Longitudinal studies are more difficult, more time-consuming, and more costly, but they generally prove more informative. The classic example concerns the oft-quoted figure of only 5 percent (or one out of twenty) of the over-sixty-five population as being institutionalized at any given time. However, ongoing studies have demonstrated that three out of five older persons (or 60 percent) spend time in nursing homes at some point in their lives.

Medical care evaluation studies are clinical explorations required by the utilization review program and may take place in one facility or in several. They are clinical in that they examine aspects of patient care in an effort to improve phases of care. One possible topic might be infections of patients using catheters. If the results were to show a high proportion of infections, administrative steps should be taken to improve the situation. Thus the research would have an impact on the quality of patient care. In a different vein, a study of visitors to nursing home patients might emphasize the need for changes in the activity program to compensate for diminished visiting.

Patient care audits, a requirement of the quality assurance program of the Joint Commission, are said to evaluate the quality of care through reliable and valid measures by establishing desired outcomes of care based on given defined criteria. Outcomes are much easier to assess in the general hospital when a patient has surgery and improves; there is a beginning and an end and the outcome is clear. In a long-term-care facility, however, precise outcomes do not exist because chronically ill patients are not cured; rather, they are treated over a prolonged period and each improves and/or deteriorates differently with no predetermined schedule. In the nursing home setting, the audit may be useful to determine that everything that might help this patient has been done.

Attention should be given to the changing nature of the skilled nursing facility population—medically, economically, and culturally—in order to plan for the future. The geographical sources of patients should be examined. For example, are residents placed in nursing homes near their own homes or near the homes of their relatives? It might be useful to analyze candidates for placement who have not been admitted or who have withdrawn.

An important goal of the long-term-care facility is the maintenance of a positive and creative environment. It is essential for staff working with the chronically ill to continue to function aggressively and inventively. To assess staff and resident morale, attitudinal studies can be helpful. Periodic studies of staff satisfaction or dissatisfaction may serve to point up some problem areas. The same is true for residents, volunteers, and families. Only by observation and exploration can problem areas be identified. Once identified, steps can be taken to improve the situation.

Studies of facility services should incorporate the concept of action research, which uses the research skills of the social scientist to proceed with organizational change.[1] It really means applying scientific information to problem solving or developing sound information to apply to practical problems to effect social change. Action research is similar to organizational development, as it assists in making sound administrative decisions. In action research, as in medical care evaluation studies, follow-up and implementation are crucial. Action research does not replace good administrative practices, but it can underscore logical and systematic strategy for change and improvement.

Frequently, student interns or health care residents can be assigned to various research projects. Research studies can enlarge students' frames of reference and offer them an opportunity to do original work and make an impact on the facility.

All studies should be formally tabulated and reported to the staff, to the utilization review committee, and to other nursing home constituencies when appropriate. If the results appear helpful to others, every effort should be made to publish them in appropriate professional journals.

An institution that supports extensive research should consider developing its own professional bulletin for annual distribution, which gives a synopsis of each published staff study or article. This offers an overview of the research conducted at the nursing home for communication to interested persons and agencies.

SUMMARY

Education is the single most important factor in determining the quality of care provided by the nursing home. Patients can only be helped if staff are educated to their needs. Personnel and volunteers will have a positive attitude if they feel they are growing and developing. Families can help in the rehabilitation process only if they are informed about their relatives' problems. Informed families can help to bridge the gap between the institution and the community.

Research identifies the present problems and thereby lays the framework for planning future programs. The growth of educational opportunities in geriatrics and gerontology on a baccalaureate, graduate, and continuing education level can only help to improve the care and quality of life of the nursing home patient population.

NOTES

1.   Newton Margulies, "Managing Change in Health Care Organizations," *Medical Care* 15, no. 8 (August 1977): 695.

Epilogue

While the first book used the term "extended care facility," this book discusses the "skilled nursing facility." Names may change, regulations may change, government involvement may change, family relationships may change, needed services may change, society's interest may change, and even the nature of the patient population may change, but the skilled nursing facility will continue to be an integral part of the network of community health agencies. We firmly believe that whatever its name, the skilled nursing facility is needed and will continue to be needed.

Some planners anticipate an explosion in noninstitutional long-term-care services, thereby effecting a decrease in the number of long-term-care beds. In Great Britain, however, where home health services grew by 25 percent in a six-year period, the number of people entering long-term-care facilities still rose from 2 to 2½ percent.[1]

Others emphasized the earlier discharge pattern from the acute hospital due to improved control of the use of hospital beds, causing a more rapid transfer to the skilled nursing facility and a continued need for such beds.[2]

Demographers cite an expected 60-percent growth in the over-seventy-five population by the year 2000,[3] thereby resulting in the need for inpatient care for more older persons as the proportion of the very sick increases from 9 percent for those aged sixty-five to seventy-five to 14 percent for the over-seventy-five group.[4]

In all probability, in this ever-growing urban society, families will continue to be smaller, more dispersed, and geographically mobile, and thus will be less apt to have ill elderly relatives living with them. Added to the increased number of working wives, and the lessening sense of obligation toward elderly relatives, this should influence the need for long-term beds.

It is generally agreed that community control will dominate the future organization and sponsorship of long-term-care facilities with greater reliance on government financing. And there is complete agreement that "there is no alternative to institutionalization when it is really needed."[5]

NOTES

1.   E. Shanas, "Factors Affecting Care of the Patient, Client, Government Policy, Role of the Family and Social Attitudes," *Journal of the American Geriatrics Society* 21, no. 9, (1973): 395.
2.   M. Pulling, "Long Term Care Trends," *Concern* 3, no. 4, (February–March 1977): 35.
3.   H. Brotman, "Population Projections: Part One—Tomorrow's Older Population (to 2000)," *The Gerontologist* 17, no. 3 (1977): 209.
4.   O. Anderson, "Reflections on the Sick Aged and Helping Systems," in B. Neugarten and R. Havighurst, ed., *Social Policy, Social Ethics and the Aging Society*, the Committee on Human Development, the University of Chicago (Washington: Government Printing Office, 1976).
5.   Pulling, "Long Term Care Trends," p. 35.

Index

Accidents/incidents
  prevention, 333–339
  records, 138, 339
Accrual system, 353, 371
Activities and volunteers, general,
    210–241
  committee participation, 412,
    417–418
  facilities, equipment, and supplies,
    238–240
  interdepartmental cooperation, 408
  patient participation plan, 221
  program, 212–221, 222–223
  records, 232, 234–238
  staffing pattern, 210–212
  volunteers, 227–232; family, 252;
    records, 238
Activities of daily living, 187, 197
  self-help devices, 201
ADL. See Activities of daily living
Administration, general, 1–28
  committee participation, 411–412,
    415–418
  intra- and interfacility
    relationships, 25–27, 403
  policies, 12–16, 420
  records, 16–17
  staffing pattern, 7–10;
    administrative director, 7–8
Administrative director, 7–8
Administrative resident, 437–438

Administrator-in-training. See
    Administrative resident
Admission
  contract, 182, 384
  policies, 12–13, 62, 148–149
  process, 57, 164–169
Advocates, resident, 250–258
  ombudsman, 254–256
AIT. See Administrative resident
Alcoholic beverages, 270
Architecture. See Building design and
    maintenance
Assessment, patient, 121
Audiology. See Speech pathology
    and audiology
Autopsy, 68

Biological waste disposal, 149, 160,
    297–298
Board of directors, 3–4, 252, 411, 435
Budget, operating, 5, 354, 411
Building design and maintenance,
    general, 306–330
  architectural design, 311–315;
    related to rehabilitation, 185,
    310–315; safety features,
    332–333; worship facilities, 226
  infection control, 155
  maintenance: committee
    participation, 416–418;
    equipment systems, major,

320–321; facilities, equipment,
and supplies, 329–330;
interdepartmental cooperation,
408–409; preventive, 316–319;
program, 315–321; safety,
335–336; staffing pattern,
307–310
records, 326–329
security, 339–342
site of nursing home, 310
Business, general, 352–385
accounting definitions and
principles, 353–363
accounts payable, 371–372
accounts receivable, 370–371
bank accounts, 378
committee participation, 411, 418
facilities, equipment, and supplies,
384
insurance, 375–378
interdepartmental cooperation, 410
payroll, 372–373
purchasing, 373–374
records, 381–384
staffing pattern, 363, 366, 368
stores control, 375
technology, 379–381
Bylaws
of the medical staff, 59–61
of the nursing home, 4–5

Capital expenditures plan, 354
Carpet. See Floor coverings
Catheters, foley, 105, 334
Central storage. See Business, stores
control
Civil rights
Civil Rights Act of 1964, 24
selection of employees, 31–32
Clergy. See Religious activities
Clothing, patients', 104–105, 296–297,
299–300, 302, 304–305
Committees. See Therapeutic
organization, the
Communication
systems, 17–19, 138–139
written, 19–21
Community relations, 25–26, 27, 180,
228, 231, 254–258, 429–430,
438–439
Computer. See Business, technology

Conditions of participation, 23
Consultants, 10–12
accountant, 368, 411
activities, 197, 212
contracts, 11
dentist, 68–70
dietitian, 262–263
interior designer, 283
medical, 65, 115
medical records administrator, 387
optometrist, 68–70
pharmacist, 79–80
podiatrist, 68–70
safety, 417
social work, 163
speech pathologist/audiologist, 205
Consumerism, general, 242–258
community intervention, 254–258
families as consumers, 251–253
residents as consumers, 242–251;
resident advocates, 250–258;
residents' council, 243,
247–250
Continuing education. See Education
and research
Continuity of care, 33, 34, 59, 62,
104, 111, 119, 145, 188–189, 205,
225, 392, 438
Contracts
admission, 182, 384
consultants, 11
outside services, 6, 259, 282–283,
298–299, 315–316, 320, 376
Contributions, 355
Corporations
non-profit, 2, 6
proprietary, 2–3, 6
Cost allocation, 362
Cost-finding, 356

Data processing, 379–381
Death, 67, 114, 116–117, 180, 226
records, 137–138
Decubitus ulcers, 113, 393
Dentistry, 70–71
equipment, 92
financial arrangements, 84
records, 86
Dentists, 68–70
Departments, 8
Dietary, general, 259–281

committee participation, 411–412,
    417–418
diet manual, 266
diets, 266–269; kosher, 269;
    nasogastric tube feeding,
    267–268
eating problems of patients,
    260–262
facilities and equipment, 275–278
feeding patients, 96, 107, 109,
    271–272
food ordering, 278–279
foods, convenience, 279–280
infection control, 155–156,
    265–266, 275, 279, 280
interdepartmental cooperation, 408
meal service: employee, 272–273;
    guest, 280; resident, 270–272
menus, 269–270
records, 273–275
safety, 335
staffing pattern, 262–266
unique aspects of, 218, 260
Disaster plans. See Safety
Discharge, 67, 115–116, 179–180
    plan, 64, 179, 412
    record, 67, 393, 398
Disclosure of ownership, 6, 353
Drugs. See Pharmacy

Education and research, general,
    419–443
    budget, 439–440
    education: community, 256–258,
        438–439; family, 251–252,
        304–305, 434–435; patient,
        152, 331; professional, 420;
        records, 431–434; staff, 34–35,
        38–39, 191, 200, 206, 231, 284,
        331, 343–344, 421–431;
        students, 436–438, 439–440,
        442; volunteers, 435–436, 439
    equipment, 429
    library, 440–441
    research, 395–396, 415, 441–443
    staffing pattern, 420–421
Electrocardiography
    equipment, 86
    services, 74
    technician, 74
Emergencies
    drug box, 83

first aid kit, 337
medical care, 55
nursing cart, 142–143
telephone numbers, 17, 19, 139
Energy conservation, 321–322
Epilogue, 444–445
Equipment. See Facilities, equipment,
    and supplies
Ethics, 117, 191, 213, 215, 244, 246
Evacuation plan. See Safety

Facilities, equipment, and supplies
    activities and volunteers, 238, 240
    business, 384
    dietary, 275–278
    education and research, 429
    housekeeping, furnishings, and
        laundry, 302–304
    maintenance, 329–330
    medical, 86, 92
    nursing, 139, 141–143, 145
    occupational therapy, 201, 204
    pharmacy, 81–82, 83, 143
    physical therapy, 191, 195, 334
    records, 398–400
    social service, 182
    speech pathology and audiology,
        208
Family
    future, 2, 444
    perception of relative, 165–166, 171
Family relations
    with administration, 25, 26
    with dietary, 280
    with housekeeping and laundry,
        304–305
    with nursing, 114
    with patient, 171, 176
    with personnel, 38
Financial arrangements
    changes in patient status, 177, 179
    dentistry, 84
    medical care, 84
    occupational therapy, 200–201
    optometry, 84
    physical therapy, 192
    podiatry, 84
    speech pathology and audiology,
        207–208
Fire safety program. See Safety
Floor coverings, 288, 293
Food. See Dietary

Functional accounting, 362
Furnishings. *See* Housekeeping,
   furnishings, and laundry

Governing body. *See* Board of
   directors
Gratuities for staff, 38
Grievances, patient, 247
Grounds, 310–311
   security, 339–342
Group process, 176–177, 221

Handicapped persons
   Rehabilitation Act of 1973, 24–25
   selection of employees, 24, 31–32
Health records. *See* Records, health
Health Systems Agency, 21–22
Housekeeping, furnishings, and
      laundry, general, 282–305
   clothing storage, 296–297, 302
   committee participation, 416–418
   facilities, equipment, and supplies,
      302–304
   furnishings, 287–293, 296; floor
      coverings, 288, 293
   housekeeping procedures, 293–298
   infection control, 153, 160, 296,
      300
   interdepartmental cooperation,
      408–409
   laundry, 298–301
   odors, 256, 293, 298, 300
   records, 302
   safety, 296, 334, 335
   staffing pattern, 283–285, 287
   waste disposal, 297–298

Incidents. *See* Accidents/incidents
Infection control, general, 146–161
   building structure and
      maintenance, 155
   committee, 152, 158, 416–417
   dietary, 155–156, 265–266, 268,
      275, 279, 280
   housekeeping, 153, 160, 296
   isolation, 149, 158, 160
   laundry, 153, 300
   policies, 148–149, 152
   prevention, 147–148, 334
   residents' personal care, 152
   surveillance, 156–158, 160

Infections, nosocomial, 147, 157
In-service education. *See* Education
   and research
Inspections
   government, 23–25, 323–324, 339
   insurance, 323
   safety, 333
Insurance, 375–378
Interdisciplinary team. *See*
   Therapeutic organization, the
Interior design, 287–293, 296,
   302–303, 327
Inventory, 75, 145, 276, 329, 373, 375

Joint Commission on Accreditation of
   Hospitals, 14, 16, 57, 59, 324

Laboratory
   equipment, 92
   services, 74
   technician, 74
Laundry. *See* Housekeeping,
   furnishings, and laundry
Library
   professional, 440–441
   residents', 222
Licenses
   nursing home administrator, 25
   operational, 5–6
   personnel, 32, 33, 59, 138
Life Safety Code, 22, 343

Maintenance. *See* Building design and
   maintenance
Medicaid, 22–25
   reimbursement, 369–370
Medical care evaluation studies, 415,
   441
Medical director
   alternatives, 54–55
   committee participation, 411–412,
      415–418
   contract with, 61
   duties, 55–57
   interdepartmental cooperation, 403
Medical records. *See* Records, health
Medical staff
   closed, 57–58
   committee participation, 411–412,
      415–418

consultants, 65
facilities and equipment, 86
financial arrangements, 84
interdepartmental cooperation, 403
nomination of attending physician,
    168–169
office visits, 65
open, 57
organizational plan, 57
panel, 61
records, 84–86
responsibilities, 61–68; annual
    physical examination, 64;
    change in patient status, 67;
    telephone orders, 65
Medicare, 22–25
    reimbursement, 369–370
Medications. *See* Pharmacy
Medicine and allied health
    professionals, general, 53–92
Memberships, professional
    institutional, 16, 440
    personal, 16, 430, 440

Nonprofit corporation, 2
Nursing, general, 93–145
    committee participation, 411–412,
        415–418
    facilities, equipment, and supplies,
        139, 141–145
    interdepartmental cooperation,
        404–405
    procedures, 104–119, 152
    records, 119–138, 393
    safety, 334–335
    staffing pattern, 95–96, 98–104;
        director of nursing, 100;
        master staffing plan, 98–99
    unique aspects of, 93–95, 105, 107,
        115
Nutrition. *See* Dietary

Occupational Safety and Health
    Administration, 324, 339
Occupational therapy, general,
    196–204
    committee participation, 411–412,
        417–418
    facilities and equipment, 201, 204

financial arrangements, 200–201
    interdepartmental cooperation,
        407–408
    program, 197, 199–200
    records, 201
    staffing pattern, 196
Odors, 256, 293, 298, 300
Off-premises patient activities
    patient disappearance, 113–114, 340
    patient outings, 219
    policies, 13–14, 113–114
    records, 137, 237
Ombudsman. *See* Advocates, resident
Optometrists, 68–70
Optometry, 71
    financial arrangements, 84
Organizational plans, 14, 57
Orientation. *See* Education and
    research

Patient care plan
    activities, 221–222, 234
    medical, 64
    nursing, 127
    nutrition, 273–275
    occupational therapy, 200
    physical therapy, 190
    social service, 170
    speech pathology and audiology,
        207
Patient population
    future, 1–2
    nature of, 1, 93, 185, 204–206, 213,
        260–262, 331
Patients' rights, 117, 182, 242–247,
    295, 379
    community advocates, 254–258
    family advocates, 251–252
    married inpatients, 168
    patients' personal funds, 14,
        243–244, 246, 341–342,
        378–379
    permission for news releases, 237
    resident advocates, 250–251
    residents' council, 243, 247–250
    sexual activity, 244
Periodic medical review, 23
Personnel, general, 28–52
    committee, 38, 412
    education, 34–35, 38–39, 191, 200,

206, 231, 284, 331, 343–344,
    421–431
meal service, 272–273
part-time employment, 33
policies, 34–39, 337, 339, 378, 403,
    439; attendance bonus, 37;
    compensation, 36, 411;
    evaluation, 37; infection
    control, 149; recognition,
    38–39
private duty staff, 33–34, 103
records, 39–43
recruitment, 31–33
safety, 337–338
security, 340–342, 363
staffing pattern, 30
turnover, 31
Pharmacy, general, 74–84
charges, 79, 84
committee participation, 416–417,
    418
community, 76–79
consultant pharmacist, 79–80
facilities, equipment, and supplies,
    81–82, 83, 143
in-house, 74–75
medication administration,
    117–119; records, 127, 138
policies, 80–84; emergency drug
    box, 83
records, 81, 137
unit dose, 75–76
Physical therapy, general, 185–195
committee participation, 411–412,
    415–417, 418
facilities and equipment, 187–188,
    191, 195; patients' personal
    use, 191
financial arrangement, 192
interdepartmental cooperation,
    407–408
program, 189–192
records, 192, 195
staffing pattern, 188–189
supplemental nursing
    rehabilitation, 109, 111, 187,
    190–191
Physician. See Medical staff
Podiatrists, 68–70
Podiatry, 71
financial arrangements, 84
records, 86

Postmortem examination. See
    Autopsy
Private-duty staff, 33–34, 103
Professional Standards Review
    Organization, 25, 416
Proprietary agency, 2–3
Protective devices
chemical, 111, 246
physical, 65, 111, 246, 334
Public agency, 2
Purchasing, 145, 238, 240, 278–280,
    302–304, 324, 326, 373–374

Quality care, evaluation of, 16, 23,
    60, 92, 119, 222–223, 232, 251,
    254, 257–258, 259, 339, 390, 395,
    398, 415, 418, 441–442

Rates, daily, 368–370
posting, 14
prospective, 369–370
retrospective, 369–370
third-party payer, 369–370
Reality orientation/remotivation,
    184, 197, 199, 225
records, 201
Records, 386–400
committee participation, 415–417,
    418
facilities and equipment, 398–400
general records and forms, 388–390
health, 390–396; confidentiality,
    119, 227, 394–396; indexes,
    396–397; problem-oriented,
    393–394; serial numbering,
    392; source-oriented, 393; unit
    numbering, 392
interdepartmental cooperation,
    409–410
retention, 388
staffing pattern, 386–387
Records, departmental
activities and volunteers, 232,
    234–238
administration, 16–17
business, 381–384
dental, 86
dietary, 273–275
education and research, 431–434
housekeeping, furnishings, and
    laundry, 302
infection control, 157

maintenance, 326–329
medical, 84–86
nursing, 119, 121–127, 129–138, 393
occupational therapy, 201
personnel, 39, 43
pharmacy, 81, 137
physical therapy, 192, 195
podiatry, 86
social service, 169–170, 180–182
speech pathology and audiology, 208
Rehabilitation services, general, 184–209
occupational therapy. See Occupational therapy
physical therapy. See Physical therapy
speech pathology and audiology. See Speech pathology and audiology
Religious activities, 223–226
Relocation stress, 169
Representative, patient's, 13
Research. See Education and research
Residents' council, 243, 247–250
Restraints. See Protective devices
Risk management, 375, 377
Roommates, 104, 170, 244

Safety, general, 331–350
accident/incident prevention, 333–339
building and grounds security, 299, 339–342, 417
building criteria, 332–333
committee, 331, 417–418
disaster plans, 348–350; bomb threats, 349; civil disturbance, 349–350
evacuation plan, 345–346, 348
fire safety program, 324, 342–345
housekeeping, 296
patient, 113–114, 335, 340
patients' personal belongings, 243, 244, 246, 341–342, 378, 379
utility interruption, 346–348
Security. See Safety
Sexual activity of residents, 244
Social service, general, 162–183
admissions, 164–169

changes in patient financial status, 177, 179
committee participation, 411–412, 415–417, 418
discharge, 64, 67, 115–116, 179–180, 393, 398, 412
facilities and equipment, 182
group process, 176–177
in-residence phase, 169–171
interdepartmental cooperation, 405–407
records, 169–170, 180–182
staffing pattern, 162–164
Speech pathology and audiology, general, 204–209
committee participation, 411–412, 418
facilities and equipment, 208
financial arrangements, 207–208
interdepartmental cooperation, 407–408
program, 205–207
records, 208
staffing pattern, 205
Sponsor, patient's, 13
Staff development. See Education and research
Staffing pattern
activities and volunteers, 210–212
administration, 7–10
business, 363, 366, 368
dietary, 262–266
education and research, 420–421
housekeeping and laundry, 283–285, 287
maintenance, 307–310
medical: attending medical staff, 57–61; director, 55–57; director, alternatives to, 54–55; panel, 61
nursing, 95–96, 98–104
occupational therapy, 196
personnel department, 30
physical therapy, 188–189
records department, 386–387
social service, 162–164
speech pathology and audiology, 205
Stores control, 375
Strike, 50–52, 349–350
Suicide, 107
Supplies. See Facilities, equipment,

and supplies
Surveys. *See* Inspections, government

Team, interdisciplinary. *See*
    Therapeutic organization, the
Therapeutic organization, the,
    401–418
  activities and volunteers, 408
  administration, 403
  business office, 410
  committees, 410–418; budget, 411;
    family, 251–252; governing
    body, 5; infection control,
    152, 158, 416–417;
    interdisciplinary, 411–412, 426;
    joint conference, 60, 411;
    patient, 216, 218, 243,
    247–250; patient care policy,
    412, 415; personnel, 37–38,
    412; pharmacy, 416; residents'
    council, 243, 247–250; safety,
    417–418; utilization review,
    415–416
  dietary, 408
  housekeeping, 408–409
  maintenance, 408–409
  medicine, 403
  nursing, 403–405
  occupational therapy, 407–408
  physical therapy, 407–408
  records department, 409–410

  social service, 405–407
  speech pathology and audiology,
    407–408
  team organization, 401–402, 410
Transfer agreements, 13, 257, 415
Transfers
  out of the facility. *See* Discharge
  within the facility, 170–171
Transportation, 31, 256, 322–323
Tube feeding, 109, 262, 267–268

Uniforms
  personnel, 36–37
  volunteers, 229
Unions, 43, 48–52, 255, 283
Unit dose, 75–76
Utility interruption. *See* Safety
Utilization review, 16, 415–416

Visiting, 13, 149, 215, 252, 280,
    340–341
Volunteers. *See* Activities and
  volunteers

Waiting list, 166
Work sampling, 293–294, 326

X ray
  equipment, 92
  policies, 64
  services, 74
  technician, 74